T0133870

Sacrificing the WHO to the Highest Bidder

# Sacrificing the WHO to the Highest Bidder

**Théodore H MacDonald** PhD, MD, FRSM

*Professor (Emeritus) and Member of Research Institute for Human Rights
and Social Justice, London Metropolitan University
Former Director of Postgraduate Studies in Health, Brunel University
Consultant to the World Health Organization, International Development
Agency and various NGOs in developing countries*

*Forewords by*

**David Player** MBChB, FRCPE, FRCPsych, FRCM

*Former Consultant to the Far East in Dermatology and HIV/AIDS
with the Royal Army Corps Registrar in Psychiatry, and Medical
and Psychiatric Adviser to the Secretary of State for Scotland*

and

**Mathura P Shrestha** MBBS, MComH

*President, Physicians for Social Responsibility, Nepal
Laureate Nobel Peace Prize 1985
Chairperson, Resource Centre for Primary Health*

Radcliffe Publishing
Oxford • New York

**Radcliffe Publishing Ltd**
18 Marcham Road
Abingdon
Oxon OX14 1AA
United Kingdom

**www.radcliffe-oxford.com**
Electronic catalogue and worldwide online ordering facility.

British Library Cataloguing in Publication Data

A catalogue record for this book is available from the British Library.

ISBN-13: 978 1 84619 252 4

Typeset by Pindar NZ (Egan Reid), Auckland, New Zealand
Printed and bound by TJ International Ltd, Padstow, Cornwall

# Contents

# Foreword

This is the most recent book by Théodore MacDonald, a true polymath, who has worked in many countries, in both the First and Third Worlds. As always, it is provocative and well researched, and could be regarded as a brilliant and thoroughgoing Marxist analysis. The title itself prepares the reader for the forced march – truly educational at every stage – through the following coherently argued nine chapters. The underlying theme is the present crisis in capitalist globalization, its progress fired and sustained by neoliberalism and unrestricted competition, which has been gathering strength since Nixon's dissolution of Bretton Woods in the early 1970s.

At the end of World War Two, the United Nations was set up with the mandate to fulfil its Universal Declaration of Human Rights. To facilitate this, it established such agencies as the World Health Organization (WHO), UNICEF, UNESCO and others.

Other agencies, such as the World Trade Organization (WTO), technically not actual agencies of the UN itself, have also been initiated. The WTO mediates its activities through a variety of such instrumentalities as GATT, GATS, etc. and, most crucially, TRIPS (Trade-Related Intellectual Property Rights). Initially the WHO played a key rôle in promoting health as a basic human right, but since 1988 it has been increasingly sidelined by various global trade and competition rules. In this way health, and some other human rights, have come to be regarded as 'desiderata – subject to availability of finance', rather than as basic non-negotiable 'rights.'

MacDonald leads us on to consider what amounts to the 'selling off' of various functions of the UN. With others, he points the finger of blame at the former Director General of the UN, Kofi Annan, because of his call in 2005 for UN agencies to cooperate with private enterprise to achieve the Millennium Development Goad (MDG) objectives. Others blame the World Economic Forum – famous for its annual meetings (under prodigiously tight security) at the ski resort of Davos in Switzerland, and attended by wealthy corporate finance leaders and some selected representatives of non-governmental organizations (NGOs).

He also identifies some supporters of the neoliberal backlash, such as the John Birch Society, and US and UK Tobacco Corporations (especially Philip Morris in 1989), who described the WHO as their most dangerous opponent. Others include the Heritage Foundation, the Cato Institute, the *International Herald Tribune* and the

*Wall Street Journal.* Under persistent pressure, the US government cut its financial contribution to the UN by 20%. We are then led to examine serious attacks on the guiding principles of the UN, such as the global privatization of water. Particularly shocking is the concurrence of both the UN and the WHO in these attacks, their main rationale for such complicity with privatization being that IMF loans to very poor nations contain conditional Structural Adjustment Policies.

In 2005, millions of babies died as a result of consuming polluted drinking water while gallons of good-quality water were used to irrigate the golf courses of wealthy elites in the same countries. It is estimated that within the next 20 years, two-thirds of the world's population will be faced with acute water shortages. At present the annual profits of the water industry worldwide are equivalent to 40% of the oil industry. The building of dams worldwide also represents continuing catastrophes on the near horizon, such as the fate of the Aral Sea in the former Soviet Union, the Three Gorges Dam in China, the Yacyveta Dam in Paraguay, the Chixoy Dam in Guatemala, the Lesotho Highlands Water Project (which involves five dams), the Bujagali Falls Dam on the Nile, and the Sardar Sarovet Dam in Narmada Valley in India. MacDonald quotes John Maynard Keynes in this context: 'Capitalism is the extraordinary belief that the nastiest of people, for the nastiest of motives, will somehow work for the benefit of all.'

Impressive local resistance to these water projects has developed, and MacDonald himself writes that reflex anti-Americanism is a mistake, because much of the thinking and action that prevent excesses of neoliberalism actually originates in the USA by virtue of that country's emphasis on the importance of the individual conscience. The author's next wake-up call concerns the auctioning of viruses! This refers to the UN and its agents developing vaccines against, for example, avian flu, using TRIPS as a means of allowing pharmaceutical corporations to gain patent rights over vaccines. Of course, most of these cannot be afforded by the very countries which supplied the WHO with the viruses in the first place. Yet another prescient point that MacDonald brings to our attention is the suspicious relationship between the UN and its International Atomic Energy Agency. His analyses are extraordinarily insightful, as he deals with the financial, political and psychological aspects of the Chernobyl accident as a template. His ability to explain complicated scientific theories and consequences is both educational and encouraging. MacDonald does not despair that many of his critics regard his commitment to human rights as 'pie in the sky.' This is best demonstrated in a direct quotation from Chapter 8:

> As we have seen in the preceding chapters, this has consistently been the view of the rapidly burgeoning forces of neoliberalism. In fact, in a recent issue of the *Lancet*, one of that journal's book reviewers describes how she had been so angered at an editorial in *The Economist* dismissing much chatter about social and economic rights as nonsense, that she wrote to them, opposing their view and asking if they had ever heard of the Universal Declaration of Human Rights.

She goes on:

> 'The response I got from one of the editors left me stunned. "I am of course aware that economic and social rights feature in the UDHR and elsewhere. The "right" to a job, education, health, etc. sounds superficially attractive, but in practice it is either pernicious or meaningless. It would be more honest if the defenders of these economic, social and cultural rights would come straight out and say that they believe that socialism is the answer, and campaign for it, rather than dressing up their demands for more state intervention in the legalistic language of rights."'

The author then goes on to describe the success of the Cuban Health and Education Services, which is a marvellous and uplifting reminder of what can be done, and full of hope.

**Dr David Player** MBChB, FRCPE, FRCPsych, FRCM
**Former Consultant to the Far East in Dermatology and HIV/AIDS with the Royal Army Corps**
**Registrar in Psychiatry**
**Medical and Psychiatric Adviser to the Secretary of State for Scotland**
*January 2008*

# Foreword

I came to know Théodore MacDonald through his numerous thought-provoking books (about 40 in number) and nearly 200 refereed and research-based journal articles, but also personally at a get-together during a People's Health Assembly in Cuenca, Ecuador. Théodore has chosen the hard life of a persistent fighter, with his powerful pen, for conscience over super-power chauvinism, socially irresponsible neoliberalism that has 'no national or cultural loyalties' and with profit as its only goal, and indecisive leadership in the UN and in many of its agencies. All of these influences contravene the spirit of the UN's mandate, as do the interests of the nuclear power players with which they now cooperate. His writings deal critically and extensively with many layers of social injustice as they impact on the health and rights of peoples in the Third World. His approach exhibits an analytically scrupulous account of the epidemiological issues, combined with an irreproachably scholarly account of how neoliberal global finance – largely controlled from US and EU corporations, banks and power centres – lies at the root of health inequalities worldwide. His rich experience, gained while working as a doctor in many Third World countries and interacting with different cultures, has obviously opened such important and credible intellectual resources to him. These he employs to equip social advocates, and the suffering peoples themselves, to understand the political, socio-cultural and economic determinants of the social injustices that they suffer. This book, *Sacrificing the WHO to the Highest Bidder*, is both timely and appropriate.

Many readers may be troubled by doubts about a variety of things, but the integrity of the UN is not likely to be one of them. After reading this account, however, one can but hope that they will realize that their faith may perhaps have been misplaced! Why is this so? Because the UN and many of its agencies have effectively been privatized and beguiled by the same forces of neoliberalism that have subordinated so many of our social values, along with the economic ones, to the antisocial and profit-driven exigencies of the marketplace. Indeed, the Universal Declaration of Human Rights (UDHR) was initially the UN's guiding document but, as this book makes plain, 'human rights have in many cases been replaced by needs that might be met if this can be achieved in the context of business efficiency.'

Théodore, who has been involved with a range of projects run by the WHO, recognizes that the UN is widely perceived as the world's only real hope for the future, and that losing its reputation for integrity would be a moral disaster. He regards it as vital that we defend such precious ideals as the UDHR, the principles implicit in the WHO, the momentous Alma Ata Declaration and other mandates to keep the world healthy, green and peaceful. These embody a responsibility to protect peoples, especially women and children, disabled, deprived and marginalized people of all races and classes, and those living in Third World countries and forgotten ghettos in developed countries.

However, many of these principles have 'effectively been sacrificed to the thrusting financial appetite of neoliberalism', becoming subservient to the moneylenders and international financial institutions – including the International Monetary Fund (IMF) and the World Bank. This book analyses how the UN agencies have been progressively penetrated by neoliberal interests and even by hostile media thrusts. This has in fact involved bugging of UN websites and information systems, and financial blockades by First World consortia and by other allies of neoliberalism.

To address the full spectrum of these issues individually would not be feasible in the compass of one book, as well as representing an unremittingly tedious barrier for the reader. Therefore the author has adopted the strategy of classifying the problems in terms of typology. He has eclectically chosen a small sample of nations where human rights problems illustrates what the author identifies as the sort of inconsistencies and contradictions of policy reflected in UN responses generally. This approach is very much strengthened and validated by MacDonald's wide personal experience in dealing with the health problems arising as a consequence of neoliberalism on health in the countries selected.

Thus, he is able to give a comprehensive account of how the World Trade Organization (WTO) is able to act in such a way as to reflect the needs of the First World's corporate sector, even if doing so compromises health, and other human rights, in various Third World countries. He thus has acted not only as a medical man pure and simple, but as one with an acute insight into international finance. As the author so coherently argues, the WTO does not have to be an actual agency of the WHO to be able to determine the impact of the IMF and other UN agencies in their actions on Third World countries. This has inevitably led to the WHO and the IMF conflicting with the UN mandates they are intended to uphold.

Those considerations set the leitmotif for the detailed accounts given in succeeding chapters of the book. Indeed, in such a context, one is not entirely surprised that the IMF and the World Bank are not the only UN agencies that have become enmeshed in the subsequent matrix of conflicting interests. As the author goes on to show, the International Atomic Energy Agency (IAEA) is also deeply involved and this carries immense and immediate implications for First World nations.

Despite the author's assertion of optimism, this book – which demands the attention of all intelligent readers and policy-makers – starkly raises alarming issues which should worry us. More to the point, it should energise us to an urgently increased involvement in the political issues which we have for too long taken for granted, regarding them as background only to more pressing practicalities well outside of our capacity to influence.

Mathura P Shrestha MBBS, MComH
President, Physicians for Social Responsibility, Nepal
Affiliate of International Physicians for the Prevention of Nuclear War
Laureate Nobel Peace Prize 1985
Chairperson, Resource Centre for Primary Health
*January 2008*

# Preface

This morning most readers of this book awoke with doubts about many things, but the integrity of the United Nations is not likely to have been one of them. However, after reading this account, it is hoped that the reader's customary trust in that organization, and its various agencies, will have been replaced by the feeling that perhaps their faith may have been misplaced! Why is this? It is because the UN and many of its agencies have effectively been privatized, beguiled by the same forces of neoliberalism that have subordinated so many of our social values, along with the economic ones, to the rules of the marketplace. Indeed, the Universal Declaration of Human Rights (UDHR) was initially the UN's guiding document but, as this book makes plain, human rights have in many cases been replaced by 'needs that might be met if this can be achieved in the context of business efficiency.'

As one who has been privileged to serve in many Third World countries, including working on several projects run by the WHO, this author had also regarded the integrity of the UN as unimpeachably obvious and, moreover, as the world's only real hope for the future. However, in recent years closer analysis of the matter has persuaded him that the UN, through the WHO, is no longer able to be concerned primarily with the promotion and defence of health as a basic human right. Instead, it has been compelled to cooperate with agencies that are funding loans to less developed countries in situations where such loans are tied to conditionalities which actually undermine the health of the citizens of the debtor nations. Clearly this can only serve to widen the health rights gap between the developed world and less developed countries (LDCs). However, dear reader, worse is to come, for prominent among these lending agencies are the International Monetary Fund (IMF) and the World Bank, both of which are themselves also UN agencies!

The above-mentioned conditionalities are referred to as Structural Adjustment Policies (SAPs), and are generally geared to ensure repayment of the loan, and the money itself becomes designated for infrastructural developments run by private enterprises in order to render the debtor nation more fit for international trade. Much of the profits from this will line the pockets of corporation and bank stockholders in the First World. Frequently the impact on the health of the people concerned is a low priority for consideration. In other words, business efficiency trumps the UDHR.

To address all of the evidence for this shocking state of affairs would require a library of books. The compromise struck here is to provide introductory chapters on how the relevant UN agencies, and their almost esoteric legal instrumentalities, work. As the book's title implies, the focus is largely on the involvement of the WHO. It is through the IMF and the World Bank, the author claims, that the WHO finds itself sacrificed to the dictates of neoliberalism. The reader is also probably aware of the World Trade Organization (WTO). This powerful organization is not itself technically a UN agency, but it might as well be for, as the author shows, the IMF and the World Bank could not operate nearly so efficiently without the WTO, and without the IMF and the World Bank, the WTO would have no *raison-d'être*.

In succeeding chapters, the author shows how privatization of the WHO's activities has had extremely negative impacts on health, especially in the LDCs. Among the issues cited in support of this Gothic claim are water privatization and the privatization of vaccine production. The latter, in fact, although mediated by the WHO, has been shown to have been done in such a way that many of the poorest people – and often the very people who provided the serum material necessary for production of the vaccine – will not be protected should a global pandemic, calling for the application of the vaccine, break out! The author then moves on to consider the WHO's appalling collaboration with the nuclear power industry to cover up the true and ongoing impacts of the Chernobyl disaster, and how this abandonment of its principles has vastly enriched those corporate interests that are marketing nuclear power in the First World. It wouldn't do to have too many people aware of the potential dangers of the nuclear option!

As the book draws to a close, the author raises the following rhetorical question: Is neoliberalism good for our health? After arguing the negative, the author demonstrates the foolishness of asserting that neoliberalism is 'inevitable' and that we have no choice but to live with it. He does this by discussing the remarkable achievements of Cuba in the field of healthcare, and how this was all accomplished by adherence to social policies which put humanity and community values ahead of profit, and cooperation ahead of competition, asserting that the former binds communities together, whereas the latter divides them.

**Théodore H MacDonald**
**Littlehampton**
**UK**
*January 2008*

# Acknowledgements

As the dedication page makes clear, I acknowledge – in the writing of this and of all my books – the debt of love and gratitude I owe my father. A newspaper editor and a poet himself, it was he who, having introduced me to great literature, then proceeded to instruct me in the craft of writing. Each day he set me a theme on which I was expected to have prepared an essay by the time he returned from work in the evening. In his methodical analyses of my efforts, after dinner, my grammatical and syntactical errors would be corrected and my skills in argument honed. He constantly impressed upon me the idea that one purpose of writing was to persuade readers and, in this way, to help to make the world a better place.

At a more prosaic but equally crucial level, this book would not have seen the light of day had not my hundreds of sheets of handwritten script been so efficiently word processed by Beth Archer. She also detected various inconsistencies in reference numbering and other minor errors.

Finally, I wish to thank the staff at Radcliffe Publishing, particularly Jamie Etherington, Editorial Development Manager, and Gillian Nineham, Editorial Director.

Finally, and as always, I thank my wife Chris for her immense forbearance in the face of the general disruption to the even tenor of domestic life caused by book authorship. Even I can't stand the mess that it generates!

Théodore H MacDonald
Littlehampton
UK
*January 2008*

This book is lovingly dedicated to the memory of my father.

CUTHBERT GOODRIDGE MACDONALD

1897–1967

Trouble-shooting journalist and one of Canada's leading poets, who taught me my craft more thoroughly than any school or university ever did.

# Chapter 1

# The UN: its origins, problems and contradictions

## BRETTON WOODS – AND CONSEQUENCES

This author can recall the dark days of World War Two in a fair amount of detail and, as it became increasingly obvious that fascism would be defeated, one often heard earnest conversations about how such insanities as global warfare might be prevented in the future. The League of Nations was pretty well wholly concerned with the negative task of 'preventing' nations from fighting, but lacked a strong matrix of agencies, each charged with some specific task that would – if success-ful – obviate such primary underlying causes of war as inadequate attention to equity in food distribution, the prevention of disease, mechanisms for ensuring a 'balanced' approach to international trade, and some means of preventing undue exploitation such as would advantage one country over others. That is, I think it fair to say that while the League was concerned to prevent militarism from break-ing out, what was needed was a transnational body concerned with preventing the kind of circumstances that would be likely to lead to militarism.

Thus, when the leadership of the USA, the UK, the former Soviet Union, France and China gathered at the delightful little town of Bretton Woods in the US state of New Hampshire in 1944 to plan for such a world body – in this case, to be called the United Nations – they set about creating agencies aimed at specific aspects of the UN's mandate to forestall international conflict by preventing various root causes of it. Thus the World Health Organization (WHO) was founded with a mandate to 'promote and defend' a defined 'right' of access to primary healthcare. As we shall see, the latter became a political obligation of the UN as a whole. However, that question of 'rights' is important because basic to the UN's mandate was its obligation to 'promote and defend' human rights globally. This mandate subsequently became enshrined in the UN's defining Declaration – the Universal Declaration of Human Rights (UDHR).

A number of the UN's other agencies specifically uphold the UDHR and create mechanisms for fulfilling this Declaration. One could list the WHO, UNICEF, UNESCO and various others. However, in order to be effective, the UN has to have moral authority. For example, member states must feel an obligation to acquiesce to the health research findings of the WHO in their own countries, and be willing to bring their individual national legislation into line with them. In doing so, they would be giving substance and transnational authority to the UDHR. It goes without saying that such a degree of commitment on the part of each member state to make the UDHR a reality would render international war (or even civil war) unthinkable.

However, there are a number of problems. For instance, what if one nation or a bloc of nations decided to pursue a less inclusive agenda based on some short-term advantage, such as control over oil supplies, grain-producing fields, etc.? This question also arose in planning for the old League of Nations, and the assumed solution was purely military. The UN response has been less rigid because of the existence and influence of such agencies as the WHO, UNICEF, etc., but it has still all too often involved military responses. Moreover, in recent history, such military responses (we cannot call them 'solutions') have become increasingly transparent as satisfying some self-serving economic purpose of the invading nations. This author takes the optimistic view that most people now can see through such ploys and are less inclined to allow their governments to acquiesce to them. Methods based on trade embargos, etc. are generally much more effective.

However, a series of persistent problems beset our UN as a 'transnational mediator of human rights', and these have been considered in detail by the author in a previous book.[1] Only some of them need to be alluded to in the present discussion. At the above-mentioned Bretton Woods Conference, many issues other than human rights were discussed. For instance, the participants were all important allies in the fight against fascism. Not unnaturally, their concern to prevent a further outbreak of international strife tended to focus on ways and means of preserving their own hegemony. The USA was by far the wealthiest of these victor nations, and its president, Franklin Delano Roosevelt, tended to carry the most weight in the discussions. However, a few words are warranted at this point about such a remarkable man.

Even today, many Americans still view Roosevelt with almost reverential admiration. Although many nations and 'individuals' had been brought to the edge (and over it) of economic ruin by the Great Depression, he introduced the New Deal and the Tennessee Valley Authority. Thus his legislation not only dramatically reduced unemployment, but it also laid the groundwork for even further industrialization and business. At the age of 39 years, and at the height of his innovatory powers, he was suddenly stricken with polio. From that time onward he was wheelchair-bound, but this did not prevent him from becoming President (as a Democrat) in 1932, and from being re-elected three more times in 1936, 1940 and 1944. He died of a brain haemorrhage in 1945.

Consistently, his administration had reflected his devotion to the ideal of the rights of ordinary people, and his almost visceral detestation of royalty or anything that smacked of privilege gained by unearned wealth or social class. For that reason, as well as strategic ones relating to US trade, he felt an intense animus toward the British Empire. At that time the latter constituted a serious check on US international trade, by virtue of the complex matrix of tariffs and trading arrangements within the British Empire. Hence on coming to office for the first time in 1932, Roosevelt aggressively promoted US trading interests.

It was in this context that he, along with the famous English economist, John Maynard Keynes (1883–1996), played such a pivotal rôle in setting up the two major economic bodies which today are important levers controlling international finance and trade. These two bodies are the World Bank (WB) (officially known as the International Bank for Reconstruction and Development) and the International Monetary Fund (IMF). They, at Keynes' insistence, were also about to set up a World Trade Organization (WTO) to ensure equity in international trade, but Roosevelt eventually vetoed this idea because it would have imposed restraints on US economic power. Also, as will be explained later, the WTO was eventually set up in 1995, but in such a way as to embrace US control over global trade, rather than the reverse. Keynes' WTO would have been an agency of the UN, but the current WTO is not. This makes a great difference.

## RÔLES OF THE WORLD BANK AND THE IMF

The relationship between these two bodies is of immense importance to a consideration of what follows. Briefly, for now, it can be summarized as follows.

The IMF agrees on broad lines of policy in matters such as establishing and maintaining currency convertibility, and trying to avoid competitive exchange depreciation. In that sense, and unlike the World Bank, its main rôle was as a fiscal think tank and not merely a financial institution. Initially its basic financial policy was to adhere strictly to the gold standard in adjudicating loans to member countries. However, the USA came off the gold standard in the early 1960s. Thus the IMF was restrained from high-risk lending. Indeed, it only lends to treasuries and central banks of member countries, and generally over only 5 years. Originally, then, the IMF saw its function as being to help member states in the short term should they run into temporary balance-of-payments problems.[2]

However, it is the issue of which countries were 'member states' at Bretton Woods, and which ones were not, that has brought about a sea change. That is, the World Bank and the IMF were never intended to lend money to desperately poor peasant economies of perennially low industrial capacity, but to nations – such as those in Europe – whose infrastructure had only been badly damaged by the war.

Before discussing how the IMF could moderate short-term loans to temporarily cash-strapped nations, let us consider the IMF's twin sister, the World Bank. The World Bank has virtually the same membership as the IMF, but is endowed with much greater financial flexibility. For instance, it can make long-term loans over periods of, say, 20 years and can now even lend to private projects in less developed countries. As we shall see, it can – and frequently does – finance such private projects as the setting up of water purification facilities, which in turn has meant that users can only access safe drinking water by paying for it. Thus it is seen as directly influencing the running of poorer countries. The World Bank makes very widespread use of private banks in both the developed and less developed world as principal and intermediary lenders. Furthermore, it can even sell outstanding debts on the financial markets. Indeed, it is this capacity of First World banks to 'sell outstanding debt' that keeps them safe, while mortgaging the less developed countries (LDCs) even further.

As to how the IMF and the World Bank became involved in lending money to very poor LDCs whose economics had never been strong, and had not been ruined suddenly through war, the scenario unfolded as follows. From 1944 to 1972–73, the World Bank and the IMF loaned very little money to impoverished LDCs, especially those with no domestic oil reserves. However, the Organization of Petroleum Exporting Countries (OPEC) began to put pressure on the oil-hungry heavily industrialized nations in Europe and North America by raising the price of oil. This brought huge profits in US dollars to the OPEC countries, which then invested them in banks in developed countries. These banks would then have to pay heavy interest rates on the deposits. They, linked with the World Bank and the IMF, had to find some way of reinvesting the deposits to extract a higher interest rate than they would have to give to the original depositors. In effect the LDCs, especially those which had no access to domestic supplies of oil, saved the banks in the developed world. The World Bank and the IMF shifted their interest to the LDCs, offering to make them development loans without too great a regard as to whether or not the loans could ever be paid back without jeopardizing the recipient country.

In order for the LDCs to repay, they needed to industrialize rapidly. This required the importation of oil from OPEC countries at high costs, which drove them to default on loan repayments and to ask for extensions on existing loans at even higher interest rates. Of course, the banks were now awash with US dollars that had to be reinvested quickly, so they were only too glad to help out in this way. Over time, this has led one LDC after another into unbelievably perilous financial circumstances. For instance, some African countries are actually spending more on compound interest rates (not the principal!) than they can spend on health and education. And it is here that the question of how the World Bank and the IMF can ensure that debt repayment comes in.

As soon as a loan is made by the World Bank or the IMF, the debtor nation has to agree to certain Structural Adjustment Policies (SAPs). These are conditions imposed by the banks on the country in order to ensure that its economy can maintain the repayments. Thus a common SAP requirement is that the debtor nation must drastically reduce its expenditure on government services. In any government, two major services are health and education. Thus the debtor nation is compelled to privatize such services as far as possible. This means that there follows a great reduction in these services in the debtor country. Teachers and healthcare workers who were once employed in the public sector are dismissed and driven to seek employment in newly established private enterprises, which of course have to make a profit (which a public service is not required to do), and all of this results in poorer working conditions in health and education at the same time as it excludes a large proportion of the population from accessing these services.

This is routinely coupled with what is referred to as 'verticalization', which means the tendency to concentrate medical and educational services in the main urban/industrial areas, near to ports, in order to further sustain the growing need of the debtor country to export goods for foreign sale in US dollars. All World Bank and IMF loans have to be paid off in US dollars. A country that is free to spend its resources running health and education as public services will try to 'horizontalize' those services, the obvious aim being to reach all of its citizens. Thus, increasingly after 1973, the IMF and the World Bank became accused of widening the gap in health rights between the developed countries and the LDCs.

## RÔLE OF THE WTO

The author will now show how the WTO ties in with the World Bank and the IMF, and how its own mechanisms operate to ensure compliance with SAPs. As we have seen already, the type of WTO advocated at Bretton Woods by Keynes was rejected by US President Roosevelt as an impediment to America's need to provide a global outreach for its huge and growing domestic industrial capacity, unchanged until then by the ravages of war or armed invasion. However, the WTO was reinstated in 1995, under terms that were more in harmony with US corporate interests, and not as an agency of the UN.

This was done as follows. Each country is, theoretically, represented in the WTO, and the latter mediates trade regulations between countries, the emphasis being on unfettered free trade. In pursuit of this the WTO encourages various bilateral and multilateral agreements between countries to open up access to one another's markets – for instance, the North America Free Trade Agreement (which encourages Canada, the USA and Mexico not to tariff one another's industrial output), and the Caribbean Free Trade Association (CARIFTA), which similarly applies to the small Caribbean countries, etc. However, two unilateral agreements that have been mediated and enforced by the WTO will be mentioned here as being of particular significance. These are the General Agreement on Tariffs and Trade (GATT) and the General Agreement on Trade in Services (GATS). GATT essentially gives the WTO the right to insist on any country's rights to export its goods to any other country. No country in the WTO has the right to try to protect its own products by imposing tariffs on imports. Even more draconian in its impact on health inequities between nations is GATS, which gives any WTO member the right to compete in selling services (such as health and education) to any other member state.

Both GATT and GATS have attracted a great deal of adverse comment over the last few years with regard to their negative impact on health, but any account of the WTO's arsenal for enforcing free trade would be incomplete unless it mentioned Trade-Related Intellectual Property Rights (TRIPS). TRIPS is really a radical reinterpretation of patent law. One implication is that if a region is known to have traditionally been particularly successful in producing a particular crop, and if agronomists over time succeed in isolating the particular gene complex and, better still, in reproducing it, they can patent it. Even if the original local producer wants to continue exporting its unique product, it can be charged a fee to do so under TRIPS regulations. This also applies to pharmaceuticals isolated after years of research by large multinational houses. A telling example that has recently appeared in the news is the production of antiretroviral drugs (ARVs) for the control of HIV/AIDS. Such pharmaceuticals are extremely expensive and cannot be routinely purchased by the vast majority of patients with HIV/AIDS in the LDCs. However, both India and Brazil have recently earned a reputation for being able to mass-produce generic copies of these expensive ARVs at as little as 4–5% of the cost demanded by the pharmaceutical companies. Yet TRIPS regulations under the WTO may well prevent the widespread sale of these generic copies to countries in Africa or elsewhere. This issue will be dealt with in detail in subsequent chapters of this book.

An even more negative aspect of TRIPS will be discussed in Chapter 4, where we deal with the issues involved in using the specific viruses that cause disease in LDCs, and the WHO's rôle in extracting these viruses in order to develop vaccines to counter those diseases. The WHO is free to pass these samples out to private agencies which, once they have developed an effective vaccine, then patent it. The upshot is that the LDC which originally provided the virus has no authoritative rights to the vaccine to protect its own people because, under TRIPS, the vaccine now belongs to the private agency concerned and must be purchased from them. As the reader will be aware, there are several varieties of bird flu, which vary slightly according to where they are active. Indonesia, in good faith, provided the WHO with samples of the bird flu pathogens active there. Only sometime later did they become aware (as discussed in detail below) that the WHO had handed the sample over to a private laboratory for analysis without any precondition that Indonesia should have prior access to any vaccine developed to counter the infection.

The question arises as to whether the WHO – given its mandate to promote and defend universal access to healthcare as a human right – even recognizes TRIPS. To do so would surely constitute privatizing the WHO.

Another major criticism of the WTO is that despite its democratic pretensions, its successive meetings have failed to address the LDCs' objections to the adverse impact on health and other human rights of its rulings with regard to trade, and the application of TRIPS to medicine, agriculture, etc. To set the scene for further analysis of these pivotal issues, let us now summarize the state of play.

## A QUICK HISTORY OF WTO RESOLUTIONS

As already stated, the purpose of the WTO is to bring about global free trade, and to this end the Technical Barriers to Trade (TBT) Agreement was negotiated at the Uruguay round of GATT and then culminated in the Marrakech Agreement, from which the creation of the WTO was actually negotiated (in 1994). The WTO formally came into existence on 1 January 1995. At the very first of its ministerial conferences (in Singapore in 1996), disagreements arose over the issues discussed previously between the delegates from developed countries and LDCs. They were not satisfactorily resolved, and were reserved for resolution at the Second Ministerial Conference (in Geneva in 1998). The debate was acrimonious, and it was decided to defer the issue until after a new Director General had been elected. On 1 September 1999, Mike Moore (from the USA) assumed the post, but not without protracted argument. Another contender was Supachai Panithpakdi (from India), and a compromise was reached with the two sharing the post for 3 years each, Mike Moore holding it first. Again, attempts to settle the concerns of the LDC delegates were deferred until the Third Ministerial Conference (in Seattle in December 1999). It was during those deliberations that the now famous riots occurred, as popular antagonism to the WTO began to mount. The Seattle conference was followed in November 2001 by the Fourth Ministerial Conference in Doha, Qatar. At this conference the Doha Declaration was drawn up. This is a pivotal document that contains clauses purportedly designed to protect less developed nations from the detrimental effects on health and trade arising from WTO rulings relating to TRIPS, etc. These clauses did not themselves have the force of law, and were sufficiently general in their formulation as to make their enforcement ambiguous. For a more complete discussion of the Doha Declaration, the reader is referred to an earlier book by this author.[3]

Since the Doha Declaration, the WTO has been a primary concern among people working for global equity in human rights, and its subsequent ministerial conferences have been anticipated with a mixture of cynicism that nothing will change, and the hope that protective clauses will become binding. The Fifth Ministerial Conference took place in Taiwan in January 2002. However, the Doha Declaration barely got a look-in there, as the debate focused on the issue of customs and trading rights vis-à-vis China and Taiwan. China had finally become a member of the WTO a year previously, in January 2001. The conference was on this occasion under the chairmanship of Supachai Panithpakdi, so there was an expectation that perhaps the concerns of the LDCs would be given greater priority. Instead it was resolved that they would be discussed at the Sixth Ministerial Conference, which was scheduled to take place in Cancún, Mexico in September 2003!

At that meeting, an alliance of 22 delegates representing LDCs led by India, China and Brazil resisted developed-world trading interests. In particular, they called for an end to agricultural subsidies within the EU and the USA. However, these talks also broke down, although there was an agreement to solidify the

Doha Declaration clauses at the next meeting. These delays of course continued to exacerbate the problems in the LDCs and – as we shall see – the inequities in health rights between the developed and less developed nations widened. Progress seemed to be made at the Seventh Ministerial Conference in Geneva in August 2004. Roughly the agreement was that the EU and the USA, along with other developed countries, would lower tariff barriers to manufactured goods from the developed world.

The significance of these concerns may seem to the casual reader to be remote from health rights issues. However, this is far from the case. Consider Burkina Faso, one of the world's poorest nations and a former French colony in Africa that achieved independence in 1960. Its soil and climate are such that it produces prodigious crops of cotton cheaply and easily, and this is its principal export. However, in the USA, cotton farmers in Mississippi receive agricultural subsidies that allow them to use expensive fertilizers to produce cotton, not as easily as Burkina Faso does, but because of the subsidies, the USA can sell what it does produce on the international market at an even lower price than Burkina Faso can. As Burkina Faso's cotton farmers face economic ruin, a precipitous derogation of domestic, health and other human rights, there is an obvious consequence.

## THE WORLD HEALTH ORGANIZATION

The WHO was formally established on 7 April 1948 as the UN's specialist agency for health. In its constitution,[4] it states that the objective of the WHO is attainment by all peoples of the highest possible level of health. The constitution then goes on to define health as a 'state of complete physical, mental and social well-being and not merely the absence of disease or infirmity.' This definition obviously casts its remit very broadly indeed, for if we are not speaking only of the 'absence of disease', we are referring to much more than clinical or biomedical criteria. Indeed, we are referring to health promotion.[5] This in turn must involve – at the very least – primary healthcare (PHC). PHC is defined in slightly different ways by different health agencies. For instance, within biomedical circles, PHC is but the first rung of a three-rung hierarchy, consisting of PHC, secondary healthcare (SHC) and tertiary healthcare (THC). PHC refers to access to a general medical practitioner and possibly a nurse or health visitor, SCH refers to clinical facilities and more diagnostic tests (e.g. X-ray), and THC refers to the most esoteric levels of medical technology, specialist surgery, etc. However, that is not what the WHO meant by PHC, nor was it what the UN Charter had in mind when it referred to PHC as a 'human right.' Not only does PHC have a wider remit than the 'operational' definition given above (because it includes access to dentistry and to pharmaceuticals), but also it embraces all of the social contexts that enhance health.

The working definition of PHC in this context was elaborated by the WHO in 1978 in its now famous Alma Ata Declaration.[6] In general, it was held to be a strategy that not only responds equitably, appropriately and effectively to clinical healthcare needs, but also deals comprehensibly with social, economic and political causes and consequences of poor health. It unambiguously establishes health as more political than a purely clinical concern. At a meeting of the International People's Health University (IPHU) in Cuenca, Ecuador in July 2005, PHC was defined by David Sanders[7] as including the following:

1  It must be applicable universally and converge on the basis of need alone.
2  It must be comprehensive in that it emphasizes disease prevention and health promotion.
3  It must embrace both the individual and community involvement, and inculcate responsibility for maintaining health.
4  It must be intersectorial, involving cooperation between all of the relevant agencies (education, law enforcement, medical, etc.).
5  It must include access on the basis of need alone to all available medical or diagnostic technology that resources allow.

The WHO has continued to play a key rôle in promoting the need to make PHC realisable as a 'human right', and indeed in this it has been perfectly consistent with the UN Charter. However, since 1988 it has been running into difficulties. As the author pointed out in 2005,[8] the original guiding WHO principles of PHC as a basic human right have been increasingly sidelined as financial globalization, under such mechanisms as the IMF, SAPs and WTO imposition of policies under GATS, has predominated. Instead of health being regarded as a basic human right (as in the UN Charter), it has been becoming more and more of a 'desideratum if it can be afforded.'

The primary agencies that concern us in this context are the World Bank, the IMF and the WTO. Each of these bodies is linked to a huge array of instrumentalities for accomplishing its objectives. The principal ones are the SAPs, GATT and GATS. There follows a brief account of these agencies, showing how they interrelate. We shall then consider a much more detailed account, which forms a basis for analysing the often negative impact of these agencies on health and other human rights, even in the developed world, but especially in the LDCs.

## THE WORLD BANK AND THE IMF

The World Bank and the IMF are sometimes referred to as 'twin sisters', because they both emerged from the Bretton Woods Conference that was convened in July 1944. However, the context in which both of these agencies emerged, and the roots of their subsequent highly controversial rôles in restraining the WHO, must be briefly revisited if the reader is to make any sense of the current dominance of neoliberal influence in the UN. This will also provide a better insight into those factors which render it necessary to reform the UN if it is to regain authority as a transnational mediator of human rights.

Not only did the horror and devastation of World War Two itself impose a sense of urgency on the project, but also overwhelmingly the opinion among delegates was that pre-war problems had to be resolved in order to bring about an administratively feasible procedure for exercising transnational control over future events. Specifically, it was a majority view at that meeting that the emergence of fascism itself, especially in Italy, Spain and above all Germany, had been caused by the collapse of international trade and the tendency, especially in the USA, to indulge in isolationist economic policies. The Great Depression itself was held to have had its origin in the same causes.[9]

The US delegation played a hugely dominant rôle in the discussions and in determining the agenda for debate. In that sense, the presence of John Maynard Keynes from the UK proved to be somewhat of an irritant to the negotiations. He wanted to establish a world reserve currency administered by a Central Bank that would itself be set up by the Bretton Woods delegates. His argument was that this would create a more stable, and certainly more impartial, global economy by automatically recycling trade surplus in order to compensate for trade deficits. Such an idea was anathema to US interests. The US delegates wanted to run and referee global trade alone, and insisted that the only recognized tender be the US dollar, not some 'artificial world reserve currency' produced by a transnational central bank. Before dealing with this, however, it is imperative to remember just how robust the US economy had become during the isolationist pre-war years. The wealth and welfare of citizens were tied to its huge industrial capacity and to its flexibility and inventiveness in adapting to new industrial needs. Without unhindered global access to trade, its economy would be stifled. We shall explain later how Keynes' system would have worked.

Just to give an idea of how thrusting and vibrant that economy was, we are talking about a country that, towards the end of World War Two, was turning out one fully equipped battleship a day![10] US fears back then were perfectly in keeping with the strongly isolationist tendencies which grew and fed into domestic politics between world wars. (In the author's view, it is important to appreciate this because it renders current US resistance to such initiatives as an International Court of Justice, Kyoto Environmental Global Protocols, etc., much more understandable. These are not instances of some newly hostile trend in US politics, but are deeply rooted in the country's cultural consciousness.) Instead, the Conference made the fateful decision to impose a system based both on the freedom of movement of goods between countries and on the use of the US dollar as the international currency. As we shall see, both of these policies underlie the global inequity with regard to health and human rights which so urgently needs to be addressed. Out of those decisions arose the agreement that the IMF and the World Bank should be restricted to managing problems related to currency and capital shortage.

## ORIGINAL MANDATE OF THE IMF AND THE WORLD BANK

It should now be obvious that the foregoing discussions were based on the assumption that the primary purpose of the IMF and the World Bank was to finance the restructuring of the war-wrecked economies of Europe. The idea of their rôle being to provide basic financial aid to the LDCs was not even considered. Indeed, the rôle of the LDCs as debtors to the Bretton Woods institutions only came about through factors outside the control of the Conference.

The lack of a transnational central bank (as suggested by Keynes) meant that the IMF and the World Bank were not really 'banks' themselves with money to lend. They worked (and still do) largely through private banks in the USA and the UK. The application for a loan would be considered and handed over to one of the private banks involved for their discussion. The discussion was usually positive because, unlike personal loans, for which the bank manager has to decide whether the putative borrower is a good risk, a debtor country is almost always useful to have on your books. There are two main reasons for this. First, the loan is made to the country, not to its leader. Thus if a country is run by a corrupt leadership which squanders the money on arms to keep its own populace down, or even fiddles and squirrels it away in Swiss bank accounts, and the government is then overthrown, the debt is still owed. The new regime, even if it is impeccably honest, is still liable. Secondly, and more to the point, in both the USA and the UK, if a debtor nation defaults, the bank's loss is made up by the Government. This is part of the arrangement that the IMF and the World Bank have with the participating private banks. Not unnaturally, bank stockholders are rather partial to lending money to poor LDCs under these circumstances.

## PRIVATE BANKS PROFIT FROM THE IMF AND THE WORLD BANK

In addition, the repayment programme to which the debtor nation agrees, and the attendant SAPs, generate even greater profits for the lending bank. The repayments must be made in US dollars. To obtain these, the debtor nations generally have to export goods to wealthy developed countries. As part of the SAPs, the debtor nation has to buy from the lender nation any infrastructural equipment and/or services that are needed to industrialize production of the goods that are being marketed. This of course includes not only the goods themselves, but also the roads required to move the produce to the ports, the fertilizers required to increase yields, etc. Large-scale deforestation is often one of the attendant results. In addition, water supplies become chemically polluted, working conditions deteriorate and union activity is suppressed in order to produce the export goods more cheaply. Typically, an LDC that is intensively producing a particular crop in order to finance repayments on its loan finds itself in cut-throat competition with other similar poor countries producing the same crop.

When such a debtor nation is unable to maintain payment of the compound interest[11] on the loan, it is usual for the loan to be rescheduled, which generates even more profit for the developed-world lender nation's bank stockholders. As a result of these arrangements, the total international debt of the LDCs to the developed world has ballooned enormously. Fidel Castro famously commented in one of his speeches that 'La deuda internaccional es una deuda impagable'

('The international debt is an unpayable debt').[12] Further information about these matters can be found in the author's book *Third World Health: Hostage to First World Wealth*.[11]

## THE WTO AND THE TYRANNY OF FREE TRADE

Greatly adding to the IMF-induced woes of LDC borrowers is the power of the WTO in enforcing free trade. Although all nations can be admitted as members to the WTO, all on a theoretically equal basis, this 'equality' is questionable. Each WTO member has one seat, certainly, but there is no limit to the number of legal advisers that any nation can call upon in making its case to the WTO Council. This is crucial, because most LDCs can only provide one 'adviser' (someone with specialist training in international law), and some have no such representation at all. The wealthier nations, on the other hand, can have several advisers, while the USA can provide dozens. The predictable effect is that, in a dispute between a small LDC and the USA over a free trade issue, the USA is in a far stronger position to prevail. Also, it must not be forgotten that, since the WTO is not a UN agency, it is not constrained by the UDHR.

However, despite this disadvantage, there are powerful voices in the developed world that seek to disempower LDC members of the WTO even further. Before dealing with this issue, though, it is important to realize that these poor nations were not entirely supine in their predicament.

## THE EMERGENCE OF UNCTAD

The LDCs had begun to organize and to demand better conditions by the early 1960s, when things were beginning to go badly in Vietnam for US interests. The latter could no longer take the LDCs for granted so easily. The cold war meant that the former Soviet Union and the USA each worked assiduously to curry favour with the less developed nations. In this context, by 1965 the non-aligned nations had formed the Group of 77 to promote their grievances in UN circles. As a result, the UN Conference on Trade and Development (UNCTAD) was convened, and there the aggrieved LDCs were able to argue for more equitable terms for financing urgent development needs. The major developed nations could do little but agree, but insisted that the Bretton Woods institutions would have to challenge any initiative arising from UNCTAD.[13] Of course, the major developed nations, and particularly the USA, controlled the Bretton Woods institutions!

However, by 1968 the belief that the Bretton Woods committee could realistically run a global and stable monetary system, based on fixed interest rates, with the US dollar as the only permitted international currency, was beginning to appear less and less plausible. Not only was this being resisted by both France and Germany, but the US dollar was collapsing under the strain of war and budgeting deficits. Some of the smaller economies, such as Japan, were in vigorous ascendancy. Altogether some LDCs had their self-confidence boosted by comparatively high growth rates and the above-mentioned dramatic increase in the price of oil. However, even that did not alter the balance of equity to the degree that was hoped and expected. Nations of the developed world responded by making many noble declarations of good intentions at international level both within and outside the UN, but without actually committing to drastic change.

Of course, we have since seen this many times, with successive G7/G8 resolutions to address the inequities and the dilatory tactics of the WTO in implementing the Doha Declaration as cases in point. We have already referred in passing to the enormous increase in dollar reserves accumulated in 1973 by the OPEC nations, and their tactic of investing this in the USA or the EU.

The enormous oil profits made by OPEC in the 1970s – over US$310 billion between 1972 and 1977 alone – meant that the money had to be reinvested. Most of it was deposited in commercial banks which, through the IMF, lent it to the non-oil-producing LDCs. The latter needed the money badly to finance their major infrastructure projects which were being carried out for development. This increased the debt fivefold between 1973 and 1982. The amount owed reached US$612 billion, plus the high interest rates on the loans. Corruption saw to it that much of this money was filched by government personnel, and a great deal was spent on poorly planned projects. Countries such as Mexico and Peru found themselves unable to pay even the mounting compound interest bills. Banks that were already in the IMF and the World Bank sold their outstanding debts to these bodies, which then imposed SAPs on the LDCs concerned, effectively taking over their economic policies.[14]

It is undeniable now that, at the time, the World Bank and the IMF did take advantage of the situation. Indeed, this was also consistent with the prevailing right-wing political context in the developed world, characterized by the policies of US President Ronald Reagan and UK Prime Minister Margaret Thatcher. All of these factors sustained what became the dominant orthodoxies of both the World Bank and the IMF. From this grew the ideas of 'structural adjustment' and the various contradictions that have already been discussed.

By 'structurally adjusting' the economies of the LDCs, they in effect deflated them, because the SAPs required the borrower nation's government to use private services and to concentrate on production for dollar-earning exports, rather than for domestic consumption. This policy was highly profitable for the private banks – netting them US$178 billion between 1984 and 1990 – but of course the LDC debt increased rapidly, and by 1992 had reached US$1300 billion, most of which was shifted to the IMF and the World Bank.

These policies allowed firms to take over the provision of such infrastructures as the telephone and telecommunications services, and even the water supply, in one LDC after another, for which the country concerned then paid back in US dollars as part of the SAPs on which the loan was conditional. Delays in implementing reforms promised at G8 and WTO meetings only highlight the problems. What this means, in effect, is that the IMF and the World Bank were taking more money out of the LDCs than they were putting back in! People in the LDCs, aware of this, often resisted their government's alliance with the IMF by holding street riots, etc. Meanwhile, World Bank-funded mega-structures, such as dams, also encountered popular resistance due to the fact that citizens faced both eviction from their homes and loss of their livelihoods. This has caused not only antipathy to western values, but also a parallel rise in religious fundamentalism and political violence.

## THE RÔLE OF UNCTAD

This body has certainly tried to act as both advocate and mediator in trade-related issues for the LDCs, as is evident from the Third World Network comments.[15] It is obvious that 'liberalizing' trade does not create a level playing field, and certainly has not stimulated growth in service development in poor countries. In 2006, UNCTAD produced a similar paper, entitled *Trade in Services and Development Implications* (TD/B/Com.1/77), which was distributed at its Commission on Trade in Goods and Services at its Geneva meeting in February 2006.

This paper highlighted concerns about the impact of both GATS and GATT, but especially the former. These included the displacement of local providers in favour of offshore firms, particularly in health, education and broad cultural provision. Basing much of its analysis on the outcome of the Hong Kong Ministerial Conference, UNCTAD's paper emphasised that even GATS and GATT allow for more flexible arrangements than the WTO seemed ready to acknowledge. The following were mentioned in this regard:

1  Liberalization disadvantages the less favoured segments of the population, especially in essential services such as health.
2  Trade liberalization can undercut a nation's own, long evolved values in cultural and educational matters.
3  Trade liberalization creates short-term costs, which distort national planning.
4  Some services, as currently provided domestically, need time to adjust to the international market before they can become competitive.

What UNCTAD suggests is that each country has unique needs and contexts with regard to commodity and service provision, and should be allowed time to access the costs and benefits involved before being forced to comply with GATS and GATT. This must involve such issues as employment displacement vs. employment creation, provisions for technology instruction, gains in efficiency vs. negative impacts on the informal sector, raising quality standards to allow effective competition in overseas markets, etc. Barriers posed by international standards, development of infrastructures and means of facilitating market access, etc., also need time and scope for development.

The paper addresses a wide range of findings on a variety of sectors not directly related to health or other human rights, but most certainly indirectly related. For example, a study of Ecuador – which has been badly affected since 2005 by the 'dollarization' of the economy to bring it into line with the requirements of bilateral trade agreement and of GATS – showed that, in distribution of services, it is crucial to avoid a market situation in which the product (or service) of several sellers is in the interests of one buyer! That problem arose in Ecuador's wholesale services. If liberalization of trade was to take place under such conditions, it would merely replace a monopoly of domestic providers with a foreign monopoly.

## AFRICA SIGNALS EROSION OF UNCTAD

As we so often find, it is some of the African countries that seem to suffer the most at the hands of global finance. And it is African trade ministers who have been most vocal in commenting on UNCTAD's apparent loss of influence. Moreover, they strongly argue that developed-world interests are complicit in this. This issue was extensively debated in Nairobi in April 2006 at the fourth session of the African Union's Conference of Trade Ministers. Indeed, concern was so great that a special motion on UNCTAD, and possible reforms to it, was adopted by the conference.[16]

'We know that UNCTAD has come under pressure and we need a vote of confidence on UNCTAD and to send it a signal of solidarity', the Kenyan Trade and Industry Minister, Mukhisa Kituyi said. One of the Zimbabwean delegates was even less optimistic when he observed that reforms to the UN that were gathering pace in New York could even threaten the survival of UNCTAD. Proposals voicing such concerns were supported by other delegations, including those from Zambia, Lesotho and Ghana. The ministers presented a Declaration which included the statement that:

> In view of the nature of UNCTAD's programmes and activities for capacity building, we are concerned with recent proposals of some developed countries to erode the mandate of UNCTAD or even to discontinue it altogether.

Such warning signals arise in the context of a movement among corporate interests in some developed countries to radically restructure the UN so that its activities bring it more into line with neoliberal financial control. The Netherlands, Belgium and the UK, with US approval, are proposing that UNCTAD's influence be diluted by merging it with other agencies. One version of this, for instance, would see UNCTAD merged with the WTO or the UN Development Programme (UNDP), or even into a single UN Development Authority.

## THE HIDDEN FACE OF DEVELOPED-WORLD FINANCIAL POWER

What must be realized is that, catastrophic as the financial plight of the LDCs is, it fits brilliantly with the needs of developed-world business interests. Only 6 weeks prior to the 'Millennium Round' in Seattle, the US Senate had approved deregulation of the country's banking system! This would make it legal for US banks and transnational corporations to invest heavily in other countries. The implications are clear. A small cluster of US financial bodies will gain control over the entire US financial services industry. It should come as no surprise that these are the bodies that gain most advantage from financial services deregulation under GATS. These enormously powerful financial bodies will end up overseeing financial and economic development globally. They are the creditors and shareholders of high-tech manufacturing, the defence industry, major oil and mining interests, etc.

Because they would underwrite public debt, they would have an effective control on individual politicians and even of governments. They could determine whether or not it is to their financial advantage to declare war, for instance, and because of the matrix of organizational connections, they are in a position to mediate its prosecution.[17]

Furthermore, the clauses of the now defunct Multilateral Agreement on Investments (MAI), which was to provide 'national treatment to foreign banks', are in the process of becoming a fait accompli. They are fully integrated with insurance companies which themselves oversee multinational healthcare providers, such as those that the present UK government under Gordon Brown is anxious to involve in the National Health Service in Britain. In the USA, these same providers are actively lobbying for the deregulation of public healthcare under GATS. This threatens the entire welfare state, and risks nullifying most of the great social gains that have been made since 1945.

## POSSIBLE IMPACT ON THE UK'S NATIONAL HEALTH SERVICE

Since 1947, Britain has been blessed with its NHS, which was brought into being after the Second World War and has been honed over the years since. It allows every UK citizen access to all levels of healthcare, most of it free at point of contact. However, the present government, as part of its desire to become more integrated with US policies, has been making moves to gradually privatize the NHS and thus bring it under neoliberal financial deregulation. It is doing this in various ways, one of the most prominent being various Private Finance Initiatives (PFIs). Under the present NHS, whatever its inefficiencies, the entire UK population is covered and it costs less than 7% of GNP.

The USA spends more – nearly 15% of GNP – under its system, which relies largely on health cover under private health insurance funds. There are also government-funded programmes that provide financial aid for the elderly and disabled, but these are nowhere near complete, and in any case they do not cover all illness. On top of this, about 31% of Americans are without any health insurance cover at all. Basically, the British seem to get a lot more for their 7% of GNP than US citizens do for their 15%!

However, the NHS and organizations like it are anathema to neoliberal orthodoxies. The case has been well and succinctly argued by Dr Hannah Caller.[18] It turns out that the hospitals worst affected by bad management, ward closures, reductions in staff, etc. were those under the PFI. The Centre for International Public Health Policy at the University of Edinburgh has analysed the performance of eight of the PFI schemes, and showed that the proportion of their annual reserves devoted to servicing capital expenditure rose from 4.5% to 16% as a result of PFI.

Already a number of large multinational finance corporations are involved in PFI, or are hungrily waiting by the sidelines, because there are large profits to be made from healthcare under GATS. However, it stands to reason that if profits are made by it (which they are), these dividends must come out of funds that would otherwise all pay for healthcare. It is difficult to see how people can credit any argument to the contrary, but certainly a great deal of money is being spent to try to persuade them. It is in the interest of corporate power that the PFI battle is won in the UK.

Corporate involvement in Britain's NHS is comparatively slight so far, but even so, juicy profits have already been made. Caller cites an example. Two years after completion of the Norfolk and Norwich PFI hospitals, four finance corporations – Barclays Bank, Stereo, Innisfree and John Laing – decided to refinance their joint working company, Octagon. That alone allowed them to make a profit of £115 million (more than US$200 million). They gave £45 million to the hospital, and kept the rest! This increased their rate of return from 16% to 60%. The NHS Health Trust currently tied to this arrangement would have to pay £257 million to extricate itself from it. Even now, in order to pay the PFI consortia, the hospitals concerned have had to reduce beds by 25% and staff by 15%.

Two points are well made by all of the above. First, neoliberal finance does not victimize only the LDCs. The UK is most certainly a highly developed society, but once it allows itself to become so closely tied to neoliberalism, its own citizens are not spared any more than LDC citizens, nor are US citizens. Secondly, if health is to be a basic human right, there is no room for financial profits to be made from its provision. Financial deregulation in the USA threatens human rights globally.

However, it is the involvement of the UN, and the WHO in particular, with neoliberalism that is the main thrust of this book. In this regard we have given some indication of the rôles of the World Bank, the IMF and the WTO – together with such instrumentalities as SAPs, GATT and GATS – in this involvement. The reader will recall that as long ago as 1944, at the Bretton Woods conference, a WTO was first considered (along with the equivalence of GATT and GATS), as suggested by Maynard Keynes. The USA did not approve of Keynes' plans, and therefore it was rejected, but let us consider how different things would have been if his view had prevailed.

## KEYNES' IDEAS FOR A WTO

Keynes' original ideas about a WTO go even further back than that fateful Bretton Woods meeting in 1944, for he first raised the idea in England in 1942 during highly theoretical discussions along the lines of 'What should we do if we win the war?' In 1944, Keynes' ideas were eventually thrown out, and the author will now explain how this came about, and indeed what those original ideas entailed, for that history has recently assumed renewed importance. This was due to a conference (on 28 November 2006) convened by the Norwegian Foreign Ministry to consider growing global unease about the issue of conditionalities being forced on debtor nations by the IMF, the World Bank and the WTO.

The meeting involved about 100 delegates, including government officials of several European countries, along with non-government organizations (NGOs) and concerned individuals from all over the world. An excellent review of this gathering and the relevant economic issue has been provided by an NGO called 'Share the World's Resources.'[19]

The origins of the conference lie in the political platform formulated by the coalition Norwegian government, which in its Soria Moria Declaration stated that 'Norwegian aid should not support programmes that are made conditional on liberalization and privatization.' Opening the conference, Norway's Minister of International Development, Erik Solheim, said 'We are curious about what is the state of World Bank–IMF conditionality.'

'Our government came to office on a programme that there should be no conditionality forcing loan recipients on liberalization and privatization', he said. Solheim stated that the choice of such policies should be made by the countries: 'Some want to nationalize, some want to privatize. Such policies are up to the countries and should not be made by donors or creditors.' For developed countries, that had established the basis for both growth and democracy, there had been no set pattern, as there had been varying degrees of emphasis among them on the private sector or the public sector.

Explaining the reason for the conference, Solheim said that Norway had asked the World Bank and the IMF if they put forward privatization and liberalization conditionalities with their loans, and their response was 'no more.' However, the NGOs had said that in fact there had been no change. The only way forward was to determine the facts, to 'seek truth from facts.' Thus there was a need for open dialogue, as for too long the discussion had been conducted in closed circles.

Needless to say, the issue of conditionalities has assumed a high profile because of the Millennium Development Goals (MDGs) prioritized by Kofi Annan (Director General of the UN until 2007), and this motivation to rethink the issue was specifically mentioned by the UK's Parliamentary Under-Secretary of State for International Development, Gareth Thomas, who stated that the UK government took conditionalities seriously, as donors should use the right kind of conditionality. 'Imposing development from outside does not work', he said. 'Countries must formulate their own policies and donors should move away from the old neoliberal approach.' The best policies come from public debate, which donors should not prevent. As aid comes from taxes, citizens can hold the government accountable for preventing misuse of the funds.

Thomas said that the new UK aid policy is built on poverty reduction and achieving the MDGs, respect for human rights, and financial accountability. To make aid more predictable, he stated, 'we'll move from aid only if the country moves from these three principles.' Improving IMF and World Bank conditionality is important, and 'we will also press the regional development banks to review their conditionality . . . The days have moved from where the IMF and World Bank tell countries what to do.' In 2005 the UK had asked the World Bank to review whether their conditionalities had changed, and it would not release £50 million sterling to the World Bank if there was no progress. Good practice guidelines must be followed, and Thomas stated that 'we will hold the Bank to account for that.'

However, if they are to do anything about the issue, changes to the way in which the IMF and the WTO use conditionalities, and the way that they use GATT and GATS to achieve this, will be required. Thus Keynes' original ideas need to be revisited. In an article published in the Paris-based journal, *Le Monde Diplomatique*, Susan George discussed this critical historical background.[20]

As she points out, it was painfully obvious at the 1944 Bretton Woods Conference that some way must be found for all of the world's countries – but especially those extensively damaged by the war – to be able to resume reasonably secure international trade. Back in 1942, Keynes argued that the war itself was partly a result of unregulated free trade and insufficiently regulated cut-throat competition for the same markets, and that it was therefore imperative that a more carefully internationally monitored trading system be established. He suggested a new central bank which could issue its own currency (Bancor currency) to be used for trade. This new central bank would be called the International Clearing Union (ICU). Keynes' idea was for an International Trade Organization (ITO) to be established as a UN body, supported by the ICU.

If that plan had gained approval we could, according to Susan George, have had a world order in which no country could run a huge deficit (the USA deficit stood at US$716 billion in 2005) or a huge trade surplus (like that of contemporary China). Under such a system, crushing Third World debt and the devastating SAPs applied by the World Bank and the IMF would have been unthinkable, although the system would not have abolished capitalism. If we could resurrect Keynes' concept, another world really might be possible. He figured out how to make it work more than 60 years ago, so his plan would have to be dusted off and tinkered with, but its core remains relevant.

## THE POLITICS OF POWER

Why did such a good idea not become adopted? The answer is simply because those original Bretton Woods delegates were behaving like the members of the League of Nations in that they could not allow concern for anything as rational as global justice and peace to supersede national interests. And since the USA naturally had hegemony over the group, that meant paramountcy of US financial interests. However, there were other political reasons as well. As we have seen, Keynes had been promoting these ideas in the early days of the war and had tacit US support, and indeed in July 1944 he actually chaired the Monetary Sub-Committee at the 1944 Bretton Woods meeting.

However, by that time, and with US corporate interests no longer worried about losing the war, new pressures were applied to US delegates at Bretton Woods to reject the ITO and ICU ideas. Those corporations stood to make a lot of money out of world trade if the USA could be sure of controlling it. Accordingly, only the IMF and the World Bank were approved by the US Congress as UN institutions. The WTO did not see the light of day again until 1995, and then under total US control with the US dollar being the only legitimate trade currency.

The economic component, which Keynes headed, was called the Economic and Social Council (ECOSOC), and was charged in 1944 with considering all post-war proposals – especially from the UK and the USA – for actually setting up an ITO. ECOSOC scheduled a UN Conference on Trade and Employment to debate the proposals in 1946. However, things move faster than that in politics. Before the conference could actually hold the meeting, the USA adopted a two-track approach to international trade. It convened a meeting of 22 other UN member countries, which were also anxious to begin trade liberalization as soon as possible. They came together in a parallel forum to draft the General Agreement on Tariffs and Trade (GATT) as a temporary measure, or so it was thought at the time.

They signed the GATT in 1947, and it came into force in 1948. Because the participants all expected it to become a part of the ITO Charter, which would be a more permanent instrument, they included little institutional machinery in the GATT. Soon afterwards, the ITO charter was at last completed and approved at the Havana Conference of 1948. The text is now generally referred to as the 'Havana Charter', although its formal title is the Charter for an International Trade Organization.

However, by that time, US support for an ITO had largely evaporated due to corporate pressures. It was forced, once more, to behave like a League of Nations member state! Keynes died in 1946, and Cordell Hull, US Secretary of State and a strong proponent of the proposed ITO, had left government. The initial commitment to create a system of agreed international control to produce a more financially just intercourse between nations had passed. Business triumphed!

Then, in addition, there was a closely fought US election in 1948, and neither the Democrats nor the Republicans wanted to be tarred with anything as controversial as the ITO. The Democrats (under Harry Truman) in fact won the 1948 elections. It has to be said that the new president did place the ITO (Havana) Charter before Congress in 1950, but not energetically. Congress never even bothered to vote on it. Only the GATT survived, because it was still seen as temporary and it contained almost no constraining institutional arrangements. It was successful in its own way, managing over the decades to reduce industrial tariffs from an average of 50% to 5%, although steep tariff peaks remained in force in many countries. The GATT sponsored eight trade liberalization rounds, the last of which, the Uruguay Round, drafted the far more ambitious WTO agreement. The GATT – revised and updated – became the GATT 1994 within the framework of the WTO. Post-war trade arrangements therefore bore almost no resemblance to Keynes' hopes. The present WTO is even further removed from his vision.

## IS THE MODERN WTO RELATED TO THE ITO?

The reader must realize that, unlike the IMF and the World Bank, the WTO is not in any sense an actual agency of the UN. For instance, and crucially, the WTO does not even recognize the UDHR, whereas the IMF and the World Bank (as agencies of the UN) are theoretically obliged to do so. However, Keynes' ITO and WTO would have been UN agencies and hence accountable under the UDHR. The 1995 version of the WTO, for instance, is not committed (as was the ITO) to such UDHR Charter mandates as placing full employment, economic and social progress and development among its objectives. Its second section was entirely devoted to means of avoiding unemployment and under-employment. Unlike the WTO, which never mentions the subject, the ITO insisted on fair labour standards and the improvement of wages and working conditions, and it mandated cooperation with the International Labour Organization (ILO).

In fact, the originally proposed WTO could never have been the agency for the strengthening of neoliberal influences that the current WTO is. The ILO, as Susan George makes clear, took some time to realize this. It spent the first 6 years of the WTO's existence trying to obtain a 'social clause', which was only a much watered down version of the principles already included in the ITO. The unions finally gave up after the WTO Doha Ministerial meeting in 2001.

The ITO Charter formulated plans for sharing skills and technology, and it specified that foreign investment could not be used as a pretext for intervening in the internal affairs of member countries. Poorer, weaker countries were specifically authorized to use government aid, intervention and 'protectionism' for their reconstruction and development – the charter specified that 'assistance in the form of protective measures is justified.'

Special assistance 'designed to promote the development of a particular industry for the processing of an indigenous primary commodity' was especially encouraged. Many provisions of the charter also dealt with primary commodities, and were mindful of protecting small-scale producers. The ITO allowed government funds to stabilize commodity prices from year to year, and recommended the 'conservation of exhaustible natural resources.' Its measures with regard to commodities and encouraging negotiations among member countries that produced them, if taken together, led to a surprising conclusion. The ITO, without actually saying so, promoted OPEC-like arrangements – producer cartels – for primary products, and local processing to add value.

Instead of seeing such rules produce benefits, we have witnessed an inexorable decline in commodity prices. According to the UN Conference on Trade and Development (UNCTAD), average yearly decreases in these prices between 1977 and 2001 were 2.6% for foodstuffs, 5.6% for tropical beverages and 3.5% for oilseeds and oils. Only metals, which unlike food and beverages are never produced by smallholders, did slightly better, with an annual decrease of 1.9%, although this still reflects a considerable drop in revenues for producer countries.

The Havana Charter specifically permitted aid to national industries through subsidies or government procurement. It even reserved some screen time for national cinema. It allowed countries to protect local agriculture and fisheries. One of the biggest battles in the Doha round, and the immediate cause of its failure, concerned agricultural export subsidies. The ITO outlawed the subsidizing of products on foreign markets 'at a price lower than that charged to a domestic buyer.' Countries in financial difficulty were allowed to restrict imports, but had to do so proportionally, allotting fair quotas to previous suppliers.

The ITO's institutional arrangements were simple and democratic. Every state initially invited to the UNCTAD conference was to be a member, and future members were to be approved by this body. Each member had one vote (unlike the World Bank and the IMF, where votes are proportional to financial contributions, and the USA can block any important decision). Any member that was in arrears with regard to its contributions to the UN lost its vote. In the ITO, the USA would not have been a voting member in most years. As for governance, ITO members selected an executive board of 18 members – eight from countries of 'major economic importance and share in world trade', and ten representing different regions and types of economies. Votes were to be by simple majority or, in some cases, by two-thirds majority. Disputes should preferably be settled through consultations, but if these did not succeed, any member could refer a dispute to the board, which could authorize the member harmed to take retaliatory measures.

This now allows the reader to appreciate exactly how the original Keynesian version could have worked had the UN adopted it. However, having an ICU, exports produced by any nation, but particularly LDCs, earned 'bancors' instead of US dollars, while they spent bancors on imports. The idea was to mediate things so that the two were kept in balance. The effect would be that, at the end of the year, a country's accounts with the ICU would be neither in surplus nor in deficit, but 'cleared' – close to zero. Every country's currency would be assigned a fixed but adjustable exchange rate relative to the bancor. Keynes' original thinking perceived that nations with too many bancors would disrupt the system just as much as those with too few – that creditors were just as dangerous to stability and prosperity as debtors.

How could countries be forced to conform and to maintain a near-zero balance? The method was ingenious. The ICU, in its rôle as central bank and issuer of bancors, would allow each country an overdraft facility, just as ordinary banks do for customers. The authorized overdraft would equal half the average value of the country's trade over the preceding 5 years. Any country that exceeded its overdraft would be charged interest on the difference. Debtors would be charged on their deficits, but the real novelty was that creditors – countries with trade surpluses – would be charged interest on their surpluses. The greater the deficit or surplus, the higher the interest rate would be.

Countries in deficit would be obliged to devalue their currencies to make their exports cheaper and more attractive. Countries in surplus would have to revalue their currencies to make their exports more expensive and less attractive. If a trade-surplus country did not reduce its surplus, the ICU would confiscate everything above the allowed overdraft amount and put it in a reserve fund. Keynes wanted to use this fund to finance a global police force, disaster relief and other measures of interest to all members.

Susan George, whose article[20] is the source of much of the above information, is not to be taken lightly. She is President of the Administrative Council of the Transnational Institute in Amsterdam. She closes her article as follows:

> It was a neat arrangement. To avoid paying interest or submit to outright confiscation, countries in surplus would race to buy more exports from those in deficit. Those in deficit could sell more and would find it easier to return to equilibrium. Everyone would benefit. Trade would expand, the world would be more prosperous and peaceful, underdeveloped countries would have more funds to invest in development, and it would be impossible to accumulate the debts they have today.
>
> As we know, Keynes did not prevail and the post-war vision was never realized. The World Bank and the IMF have wreaked havoc through their structural adjustment policies, Third World debts can never be repaid, and Wall Street now decides the policies of democratically elected governments (as can be attested by Brazil's president, Luiz 'Lula' Inácio da Silva, along with many other leaders of indebted countries). World trade rules do not benefit the poorer members of the WTO, and the rich ones have grown more selfish as they have become richer.
>
> In these circumstances, how could the global justice movement help to make fair trade a reality, since the WTO and its disastrous rules already exist? The writer George Monbiot believes that the South could use its $26,000bn of debt as a 'nuclear threat' against the world financial system unless it consents to establish an ICU. The South could begin by creating its own smaller clearing union: perhaps Latin America could launch such a plan. Perhaps a new government in France could put it on the agenda; stranger things have happened. But it is important to realize that we need not reinvent the trade wheel: Keynes did all the work 60 years ago.

Of course, we cannot really assume that, even if Keynes' view had prevailed at Bretton Woods, it would have protected the WHO, and the UN in general, from being sold out to neoliberal interests for long. After all, the World Bank and the IMF really are agencies of the UN and, as we shall see, those two agencies have been instrumental in privatizing the WHO.

## EXTRACURRICULAR ACTIVITIES OF THE IMF AND THE WORLD BANK

Martin Khor, of the Third World Network, authored an article[21] which dealt with the meeting held on 28 November 2006 in Norway to address problems deriving from privatization of infrastructure and services in 'underdeveloped' countries under IMF (and hence UN) mandate. He cites the remarks of Charles Abugre, Christian Aid spokesman, who stated that the incompatibility of IMF and World Bank policy with stated UDHR canon related specifically to policy. The question arises as to whether those two institutions can be allowed to exercise such a high degree of control over the means used by LDCs to develop their procedure for interacting (through trade, etc.) with other countries. Do not individual nations have the right to determine appropriate policies for themselves?

A WTO based on Keynesian ITO rules would have been granted such rights automatically. However, SAPs imposed (as described earlier) by the World Bank and the IMF as a condition for development loans have completely the opposite effect. For instance, verticalization distorts economic opportunity within a country, mortgaging the very health of the many for the benefit of the few and, through them, the banks and corporations involved from the First World countries. Khor asks pertinent rhetorical questions, as illustrated by the following quote.

> The World Bank and the IMF have got it wrong as far as development is concerned, on trade liberalization (removal of protective tariffs, imposition of free trade, etc.). Given the shifting knowledge in these areas, the real question is – should these matters influence a country's policy on such domestic issues as healthcare and education?[21]

He goes on to argue that the President of the World Bank (at the time, Paul Wolfewitz), at a recent meeting with NGOs in the UK, had admitted that the World Bank realized that conditionality does not work, and that corruption caused by enforcement of conditionalities does not work either. Of course, in a critical sense he was wrong – conditionalities do work (and very effectively) in making money for wealthy First World bankers and corporations.

Khor quotes Abugre as follows:

> Another major problem is the erosion of policy space for developing countries due to conditionality, said Abugre. Although the Bank and Fund have tried to reformulate their policies, the content remains the same and they retain overwhelming power. For example, the number of conditions are said to be reduced, but in fact many of them have simply been re-grouped into fewer 'mega conditions', and instead of calling them conditions, some of these are now re-born as 'benchmarks.'
>
> Abugre said that conditionalities can be defined as 'the use of the threat of reprisal to get governments to act', and these continue, sometimes in new forms, and have even expanded. For example, the Bank and Fund have moved to get countries to adopt liberalization of services, government procurement and investment – the 'Singapore issues' were rejected at the WTO but are pushed as second-generation liberalization areas by the IMF and the World Bank!
>
> Abugre remarked that these new forms of conditionality were not reflected in the review reports of the Fund and Bank, nor in the study on conditionality

commissioned by Norway, and thus the supposed progress on reducing conditionality reported was misleading. Abugre added that 'harmonization' of donor policies, which had been stressed by the Bank, may present opportunities (for more predictability, and provide a platform for negotiations), but also the danger of establishing a creditor cartel: 'The cartellization is at national and regional levels, but there is no counterpart cartel of African debtor countries.'

For instance, these agencies are in coordination between donors and recipient countries. Unlike the Bank and Fund, the UN is not a creditor and thus there is no conflict of interest situation (as when the Bank and Fund coordinate the framework). 'UN coordination at country level helps, but there should be a shift of resources to the UN also, so there is competition too in ideas.'

James Adams, the World Bank's Vice President and Head of Network Operations Policy, said that a review of the Bank's conditionality, requested by the Development Committee, had been published, and that its findings and 'good practice principles' (GPP) had been endorsed by the Committee in September 2005.

There are five of these principles:
1 ownership (reinforcing country ownership)
2 harmonization (agreeing up-front with the government and other financial partners on a coordinated accountability framework)
3 customization (of the accountability framework to reflect the country's circumstances)
4 criticality (to choose only actions critical to achieve results as conditions for disbursement)
5 transparency and predictability.

The Vice President went on to say that in November 2006 the World Bank published a progress report involving 19 of the Bank's operations (63% from International Development Agency (IDA)-only countries). He provided figures showing that the number of conditionalities had been declining in recent years, and also that there was a shift in conditionalities away from themes such as economic management towards public-sector governance issues.

'We agree the Bank should reduce the number of conditions', he said, as the growth of conditions in the 1980s and 1990s was found to be 'inappropriate, not an effective way to respond to crises', and he suggested that there should be a focus on critical areas instead. He also denied that the 'benchmarks' introduced were an underground way to include conditions, as these are not conditionalities. On trade reform, the Bank worked with the WTO, according to Adams. The Bank also 'avoids conditions on sensitive policy areas if country ownership cannot be ascertained. Also, the Bank should not duplicate areas where the IMF has conditions.'

Khor points out that Benedicte Bull, the lead author of a report on World Bank and IMF conditionality to encourage privatization and liberalization (commissioned by the Norwegian government), stated that the World Bank and

IFM had claimed they had reduced the number of conditionalities, but that the NGOs in their studies had found instead that there was an increase in the number of conditionalities. This discrepancy was partly due to different definitions of conditionalities.

Bull said that their study included a review of 40 poverty reduction and growth facility (PRGF) programmes of the IMF signed between 2002 and 2006. There was privatization conditionality in 23 of the programmes, plus a detailed description of privatization policies in a further 10 'letters of intent.' Liberalization conditionality was also found in 11 of the 40 programmes.

In Martin Khor's paper (cited above) he goes on to state that a review on trade policy carried out under the study found that the World Bank and IMF still advocate trade liberalization, with the Bank focusing on 'behind-the-border' measures, while the IMF states that trade liberalization is part of its mandate and was found to be more 'orthodox' in policy recommendations.

The evidence is damning because in three out of four case studies (conducted in Bangladesh, Mozambique, Zambia and Uganda), privatization and liberalization conditionality was found. However, the study found that many of these conditionalities in new programmes are 'left over' from older programmes, in no case have conditionalities been efficient in ensuring policy change, and conditionalities are not the most important way of influencing policy.

This research also found that priorities set out in national development plans were reflected in the IMF–World Bank programmes. However, according to Bull, Parliament seems to play a marginal rôle in economic policies, and the use of external consultants reduces customization to local circumstances and impedes ownership.

Bull added that the case studies noted changes in World Bank and IMF practices (with greater openness, flexibility and donor harmonization), but donor harmonization also means that the donors can 'gang up' against the government. The local World Bank and IMF representatives also show little knowledge of the World Bank's good practice principles.

One of the participants at the conference was a former Finance Minister from Uganda. He commented that African countries, along with other LDCs, see themselves as supplicants without the money to buy influence from the developed countries. As he observed, it is very much a case of playing psychological games:

> The implication is that a spokesperson for an LDC, approaching the World Bank in such a context, is made to feel that, in some unexplained way, he/she is letting the home country down, especially if you contradict the IMF and the World Bank. The assumption is that they have science on their side and must be right by virtue of this power.

A considerable volume of comment from individuals working at the coalface, even in developed countries, and likewise from NGOs, brought forth dozens of actual examples showing how both the IMF and the World Bank were continuing, and even expanding, their wide use of neoliberalism in involving privatized services. The WTO was even worse, having actually been reprimanded by the World Bank for its proposals to refuse petitions of mitigating circumstances put forward by developing countries. For instance, some of their petitions concerned the disposal of special products (SPs). These are products on which the country concerned heavily depends for trade. Naturally such countries are anxious to protect such goods by tariffs and other protective mechanisms and petitioned with regard to such SPs and special safeguard mechanisms (SSMs) to try to ensure that neoliberal trade (proposed by developed nations) and the Doha Ministerial Conference would not adversely affect their small-scale producers.

In fact, a number of other examples were presented of how the IMF and the World Bank had used their power to influence developing countries' trade and investment liberalization positions and policies. For example, the World Bank and IMF had held a workshop in Geneva with African countries, which included presentations proposing that these countries should give up the principle of special and differential treatment in the WTO, as part of advice to them to undertake rapid import liberalization.

For instance, countries in Africa had suffered from deindustrialization as a result of low applied tariffs that were established previously as part of IMF and World Bank conditionality, and remain as part of their advice. The income and livelihoods of small farmers had also been hit when countries were prevented from raising their low applied agricultural tariffs (even though this was allowed by WTO rules) when cheap subsidized food imports from developed countries flooded the local market. An example of this is the above-mentioned case of cotton farmers in Burkina Faso.

An NGO from the Philippines, with the Tagalog acronym IBON, asserted that the claim that there had been a reduction in conditionalities was based on an illusion, as there had only been a change in tactics. This organization emphasized that the World Bank and IMF were 'merely clustering important conditionalities into a mega-conditionality, and then they claim that the conditions have been reduced.'

A delegate from the Jubilee Zambia group challenged the claim of increased country ownership of IMF–World Bank policies:

> When a Minister of Finance and his officials walk into the room with the IMF delegation which has come with a document from Washington, and the Minister only rubber-stamps the document, can we call that ownership?

A representative from an NGO from Uganda working on debt said that since 2001 he had not seen any serious changes in the World Bank:

> The conditions on liberalization and privatization still remain, and the results have not changed either. Poverty went down and then has gone up again. The World Bank still remains the driver in front. Who then is the owner?

An economics professor from Bangladesh said that the World Bank and IMF had to be viewed in perspective:

> We feel every day their power and privilege. The office of the IMF is in the Central Bank, and the IMF is present at the Central Bank meetings. Their privilege to set policies is not written in conditionality, but they make use of oral conditionality as part of their power and privilege.

This individual had been examining World Bank and IMF documents for three decades in Bangladesh, before and after 'structural adjustment programmes', and they remained consistent. 'Only the words change', he stated. 'Now privatization is called "restructuring public institutions." "Rationalization of prices" is used instead of raising prices. The PRSP [Poverty Reduction Strategy Papers] continues the same programme as structural adjustment.' He added that the World Bank and the IMF had built a support base in the country, and institutions had been restructured in such a way that there are beneficiaries among the elite who speak on behalf of the IMF and World Bank.

An African NGO, namely the European Network on Debt and Development (Eurodad), said that all conditionality is not acceptable as it is used as a tool of control, with adverse effects on recipient countries. A German development bank official said that lessons could be learned from the relationship of the European Union (EU) with its new member states. He questioned why conditionality is a success story in this case, but not in Africa's experience with conditionality.

Eurodad's representative stressed that the 'do no harm' principle should be adopted, and that the World Bank, IMF and donors should not experiment with people's lives: 'Stop giving policy advice that we are not certain about and that is very controversial.' They added that a major factor in the successful integration of new EU members, such as Spain (which joined in 1986), had involved a massive transfer of funding to these countries. But in this case, such transfers were based on the established principles of wealth distribution rights in the EU. This has to be seen as quite different from aid or charity, with conditions attached, as usually applies in the developing countries.

ActionAid International said that the World Bank's definition of ownership was very limited, as it considers that something is owned if the government's policy document mentions it. This raises the question of how this 'commitment' developed, as it is often the result of engagement with the World Bank. There is also the problem of the power of the World Bank and the IMF in these negotiations, especially the 'signalling power' that they have, in that other donors and the markets look to the views of the World Bank and the IMF when making their own decisions.

What, then, was the upshot of these contributions from the debt-ridden countries, and the high-flown rhetoric of the 'lending nations'? The question barely needs raising because we have so many good precedents with regard to what to expect – from G8 conferences to endless WTO Ministerial Conferences that keep forgetting to discuss the DOHA Declaration, and so on. This author is reminded of the story (no doubt apocryphal!) of a meeting in Africa between G8 leaders and a village conclave. The only ground rule was that comments should be entirely practical and not political. After about two hours of heat and wind, a little boy said to a Minister on the platform: 'I'm hungry.' Of course he was dismissed for making a political comment!

In concluding remarks at the end of the Conference, Atle Leikvoll, a senior official at the Norwegian Foreign Ministry, said that the meeting did not come up with a consensus on conditionality, and thus the debate had not ended. He concluded that there were different roads forward for the different stakeholders. The researchers would have to continue their work, as 'we will continue to need research.'

On the rôle of civil society, and specifically the Civil Society Organization (CSO), he said that this was vital, as there would be a missing element unless there is 'strong CSO engagement.' As for like-minded developed countries such as Norway, the UK, Sweden and Germany, 'we have our rôle to pursue, in the Boards of the Bank and Fund. We have responsibility to pursue it at our country level.'

## DO THE WORLD BANK AND THE IMF BELONG WITH THE WHO?

We have already said with regard to TRIPS that the discussion of 'rules' by which profits can be made from pharmaceuticals has no place on a WHO agenda. And the previous section has made abundantly clear the degree to which not only the WTO (which is technically not bound to honour the UDHR), but also the World Bank and the IMF have been all too ready to cooperate with the WTO's financial agenda and place it ahead of the basic human right to health. The question thus arises: 'What can we do?' Can the World Bank and the IMF be redeemed so as to be fit to mediate the basic mandate of the WHO with regard to primary healthcare? In an attempt to address this issue before moving on to consider more specific examples in the following chapters, I shall address a few of the more salient features of these two bodies with regard to the UDHR.

First of all, since the World Bank and the IMF must be transparently democratic internationally in order to be effective and to have global authority, as Keynes understood so well. Just how democratic are they? And how democratic is the WTO in its interactions with them? The responses of Share the World's Resources[22] to these questions have been comprehensively negative. In addressing the issue of lack of democracy and/or transparency, this NGO states that both agencies freely criticize debtor nations as being corrupt, lacking in transparency and run by undemocratic regimes.

It points out that if such countries expect to receive loans for 'development', they must reform with regard to these crucial issues before they can be regarded as sufficiently democratic even to qualify for 'debt relief.' Unfortunately, however, neither the IMF nor the World Bank reflected these noble characteristics to any marked degree themselves! The World Bank is haunted by these evils, as is the IMF. Corruption within both organizations is rife, with millions of dollars unaccounted for.

Both institutions are based in Washington, DC in the USA, and are owned by their 184 member countries. The majority (40%) of all votes are held by just eight countries (the G8). The USA holds the largest share, at 18%, which grants them the ability to veto policies that do not serve US interests. Votes are allocated according to financial strength ('one dollar, one vote'), resulting in those financially powerful countries (and the commercial interests that influence them) determining the monetary, economic and development architecture of the global economy. Thus the existing global economic system places developing countries squarely at the mercy of G8 foreign interests.

The WTO is, constitutionally, a democratic organization with an equal share of votes distributed to all member nations regardless of their economic power. Yet the poorer nations still find themselves unable to exercise their democratic rights in WTO global trade negotiations. The dominant economic powers – the USA, Canada, the EU and Japan (also known as the 'Quad' or 'Quartet') – very clearly establish the agenda before a round of trade talks. They then invite a selected group of poorer nations to a 'Green Room' meeting where the key decisions are made about which issues will be open to negotiation in the formal talks, and a declaration is drafted. During the formal talks, nations can only agree with or block the predetermined proposals.

This structure effectively excludes the majority of the world from influencing the international trade agenda. Throughout these negotiations, even within the Green Room talks, poorer nations (given their reliance upon international aid, and IMF and World Bank assistance) are at the behest of the Quad and are often unwilling to contest the declaration, due to fear of economic or financial consequences. Overall, the global south's ability to make trade work to their benefit is severely compromised.

The bias and disquiet of these negotiations are reflected by the frequent collapse of trade talks, the eventual acquiescence of developing countries in further opening their markets to the dominant nations, and the systematic inability of 'Quad' nations to live up to their pledges to remove their own protectionist measures.

Without democratic representation within these bodies, and cooperation with the south, the WTO, the IMF and the World Bank will remain unaccountable to the very people whom they claim to be assisting. In the light of the failures of the WTO, World Bank and IMF to address poverty and inequality, global protests continue to gain momentum, and citizens and nations are calling for a 'ground-up' process of globalization that is not controlled by, and for the benefit of, the ruling elites.

Needless to say, few nations make application to the IMF lightly, because of the rate at which charges on the loan mount up by compound interest. There are examples, of course, of national governments using IMF loans corruptly, but the fact is that the IMF is only too glad to hand out high-risk loans, because they are covered by First World taxation protection when debts go bad. There tends to be a great deal of corruption at this end, too! It is clear that by their insistence on diminishing government social programmes (generally health and education), the IMF and the World Bank are working hand in glove with large corporations in the First World. As we shall see later, this was made obvious recently with regard to rebuilding programmes – and funds borrowed from the IMF to mount them, after the tsunami in December 2005.

Although this assistance constitutes a crippling debt for the borrower, the IMF also insists on economic reform as a condition for the loan. In effect the IMF takes this opportunity to render the struggling economy 'free-market friendly.' Prioritizing debt repayment, market liberalization and privatization allow corporations and private interests to capitalize on these reforms. The economic consequences for the developing country are often dire.

The IMF, working in conjunction with Wall Street bankers and the US Treasury, has effectively forced many emerging economies to liberalize their financial markets. This happened to many countries in East Asia and Latin America in the 1980s and 1990s, and it often exposed them to massive financial speculation which in turn devalued their currencies, and created recession and financial crisis. Bolivia's per capita income is less than it was 25 years ago, with 63% of Bolivians living in poverty. Argentina is another well-documented recent example, as are Thailand, South Korea, Indonesia, the Philippians, Russia and Poland.

Structural Adjustment Policies (SAPs) govern the conditionalities of such loans. Briefly these tend to be as follows:

- **Reducing social spending, government budgets, programmes and subsidies for basic goods.** This allows a rapid mobilization of currency to repay the loans (debt). Meanwhile, schools and hospitals are forced to introduce or increase fees, which in turn increase illiteracy rates, disease and death rates, and perpetuate the poverty cycle.
- **Eliminating foreign ownership restrictions and increasing interest rates.** These measures increase profitability for foreign investors and enable corporations to take control of domestic resources. Meanwhile, local producers and businesses are destroyed (as they are unable to afford essential credit), unemployment goes up, and control of their resources shifts to wealthy countries. Income is transferred out of the developing country, further damaging its people and economy.
- **Eliminating import tariffs and switching from subsistence farming to export economies.** These measures benefit foreign export markets and eliminate local competition. Low-cost foreign goods, including luxury items, out-compete domestic producers, putting them out of business. Food insecurity and malnutrition increase as production shifts to cash crops for export and countries are forced into dependent relationships with northern suppliers. Increased resource exploitation causes environmental degradation and pollution.

SAPs have recently been replaced by Poverty Reduction Strategy Papers (PRSPs) as part of an effort to address the issue of 'government ownership' of structural adjustment policy, and to focus on strategies for relieving the debt of heavily indebted poor countries (HIPCs). Unfortunately, little progress has been made. Strategies are still broadly imposed on governments and are still subject to conditions that increase income disparities.

Not surprisingly, the neoliberal, open-market model preached by the IMF and the World Bank was not the model adopted by all of the existing economic powers during their industrialization and development. Instead they protected their own markets from foreign goods and investment and continue to do so, donating huge subsidies to domestic business. Indeed, the USA and the EU remain to this day highly protected economies. The hypocrisy of liberalizing emerging markets is evidently in the self-interest of economically dominant countries. Enforcing these policies on developing countries is akin to economic imperialism.

Moreover, it is highly hypocritical because we are expecting the debtor nations to have higher standards than First World countries have ever been able to muster in support of their own industrialization over the last three centuries.

The World Trade Organization, although not (in its 1995 version) itself a UN agency, has fitted in very nicely with the neoliberal agenda. Since its leitmotif is 'free trade' – as opposed to 'regional fair trade' – it must bend its policies accordingly.

Since its creation, the WTO has promoted market access for corporations with trade agreements. These agreements circumvent the democratic national rights of a country to determine domestic polices with regard to trade, natural resources and service provision.

The General Agreement on Trade in Services (GATS) was agreed by the WTO in 1994. Its aim is to remove any restrictions and internal government regulations in the area of service delivery that can be considered 'barriers to trade.' Such services include everything from marine fishing to provisions for health and education. The agreement affectively abolishes a government's sovereign right to regulate, subsidize and provide essential national services on behalf of its citizens.

The WTO's Agreement on Trade-Related Aspects of Intellectual Property Rights (TRIPS) forces developing countries to extend property rights to seeds and plant varieties. The agreement will even allow corporate property rights over individual plant genes, thereby impacting on agricultural practices on which two-thirds of the worlds are reliant for their livelihoods. It undermines thousands of years of indigenous control over local knowledge in the production of food and livestock. Six corporations now own 70% of patents on staple food crops, allowing them to set the market price for them and to block competition for 20 years.

Another serious infringement of democratic rights is that of the Trade-Related Investment Measures (TRIMS), which open domestic finance to corporate control, eliminating a country's ability to shape its policies with regard to foreign investment and capital controls.

The evidence suggests that market liberalization and intellectual property rights hinder development in poor countries and serve the economic interests of dominant countries. In 2000, an UNCTAD conference confirmed this in a report which concluded that neoliberal trade measures primarily benefit corporate interests. Even the European Commission doesn't shy away from stating that trade agreements are primarily instruments for the benefit of business.

Effectively, control over resources, services, policies and finance is granted to corporate interests through the GATS, TRIPS and TRIMS framework. Meanwhile, developing countries continue to resist the imposition of WTO agreements, and in 2006 this resulted in the collapse of the Doha round of trade talks. This opens the door to corporate pressure.

Multilateral trade rules are agreed behind closed doors between the USA, the EU and major trade partners. Around 80% of corporations reside in the USA and the EU, and through their lobbyists they enjoy privileged access to government policy makers who take part in trade talks. Over 30 000 corporate lobbyists are based in Washington and Brussels, vastly outnumbering the US Congress and European Commission staff whom they lobby! The vast majority of lobby groups represent business interests, who spend billions of dollars annually advocating their cause – typically market access in emerging economies.

Many developing countries, on the other hand, do not have the resources to send enough, if any, representatives to argue for fairer trade practices that would benefit their own economic development. In addition, these negotiations are undemocratic, with the public denied access to or information about these discussions. The same is not true of corporate lobby groups such as the European Services Forum (ESF) and many US corporations, which can directly affect and have access to Trade Committees. Unsurprisingly, therefore, corporate interests form the basis of WTO agreements. The corporate imperative is to have commercial access to all markets – whether goods, services or intellectual property – in all countries.

Unsurprisingly, the vast majority of the world's population, whose basic human needs are not met, are unlikely ever to have them met within the biased framework of the existing global economy. Now let us bring in the World Bank.

## THE IMF, THE WORLD BANK AND NEOLIBERALISM

As has already been explained, if a country wishes to apply to the IMF and/or the World Bank for a loan, it has to agree to the conditionalities implied in the SAPs. Not only does this virtually give both of those agencies carte blanche to determine domestic priorities and policies within the debtor nation, but it also imposes on that nation massive involvement with international corporate privatization. As far back as 2004, direct foreign investment by such private corporations exceeded US$1 billion a year on development projects in LDCs. It is obvious now. Such projects involved road building (and the high level of deforestation that this requires), installation of machinery (with replacement parts having to be purchased from the companies concerned), and a large increase in the use of oil and petroleum products involved. All in all, an IMF/World Bank ban to an LDC represented a bonanza to First World private enterprise.

World Bank projects in the Democratic Republic of the Congo, Rwanda, Chad, Somalia, Kenya, Mozambique, etc., in Africa and in a number of Asian and South American countries are in their way strongly directed by neoliberal interests.

In recent years the IMF has been vociferously backed by multinational corporate interests when applying for extra funding for expansion. This support was in response to the IMF bailing out big banks and foreign investors which had made bad loans to developing countries. For example, in 1995 the IMF gave almost US$18 billion to Wall Street interests who stood to lose billions with the peso devaluation. It also bailed out foreign investors in Russia with a US$11 billion package, and orchestrated a massive bailout of the big banks that made bad loans to Asian countries in the 1990s.

The interrelationship, financial opportunism, corporate mandate and US backing of the World Bank and the IMF are best exemplified by their economic occupation of Iraq. Since the occupation began, Iraq's entire economy has been fashioned by the IMF and the World Bank to suit (mainly US) foreign investors and corporate interests. The Paris Club of creditors, through the IMF, quickly approved the cancellation of 80% of Iraq's debts (approximately US$39 billion). Using this as leverage, neoliberal structural changes were swiftly enacted, including the privatization of assets and state-owned enterprises. These undemocratic economic adjustments resulted in capital flight, huge levels of unemployment and unaffordable increases in utility costs, sparking widespread protest.[23]

So far, these agencies have therefore all been very effective in promoting the economic dominance of the USA. However – and this is important – this does not necessarily guarantee the long-term hegemony of US capitalism, only of capitalism itself. In other words, even if China (nominally Communist) assumed neoliberal global hegemony tomorrow, the US system would rapidly cave in and its citizens would become victims of the system as well. Neoliberalism has no national or cultural loyalties! Neoliberalism is ruinously bad for the world's health (whoever is in hegemony at the time), and for one simple reason – competition, by definition, not only produces winners but must also produce losers. No one in their right mind would ever dream, therefore, of trying to produce equity through competition. No amount of sophistry, or rhetoric about 'democracy', 'human nature' or 'freedom of choice', can conceal the fact that neoliberalism is nothing more than competition.

In certain contexts – for example, sporting events, music fests and academic selection – there may be a place for competition, but it can never be used as a method for establishing equity! Thus it is only to be expected – as has been amply demonstrated since the mid-1980s – that the IMF, the World Bank and the WTO must actually *impede* poverty reduction. A prior requirement, therefore, for the achievement of global human rights is nothing less than the abandonment of neoliberalism.

This can only be meaningfully undertaken if we go back to Keynes' original suggestion. Moreover, the earth's natural resources belong to the global community, not specifically to the people who live beside or on top of them. That is why we need a transnational body (as the UN should be), with agencies responsible for health, etc., to mediate access to these resources and to their global exchange in commerce, etc. How can this be achieved?

## RENDERING THE UN FIT FOR PURPOSE

Some argue that the problem will be solved if we more adequately coordinate the WTO, IMF, World Bank, etc., with the mandates of the UDHR. It would seem to this author more to the point to abolish them altogether. For instance, how can it even be considered logical for the WHO to devote its time and resources to discussions about how to coordinate global health rights with the patenting of genetic engineering or the production of pharmaceuticals? Neither of these things should generate personal financial profit, because there is no way of doing this without compromising health as a global human right. In effect, then, the UN needs to be slimmed down – it has too many fingers in too many contradictory pies – but it also has to command far more authority than it now does internationally. For instance, it cannot be committed to the promotion of both human rights and national rights at the same time.

As it is currently run, the UN is far too vulnerable to manipulation by the financial interests of the 'Big Five' – the permanent members of the Security Council, and particularly the USA. As the author has suggested in a previous publication,[24] UN Security Council resolutions often reflect little more than US foreign policy. This is why, in recent years, the UN has been facing such major cash-flow problems, because the USA has cut its funding in protest at the UN's attempts to implement the UDHR through more friendly economic aid policies. Comprehensive reform of the UN along these lines is dealt with more fully in the author's previous book.[24]

Share the World's Resources, an NGO to which considerable reference has already been made in this chapter, sets out a detailed approach to UN reform.[25] This author disagrees with it with regard to whether the IMF, the World Bank and the WTO should have a place in it, but strongly endorses the general tenor of its suggestions for lessening the impact of neoliberalism on its actions. The following is a direct quote:

> UN agencies such as the Economic and Social Council (ECOSOC), the UN Conference on Trade and Development (UNCTAD) and the United Nations Development Programme (UNDP) have the necessary knowledge, information and experience to re-establish their regulatory hold on the global economy and render it more equitable. Importantly, these UN agencies are naturally democratic and representative, unlike the IFIs (International Financial Institutions).
>
> Alongside restoring democratic control of the global economy to the UN,

there must be a strengthening of the UN in general. In order to render the UN democratic, the Security Council must be dissolved (or greatly modified), and any rights to veto decisions abolished. The General Assembly must take its place as a truly representative world body. The UN must also be given greater financial power. This can be achieved through a number of possible mechanisms, such as a Tobin tax, taxes on arms, taxes on pollution, or a combination of these.

Most importantly, the UN must adopt the principle of sharing in order to fulfil its humanitarian mandate and secure basic human needs across the world. A new economic system based on sharing essential resources, such as land, food, water and medicine, needs to be urgently implemented to achieve this objective. We propose the creation of a new UN agency, whose specific task would be to facilitate this process – the UN Council for Resource Sharing (UNCRS). A system of sharing would then exist alongside an overhauled market-based economy that can continue to produce and supply all 'non-essential' resources.

Share the World's Resources, in order to facilitate such recommendations, suggests the creation of two new agencies:
1   a UN Council for Resource Sharing (UNCRS)
2   a UN Emergency Redistribution Programme (UNERP).

Fundamental to the effective operation of these agencies, and of UN reform generally, there would have to be a distinct shift from nation states tending to use the UN to enforce their national interests, instead of thinking globally. The fear of war, engendered in no small degree by the competitiveness implicit in neoliberalism, is one barrier to such a state. However, the imminent threat imposed on us all by the environmental crisis will no doubt render it easier for people to appreciate that we all belong to one very frail global village – in which civil war has no place. Share the World's Resources points out that, within this system of sharing, essential resources would be shared firstly as part of a United Nations Emergency Redistribution Program (UNERP), designed to rapidly mobilize essential food, water and healthcare to people and nations who are experiencing extreme poverty, malnutrition and unnecessary death. Thereafter, a more comprehensive system of sharing can be implemented that can ensure that basic human needs are always prioritized and met by the global community. To achieve this, the UNCRS would create a Global Sharing Network (GSN), which could monitor the ever changing levels of production and consumption of essential resources across the globe. The GSN would then be able to coordinate an efficient global redistribution of these resources according to need. Resources would be produced and consumed locally wherever possible, then shared regionally, and finally shared internationally.

In all of this the UNCRS would also play a part. A system of sharing would mean that the majority of commodities and goods that are currently traded would instead be cooperatively owned and distributed by the global public through the UNCRS. Such resources would include energy supplies and the provision of utilities such as water, essential agricultural produce required for food, cotton for clothing, essential healthcare services, equipment and medication, essential knowledge and technology, and resources for providing education. As a result, international trade in commodities and their derivatives would be significantly reduced, and confined to non-essential goods.

Sharing will ensure that essential domestic needs are largely met at the local level, reducing dependency on foreign imports of essential goods. As a result, there would be less need for developing countries to agree to prohibitive trade agreements, whether multilateral or bilateral. This would free the population to develop their own industry and economy, enabling them to compete on an equal footing with wealthier nations in the global economy. Potentially, when enough countries can effectively compete with the economic superpowers, a powerful incentive will be created for these superpowers to adopt a more cooperative approach.

Agreements relating to the remaining international trade should, where necessary, be democratically agreed through UNCTAD. The remaining international trade, under the auspices of UNCTAD, should utilize an inherently balanced mechanism similar to the International Clearing Union (ICU) mentioned above. The combination of these factors will allow the WTO to be progressively dismantled over a period of time.

This would, as the author has suggested in a previous publication,[26] eliminate the harsh requirements imposed by 'global free trade', and reasonably replace them with the flexibilities of 'regional fair trade.' The people directly affected could of course elaborate their own systems of regulations and control over the latter.

Sharing essential resources instead of trading them will mean that these resources are divorced from financial markets. This will clearly have a significant impact upon these markets, dramatically reducing the amount of stocks, and financial derivatives related to the stocks, which are traded. This in itself will help to reduce the global financial instability that many economists and analysts believe will sooner or later result in an international financial crisis.

Sharing essential resources will also mean that developing nations will require less foreign exchange in reserve, as they will be purchasing fewer goods from abroad. Balanced trading between nations (using an ICU-type mechanism) and the removal of debt burdens will also mean that there is less likelihood of countries experiencing major balance-of-payment deficits. The lack of foreign exchange is a key reason why developing countries turn to the IMF for loans, which in turn leads to crippling debt. Not only can sharing result in greater financial security for a developing country, but it will also mean that they are less likely to have to implement structural adjustments to their economy to render it acceptable to the countries that follow neoliberal principles.

When there is a need for short-term emergency foreign exchange loans, a new UN-based Finance Organization could lend money and provide the necessary expertise in a pro-development manner without crippling interest rates and without corporate or political influence. It would then be feasible for the IMF to be gradually dismantled. Its sizeable assets and gold reserves could be applied to the UNCRS and UN development projects.

At present, International Financial Institutions (IFIs), such as corporations from the First World, have a ruinous impact – through neoliberalism – on the way that the IMF and the World Bank can improve development of LCDs. However, the proposals of Share the World's Resources would disempower IFIs and render them surplus to requirements. Obviously, as the author has suggested, replacing the rôle of IFIs may require new global financial agencies. However, as has been pointed out, the present system – skewed as it is to First World banking and corporate interests – is not sustainable. The need for a national global programme for preventing environmental catastrophes makes this clear. 'Brotherly love', to coin a rather hackneyed phrase, is no longer pie-in-the-sky idealism, but an imperative.

Indeed the following quote from Share the World's Resources[27] says it all:

> Sharing the world's resources has the potential to create a sustainable economic model that puts human rights and the environment at the centre of socio-economic life. Such a system would necessitate the relegation of corporate activities to a sphere that can be managed by the global public. It will ensure that the administration of the global economy is rendered a democratic, participatory process.
>
> Together, such measures can ensure that the global economy is inherently more equitable and that it serves the interests of the people. Sharing in this way is the only way to meet the basic human needs which are currently sidelined by the need to make profit. It is also an important statement of international solidarity and an acceptance of global unity. In this way, sharing the world's resources can foster cooperation and peace between nations.

All that has been said in this chapter must leave the reader with the impression that perhaps neoliberalism itself is bad for one's health! This is an issue of huge importance, and one on which much has been written by some of the world's foremost leaders on global health equity. It will be addressed in a subsequent chapter.

## REFERENCES

1 MacDonald T. *The Global Human Right to Health: dream or possibility?* Oxford: Radcliffe Publishing; 2007. pp. 6–19.

2 Rachman J, Black E, editors. *Multinational Corporations.* Chicago: Trade and the Dollar Publishers; 1974.

3 MacDonald T. *Health, Trade and Human Rights.* Oxford: Radcliffe Publishing; 2005. p. 3.

4 World Health Organization. *About WHO*; www.who.int/about.p.1 (accessed 12 July 2007).

5 MacDonald T. *Rethinking Health Promotion: a global approach.* London: Routledge; 1998.

6 World Health Organization. *The Global Meeting on Future Strategic Directions for Primary Health Care. A Framework for Future Strategic Directions (Global Report – Alma Ata Declaration)*; www.who.int/primary-health-care (accessed 12 July 2007).

7 Sanders D. *Primary health care and health system development: strategies for regeneration.* Paper presented at the International People's Health University, Cuenca, Ecuador, July 2005.

8 MacDonald T. *Health, Trade and Human Rights.* Oxford: Radcliffe Publishing; 2005. p. 4.

9 Swift R. Squeezing the south: 50 years is enough. *New Internationalist Magazine.* 1994; July issue: 4–7.

10 Huberman L, Sweezy PM. Preface. In: *Introduction to Socialism.* New York: Monthly Review Press; 1968. p. iii.

11 MacDonald T. *Third World Health: hostage to First World wealth.* Oxford: Radcliffe Publishing; 2005. pp. 241–3.

12 MacDonald T. *A Developmental Analysis of Cuba's Health Care System.* Lewiston, NY: Edwin Mellen Press; 1999. p. 22.

13 United Nations. *Formation of UNCTAD*; http://en.Wikipedia.org/wiki/New_International_Economic_Order (accessed 12 July 2007).

14 MacDonald T. *Health, Trade and Human Rights.* Oxford: Radcliffe Publishing; 2005. p. 3.

15 Third World Network. *UNCTAD Raises Development Concerns on Services Liberalisation*; www.twnside.org.sg/title/twinfo17.htm (accessed 12 July 2007).

16 Third World Network. *African Ministers Warn Against Erosion of UNCTAD's Mandate*; www.twnside.org.sg/title?2.twinfo391.htm (accessed 12 July 2007).

17 Ibid., p. 9.

18 Caller H. Health matters. *Fight Racism – Fight Imperialism: Organ of the Revolutionary Communist Group.* 2006; June/July issue: 3.

19 Share the World's Resources. *World Bank and IMF Still Pushing Conditions*; www.stwr.net/content/view/1389/37 (accessed 15 July 2007).

20 George S. Alternative finances: the World Trade Organization we could have had. *Le Monde Diplomatique*, 17 January 2007, pp. 6–7.

21 Khor M (2006) *'Bailing Out Countries or Foreign Banks'.* Conference on Oil, Climate and Justice. Trondheim, Norway, November 2006. www.trabal.org/courses/364syllabus.html-66is (accessed 14 December 2007).

22 Share the World's Resources. *The IMF, World Bank and WTO*; www.strr.net/content/view/717 (accessed 15 July 2007).

23 Ibid., p. 4.

24 MacDonald T. *Health, Human Rights and the United Nations.* Oxford: Radcliffe Publishing; 2007.

25 *Establishing a UN Council for Resource Sharing (CSR)*; www.stwr.net/content/view/1289/36-36k (accessed 14 December 2007).

26 Carlson L, Barry T (2006) *A Global Good Neighbour Policy.* Centre for International Policy, 7 February 2006. http://Americas.inc.online.org/am/3114 (accessed 14 December 2007).

27 Share the World's Resources, ibid., p. 25.

# Chapter 2

# Selling off the UN to neoliberalism

## AN AUCTION BY STEALTH

This auction, perhaps the greatest in human history, was not advertised in the usual way, nor was any date or time set for the event. In fact, most people only gradually became aware of it either while it was going on or, more usually, after it had happened! Now while many thinking people and health/human rights-related non-government organizations (NGOs) are aware of the fact that the UN, and such of its agencies as the WHO, have effectively been sacrificed to the thrusting financial appetite of neoliberalism, there remains considerable confusion as to exactly when and – more to the point – how it actually happened.

Thus some blame the recently retired Director General of the UN, Kofi Annan, because of his call in 2005 for UN agencies to cooperate with private enterprises in achieving the Millennium Development Goals.[1] Still others point the finger at the World Economic Forum (WEF) and its bizarre meetings at the Swiss ski resort of Davos, attended by the powerful and wealthy leaders of corporate finance, to which selected NGO representatives are invited (at a very high entrance fee). However, the sale of the millennium really started long before either of these events.

The Third World Network (TWN)[2] has provided a brief summary of some of these events, explaining the WEF's original concerns about the UN's lack of coordination with business interests in Third World health and development projects. The WEF is a group of very large transnational corporations (TNCs), their lobbyists and financial power brokers. As the TWN points out, many of the NGOs originally involved have become increasingly worried by what they see as the WEF's efforts to divert the UN and some of its agencies from their original commitment to the Universal Declaration of Human Rights (UDHR) to a more profitable involvement with private enterprise.

As the TWN explains it, the WEF wanted to guide world governments into a closer cooperation with corporate agencies, and to lay down the law for such interventional groups as NGOs to 'promote neoliberal corporatist economics and globalization.' They adroitly mediate this process at the Davos 'get-togethers' through their extensive access to the media and even to advertising agencies. However, it did not take various civil society groups and some of the original NGO participants too long to sense which way the wind was blowing and to initiate protests against it. At first these were politely academic and were largely ignored by the corporate-owned media, but soon enough they attracted the less diplomatic responses of outraged public opinion. This emerged spectacularly at the World Trade Organization (WTO) Ministerial Conference in Seattle in 2001.

The response of the corporate interests was channelled through NGO-hostile media coverage, especially in the *International Herald Tribune*, traditionally a strong bulwark of economic conservatism. The International Monetary Fund (IMF), after all, is partly financed by the International Chambers of Commerce (ICC)! It strongly endorsed those UN agencies that had acceded to the Global Compact endorsed by Kofi Annan. The *International Herald Tribune* ran a series of high-profile articles, authored by ICC Secretary General Maria Livanos Cattaui, which praised the Compact and urged it to go further by emphasizing voluntary two-way agreements, open-ended and free from government or public restriction. She even called for the involvement of labour unions and selected civil society organizations to become full partners. In numerous articles she heaped praise on Kofi Annan for his 'rational stance' in advocating closer cooperation with the private sector. It cannot have escaped the notice of many that, while calling on governments to be more efficient and effective in mediating social outreach programmes under 'sensible governance', the *International Herald Tribune* made no comment at all on a parallel commitment to public accountability and efficiency in the behaviour of the corporate sector! Claude Smadja, a WEF official, wrote a column in the *International Herald Tribune* specifically arguing that the IMF, the World Bank and the WTO should *not* have to be called to account.

How did ordinary citizens and civil society generally in the USA and the rest of the First World react to this intrusion into UN policy and action? By and large they were at first predominantly uninterested, while the minority who expressed an interest were pretty much hostile to big business. The latter have generated a number of useful websites monitoring UN activities and statements which appear to suggest this neoliberal takeover.

The TWN report discusses one such website contribution by Anthony Judge of the Union of International Associations, which complains of the degree to which the Global Contract was agreed almost surreptitiously, especially with respect to reporting full details of partnership arrangements between UN agencies (or closely linked NGOs) with corporately run multinationals, often to the detriment of other UN agency involvement. As this book makes clear in subsequent pages, the WHO has often been sidetracked in this way.

Judge, it is reported,[3] asserted that the UN has been 'white anted' (an Australian expression meaning 'sabotaged from within'), allowing Kofi Annan to in effect be held hostage and be pressured into supporting schemes which are antagonistic to the UDHR and other core UN values. The details of all this are fully explained in a wonderfully informative paper by Ellen Paine.[4]

Ellen Paine works with another international group, the Global Policy Forum (GPF), which is highly suspicious of the WEF and meticulously accurate in rendering many of their practices more transparent than they would have desired. Paine is extremely thorough in her analysis of the early history of the WEF. As she points out, and as has been implied above, since about 1980 at least, First World business groups and corporations regarded the UN with some aminus, and they therefore welcomed Kofi Annan's 2005 call for involvement with business as an invitation for neoliberal initiatives in its humanitarian programmes. About 50 large TNCs signed up to this deal. However, there is a history behind even Kofi Annan's comment, because during the 1970s the New International Economic Order (NIEO) began to make itself felt as an agency committed to a fairer means of distributing the world's resources.

This aroused increased hostility and sarcastic comment about 'one worldism' and fancied leftist plots to undermine the free enterprise system globally and the 'American way of life' in particular. It was in these days, in this author's view, that a set of 'moral rhetoric' began to really make an impact on the corporately owned media, including an assumed link between unhindered entrepreneurism and a commitment to 'real' democracy. Words like 'individualism' assumed a connotation of virtue, while words like 'collectivism' or 'community action' were taken to imply totalitarian socialism. It is not difficult to go on from there to Ronald Reagan's 'Evil Empire' or George Bush's 'Axis of Evil.' Ellen Paine's account of the events sets the background for all of that, as well as indicating precisely the stages by which the UN soon found itself ensnared by neoliberal policies. Much of what follows is derived from her seminal essay.[4]

During the 1970s, many newly independent states joined the UN and began to talk about an NIEO that would distribute the world's resources more fairly. In response, big business steadily grew more critical of the organization, and Washington followed the same course. When the Reagan administration came to power in 1981, discussions about the UN in the US capital took on a tone of pious outrage. As the influential Heritage Foundation affirmed in a report of that era, 'The war against economic freedom, the free enterprise system and multinational corporations permeates the UN structure.' 'This ideology', the report continued, '. . . is antithetical to US interests and policies', and it ensures 'that developing countries remain perpetually dependent on US and Western aid and perpetually hostile to American values and principles.' For, as is explained, the partnership is not surprising in light of the fact that the USA and the UK are headquarters of 38 of the world's top 50 transnational corporations – 76% of the total by number – a share which rises still higher if profitability and market capitalization are used as measures.[5]

Heritage, one of the most prestigious Washington think tanks, helped to shape the new conservatism in the early Reagan years, and to build the framework for a deep change in economic policy. During the 1980s, Heritage produced more than 100 reports on the UN, denouncing every aspect of the organization and its agencies. Again and again, it warned that the UN favours regulation of global business and promotes 'the forced redistribution of global resources.'

Neoliberalism as a philosophy is based on opposition to Keyne's ideas, and the Heritage Foundation's fury with the UN sprang from the new post-Keynesian corporate ideology. As a global market took shape, business and financial executives abandoned an earlier view that favoured national regulation and national social protection. These new transnational conservatives sought instead to weaken the state's social and regulatory policy, lower taxes and remove barriers to capital movement, global trade and global investments. In other words, they promoted neoliberalism.

Corporate apologists and strategists at Heritage – and in other think tanks and corporate headquarters – confronted a UN that was resistant to reform along neoliberal lines. Its policies favoured state regulation, economic intervention and humanitarian social considerations, while its policy process reflected the view of many states – including the Soviet bloc, the Third World, the Asian tigers and the Western Europeans – most of whom opposed neoliberal prescriptions. By contrast, Heritage found ready supporters in the US Congress, where the conservative tide was running strong and transnational corporate influence was especially powerful. The Reagan administration warmly embraced the new conservative approach to UN reform, while in London the Thatcher government served as an indispensable partner in the global enterprise.

These right-wing and highly reactionary reformers sought to block many UN initiatives that might regulate, restrict, control and even tax transnational companies – such as the Law of the Sea (with its fees for deep seabed mining), the Code of Conduct of Transnational Corporations, the labour rights conventions, and the emerging UN-based environmental regulatory regimes. In the essentially anti-union US government of the day, these developments were anathema.

The corporate media and various industry associations established their own anti-UN campaigns or worked through groups like the International Chamber of Commerce, the principal international lobby for transnational corporations. They used their considerable influence with the media and politicians to emphasize the UN's shortcomings and to call for funding cuts and policy changes. The booming arms industry and its friends in the Pentagon wanted to undermine the UN's disarmament work, while powerful oil companies battled the UN's environment and climate change initiatives through such lobbies as the Global Climate Coalition. Many corporations opposed UNICEF's partnership with NGOs to block Nestlé's questionable baby milk formula, and they disliked the UN's investment sanctions against apartheid South Africa.

Indeed, Nestlé – along with British American Tobacco and several other corporate tobacco giants – exemplifies the situation well. In a previous book,[6] the author gives a full description of the strategies used by neoliberalism to try to discredit UN agencies and the NGOs associated with them. James Paul's findings[7] constituted another valuable source for much of the rest of this chapter.

UK and US tobacco companies were leading members of the anti-UN coalition. Thanks to millions of pages of confidential documents released in recent lawsuits, we now have clear evidence of their campaign. A lengthy report based on these documents, issued by the WHO in the summer of 2000, offers a uniquely detailed case study of the anti-UN corporate offensive.[8] The tobacco companies particularly opposed the WHO's programme on the health hazards of smoking and nicotine addiction. In the mid-1980s, the tobacco giants launched a secret campaign to attack the WHO, discredit its work and reduce its budgets. The report shows how top executives of the world's leading tobacco companies conspired together against the WHO – an organization which they saw as 'one of their foremost enemies' – and 'instigated global strategies to discredit and impede WHO's ability to carry out its mission.' The Philip Morris Company, the industry leader, held a strategy session in 1989 in Boca Raton, Florida, at which executives planned a worldwide offensive against tobacco critics, identifying the WHO as its most dangerous opponent.

As the report makes evident, the companies hid behind a 'variety of ostensibly independent quasi-academic, public policy and business organizations' whose tobacco backing was not disclosed. Using their contacts, they planted stories in leading newspapers. The *Wall Street Journal* ran a typical attacking article in 1996 entitled 'WHO Prescribes Socialist Medicine', which affirmed that the WHO 'provides justification for the never ending expansion of the welfare state.'[9]

The companies established clandestine relationships with present and former WHO staff members, hammered the organization with negative public relations, fomented disputes between the WHO and other UN agencies about tobacco-related policy, and tried to organize developing-country representatives by painting WHO policies as driven solely by the concerns of rich countries. They devoted huge resources to these campaigns and used their vast corporate networks in the food business and other non-tobacco companies to pursue their anti-UN goals. This and other corporate campaigns persuaded Washington policy makers that they must 'take back' the UN by stamping out its socialistic and redistributive tendencies, crushing its 'anti-corporate' biases and populist impulses, and making it a trusty vehicle for globalizing capitalism, and particularly for US-based investors and companies. Corporate spin doctors presented Washington's growing anti-UN spirit as reflecting public disenchantment with the world body, although poll results consistently showed the opposite – that is, strong public support for the UN, which steadily enjoyed far more credibility among the US public than Congress itself.[10]

A primary component of neoliberal propaganda is that, somehow, public services funded as government policy are inefficient, if not corrupt, because they are outside the competitive framework, whereas privatized industry, since it works out in the competition jungle, has to be 'lean and efficient.' Along with this, it operates under the assumption that the 'market' implies – providing what people want – and is therefore more democratic. Of course it omits the fact that what people decide they 'want' is – in a capitalist society – very much influenced by high power and expensive advertising, itself under minimal public control. They even employ a distorted vocabulary when describing their actions and policies. For instance, 'neoliberalism' is neither 'new' nor 'liberal.' In fact, the same phenomenon is sometimes referred to as 'neoconservative'! As Ellen Paine argues in her paper, the word 'reform' has a rather obverse meaning in 'corporate-speak', usually referring to a retreat to less protected and more dog-eat-dog financial environments. Thus 'welfare reform' means cutting taxes by withdrawing money normally allocated to aiding the less economically fortunate. Such reforms are claimed to reduce poverty – both within a nation and globally – although the evidence suggests that the opposite is true. The press and other media use such redolent expressions as 'bloated bureaucracy' to describe government expenditure on social programmes, likening it to a conspiracy of totalitarian intentions. One could give many examples of this, and many strike one as amusing except that, over time and with frequent enough exposure, people become conditioned to think in this way.

When the author was working at a university in California in the 1960s, his children's primary school had a book on its shelves called 'Tom and the Lazy Squirrel.' Tom lived in a 'big white house', and one day he found a half-starved and very cold grey squirrel in the middle of winter. He took it home and nursed it back to health. The book was withdrawn after its 'meaning' was explained by the John Birch Society – a well-known ultra-reactionary US group. What was the sinister 'meaning'? Tom's actions saved the life of a worthless squirrel that was too lazy to store nuts during the warm weather, as its colleagues had done. The 'big white house' was the US government, handing out tax dollars to lazy layabouts at the expense of hard-working fellow Americans. The book had been placed in the library to subvert the young – obviously! The author thought at the time that the propaganda effect would have been greater if the squirrel had been a red one (instead of grey), but the conspirators who planted the book in the library obviously missed that opportunity.

## THE UN AND THE NEOLIBERALS

The UN and its Charter, especially the UDHR and agencies like the WHO, are absolute grist for the mill of neoliberalism. They are large, highly bureaucratic, and in some respects resemble the popular notion of a hippopotamus – slow moving and incapable of rapid decision making (although neither of these attributes are true of real hippos!). Therefore they should be replaced by something less lethargic, leaner, and capable of thinking aggressively – a tiger, perhaps.

As Ellen Paine illustrates, the Heritage Foundation was soon joined by the Cato Institute. The latter has been particularly active in attacking the UN. It advocates 'small government' – that does not interfere with 'market forces' by improving safety regulations, taxes and other disincentives to competitive leanness and efficiency. Indeed, in 1997 the Cato Institute produced a Handbook which was distributed to every member of the US House of Representatives and Senate. It described the UN as 'a miasma of corruption, beset by inefficiency, Kafkaesque bureaucracy and misconceived programs',[11] and called for a 50% unilateral cut in US funding for the world body. In 1996 a Cato conference participant stated that 'Americans would be better off writing a check to the Red Cross than being taxed to fund the UN.' At the same conference, the chief of Cato's 'Project on Global Economic Liberty' argued that UN-based programmes of economic aid only harm developing-country economies, while another speaker attacked UN environmental programmes as 'retarding economic growth, which is absolutely vital to ecological health and cleanliness.' Cato receives its funding from many of the largest US corporations and business associations, including the State Street Bank, Chase Bank, the US Chamber of Commerce, the Investment Company Institute, the Securities Industries Association, the American Council of Life Insurance, the American International Group, American Express, HJ Heinz Co, IBM and Coca-Cola.

## CREATING NATIONAL ANTI-UN SENTIMENT

Readers will have noticed that, especially since the UN appeared reluctant to support US unilateral involvement in Iraq, even the British media have tended to denigrate the UN. For instance, any number of stories were broadcast to the effect that 'UN personnel' had been involved in corrupt activity, and even sexual assaults on children in some of the world's trouble spots. No reference is made to the fact that local governments – not the UN bureaucracy in New York – appoint local people to work in refugee camps, etc., and that these people are often themselves victims of warfare.

Most of this anti-UN rhetoric is intended for US voters, but the impact is global, because huge international media corporations tend to dominate the media in the UK and many other parts of the world. By the early 1980s – with Ronald Reagan as US President and Margaret Thatcher as Prime Minister in the UK – the UN became widely condemned as a bête noire. It was castigated for being old-fashioned, nepotistic and generally unfit for purpose, authority or international respect. In addition, it was costly and ineffective and charged that the UN opposed the spread of 'market freedoms' around the world under US 'leadership.' In 1983–85, the Congress passed several laws that selectively reduced US budget contributions to the UN, 'withholding' funds for programmes that the USA did not support. The Reagan administration also delayed the timing of US payment to the UN by appropriating funds 9 months late, in the following US budget year. US payments to the regular UN budget, due on 31 January, began arriving in October or November, at the very end of the UN fiscal year. Since the USA is the largest UN dues-payer, these and other policy manoeuvres resulted in a serious UN financial squeeze, as US debt to the organization increased steadily. The USA also forced other member states to agree to US control over the UN budget. By provision of the Charter, the budget is adopted by a two-thirds vote of the General Assembly. The USA withheld part of its annual payment, on the grounds that the budget vote should be weighted by the amount of each country's contribution. Finally, to head off the crisis, UN members agreed to a new 'consensus' approach to budget decisions. This gave the USA an effective veto over and above its automatic right to veto proposed resolutions of the UN General Assembly by virtue of its status as one of the 'Big Five' permanent members. This gave the USA the leverage it needed to cut the UN budget by 10%, to close down many of its social programmes and to dismiss 1000 staff – all of this to placate an anxious and almost hysterical US government whose members were afraid of appearing 'weak' in the eyes of their constituents.

The financial power alone of the USA over the UN is immense. For instance, the UN dues of each member nation are calculated on the basis of that member state's GNP. The USA has the largest GNP in the world and thus the highest dues. It can effectively hobble the UN by withholding dues. In 1985, the USA – after its government had taken umbrage over many of UNESCO's funding projects – withdrew from UNESCO. This by itself continues to severely restrict that agency's work. However, in addition it withdrew some of its funding from other agencies of the UN.

The UN acquiesced and made several concessions to win back the USA's favour, but this only prompted US authorities to make even more demands. When the Soviet Union collapsed, many people thought that more money could now be spent on UN humanitarian initiatives because – as the only superpower – the USA would require far less for military spending. However, the collapse of the Soviet Union did not have that effect. Indeed, the USA became even more hostile to the UN.

It appeared that, so long as there were two equally matched nuclear armed superpowers, many less developed countries (LDCs) could rely on UN aid due to fear that, if it were not forthcoming, the former Soviet Union would step in with funding. Now the USA did not have to worry about this and was less constrained with regard to what it could allow its corporations to do in the Third World. At the same time, agencies such as the IMF and the World Bank (backed after 1995 by the WTO) could – unopposed – undermine domestic policies in agriculture, trade, education and health in many developing countries. Even in Europe and Asia, this led to a range of policy changes more in line with US requirements. However, the UK was also deeply involved.[7]

In fact, the UK vigorously supported US financial authorities, including their Treasury Department, and urged a total reorientation of the global economy. Other wealthy nations joined them in this. As we have seen above, Structural Adjustment Policies (SAPs) imposed by the IMF and the World Bank were paramount agencies in neoliberalism as a condition for aid and development loans. This impacted on the health and civic life of the people of nearly 100 LDCs. Indeed, the Third World was not alone in being so affected. Pressure from the oil-rich OECD (Organisation for Economic Cooperation and Development) nations, using control of the currency market, various bilateral and multilateral agreements and a host of corporate investment strategies, was bought to bear even on countries like Australia, Canada, the USA (no loyalty there!), the UK and some other EU countries. Neoliberalism was imposed by every means possible.

Out of all of this financial chicanery the extremely right-wing Business Council for Sustainable Development was inaugurated. It liaised directly with the IMF, the World Bank and the WTO to create more profitable trading rules and arrangements – for their First World corporate supporters.

The impact on health was palpably negative, despite the WHO's original – but now unenforced (and perhaps unenforceable) mandate. When this author was engaged as a doctor in remote areas of Haiti in 1986, he actually tried to calculate the average financial return to various corporate agencies of unnecessary infant deaths by diarrhoea. The economics and social matrices involved eventually rendered impossible the precise mathematics required.

As explained earlier in this chapter, neoliberalism is based on the principles of unrestricted competition. This is why people (and agencies) that promote neoliberal agendas insist on organizing things so that UN international organizations (which should be working together to enhance compliance with the UDHR) are driven to conflict in providing services to the people in need. A number of government and non-government groups (working with the UN), designed to monitor serious distortion of trading and commercial arrangements to the disadvantage of LCDs, such as the Centre on Transnational Corporations (CTC), gradually ceased operation. The UN Conference on Trade and Development (UNCTAD) assumed a number of their tasks. One anticipated that, under that umbrella, they would carefully monitor transnational corporations, but instead they have ended up actually promoting such involvement! In their reports they even commend such TNC penetration into LDC economies. Could neoliberal interests have asked for more?[12]

The CTC developed a series of recommendations on 'Transnational Corporations and Sustainable Development' to be submitted to the Earth Summit in Rio de Janeiro in June 1992, for possible inclusion in the final conference document. Corporate lobbyists found this prospect extremely alarming, and worked hard to prevent it. They also opposed the CTC because it served to collect and publish information about corporations that were breaking the UN investment embargo against South Africa. Bowing to these pressures, the UN Director General, Boutros Boutros-Ghali, axed the Centre despite its impressive record and its important mission.

## A NEW POLICY OF THE UN IN MEDIATING HUMAN RIGHTS

Can the erosion of the UN's chief mandate, the UDHR, and the WHO's commitment to the Alma Ata Declaration, by the imposition of neoliberalism be stopped? As we have seen, the UN's origins promised much to mankind. But almost from the outset, those hopes were undermined by the corporate power brokers and by capitalism generally. It can be said that despite all the soaring Charter language, the USA and its allies never permitted the UN to assume its full powers in the social and economic fields. The visionary wartime planners soon gave way to the 'realists' – the bankers, Treasury officials, oil company executives and other managers who had their doubts about 'do-gooders' and excessive promises. Realists in the US State Department like policy planner George Kennan recognized that it would not be easy to control a world in which, as he pointed out, 5% of the world's people enjoyed nearly half the total wealth.[13] And he should know whereof he spoke, as he was one of President Harry Truman's key advisers on foreign policy and was especially interested in policies directed at 'containing' the post-war spread of communism.

One strategy that Kennan advocated was based on the (correct) assumption that, in the 'non-aligned' nations, there was an increasing call for some kind of global control – even if it involved totalitarianism – which would guarantee availability for all of sufficient food, etc., and protection against disease. Communism – at that time represented by a second superpower (the former Soviety Union) – was ready to take advantage of this yearning for world peace and sufficiency. Out of this arose the doctrine of 'containment' by which the USA and its advocates sought to 'win the hearts' of as yet non-aligned peoples to the view that the way forward for them was 'democracy' rather than any kind of totalitarianism. One strand of this policy involved aid to countries under imminent threat of communist takeover (Kennan's view), and another strand involved direct military action against communism (e.g. in Korea), which Kennan did not regard as feasible as a long-term policy. In this context, the UN became regarded by right-wing activists of this second policy as 'suspect.'

We have already seen how Heritage and other corporate agencies attacked the UN and its UDHR, and tried to undermine its efforts with regard to neoliberal policies and propaganda.

As James Paul points out, the Heritage and tobacco company attacks on the UN are textbook cases of neoliberal propaganda assaults on public institutions. The doctrine claims that the market represents freedom, flexibility, dynamism and democracy, whereas public institutions are constraining, rigid, immobile, uniform and autocratic. It also promotes the view that private actors are more efficient, better managed, less costly, less corrupt, more technologically up to date and more responsive to public needs through market-derived signals.

Neoliberal propaganda frames the public sphere as the opposite of the private – that is, inefficient, badly managed, expensive, corrupt, technologically out of date and unresponsive to public needs. Paradoxically, perhaps, it presents the market as the most effective vector of democratic control over the distribution of all (or nearly all) forms of social well-being – the ultimate act of (democratic) self-expression being the purchase of commodities in the marketplace. By contrast, political processes involving citizens' cooperative action, voting, representation, government and the like have been framed as alien, boring, futile and irrelevant.

Note how this propaganda uses the word 'reform' to mean reorganization of institutions, and even whole societies, in a neoliberal direction. It calls instead for privatization of public institutions, reduction of government budgets, and reduction of taxes, along with 'welfare reform' and 'social security reform' approaches to national budget decisions, thus giving the USA an effective veto. However, to make this strategy really work, it was necessary to get rid of UN attempts to 'mediate' in modifying market forces or in aggressively promoting human rights. In Boutros Boutros-Ghali they found the right UN Director General for the job.

Boutros Boutros-Ghali of Egypt assumed office in January 1992 as the UN's first post-Cold War Secretary General. Under heavy pressure from the USA and from lobby groups like the International Chamber of Commerce, he immediately set to work to reform the Secretariat and eliminate programmes that aroused the most intense corporate ire. His advisers warned that the World Bank and the IMF – both based in Washington and under great influence by the US Treasury – had a 'comparative advantage' over the UN in the economic policy domain, and that the UN would lose credibility if it did not scale back its efforts in this area. Competition, especially in the vade mecum of neoliberalism favours the IMF and the World Bank over other international organizations. In fact, as things stand now, various UN organisations must end up competing with one another rather than working together to uphold the UDHR. Boutros Boutros-Ghali fulfilled expectations! By March 1992, with only minimal staff consultations and virtually no input from the General Assembly, the Secretary General had eliminated many Secretariat posts and programmes dealing with social and economic policy. A newly formed Department of Economic Development had an acronym so apt and embarrassing (DED) that its name had to be hastily changed. Most significantly, the Secretary General closed down the respected CTC, a Secretariat research programme that supported UN negotiations to prepare a Code of Conduct for TNCs. Along with the Heritage Foundation, the International Chamber of Commerce had long criticized the CTC and the Code, and had mobilized its membership to weaken or destroy them.

## THE UN'S INITIAL ATTEMPTS AT RESISTANCE

However, as we shall see, Boutros Boutros-Ghali's cooperation soon wasn't definitive enough for US corporate interests that needed more control of trade and commerce. Things got under way in 1993. Following on from the 1992 UN reforms, corporate chieftains and Washington-based neoliberal policy makers pressed forward with their campaign. They remained as keen as ever to erase its institutions of public oversight and accountability in favour of private, voluntary forms of corporate self-regulation. The UN system remained deeply engaged on global environmental issues, a matter of special concern to oil companies, auto firms, chemical corporations and many others with strong voices in the US capital. The UN's work on human rights also touched the nerve of many companies, since human rights campaigns were beginning to focus on corporate malfeasance – in Nigeria, Myanmar and other countries – interfering especially in the politically powerful oil industry and its investment plans for exploration, drilling and pipeline construction. For instance, consider the plight of the people of the Ogoni Province in Nigeria, under an ungodly alliance between Shell Oil and the Nigerian Government in activities heavily funded by such UN agencies as the IMF and the World Bank.

The UN had proved remarkably resilient to the first round of reforms. UNICEF's progressive research unit in Florence, headed by Giovanni Cornea, vigorously criticized structural adjustment, the main policy tool of the World Bank and the IMF, and raised questions about poverty and mortality in the economies 'in transition.' At the UN Development Programme (UNDP), the popular annual Human Development Report (first published in 1990) advocated development based on human needs, not just on GNP growth. The Secretary General himself outraged the new conservatives by proposing global taxes as a solution to the UN's financial crisis, in a major speech delivered at Oxford University on 15 January 1996. At the same time, the UN also began a global conference series that addressed the great social and economic issues such as the environment, population, women's rights, human rights and social development – all of which produced platforms and programmes of action that unsettled the corporate lobbyists. Thousands of active NGO representatives attended the conferences as well, with UN encouragement, making demands and creating networks that were still more worrying to the magnates of global capital. However, as we shall see, the Empire struck back! To some extent, many in the UN were eager for signs of conservative trends within the UN, and these were not hard to find. The annual Human Development Report drifted slowly to the right after 1994, and began to promote economic growth as the main engine of human development. The Department of Public Information abandoned its famous progressive film-making programme under the effect of deep budget cuts. UN agency reports increasingly referred to private investments as the only viable approach to development and poverty reduction. Penetration of the public good for private profit now had a toehold.

## THE BUSINESSMAN'S FRIEND: KOFI ANNAN

Kofi Annan assumed the post of Secretary General in January 1997. Washington had summarily vetoed Boutros-Ghali's campaign for a second term, stating that it wanted a more reform-minded helmsman for the UN. Annan, a graduate of the Sloan School of Business at Massachusetts Institute of Technology, had spent the majority of his career in the UN's administrative and financial departments. Keenly aware of the organization's financial crisis, he saw the need to resolve it though strategic concessions to the largest dues-payer. We can say that at this point the auctioning of the UN and its agencies to the highest bidder in the neoliberal establishment really started to speed up.

After just 3 weeks in office, Annan made a pilgrimage to Washington to meet with members of Congress, particularly with powerful conservative Senator Jesse

Helms. He assured the legislators that he would 'streamline' the UN, bringing modern business practices to its management and setting 'realistic' goals for its work. He committed himself to further budget and staff cuts. Almost immediately thereafter, Annan travelled to Davos, Switzerland, to the annual meeting of the World Economic Forum (WEF), a grouping of the world's foremost corporate chief executives. While in Europe, he also held talks with senior officials of the International Chamber of Commerce.

WEF executives soon offered to connect the Secretary General and a few of his top officials to the Forum's new private video-conferencing system, enabling Annan and his team to converse with the Forum's Chief Executive Officer (CEO) members as well as a few select political leaders and the chiefs of international institutions such as the World Bank. Annan warmly accepted the offer, and the Forum installed its WELCOM (World Electronic Community) system at UN headquarters in April 1997. Although the new technology provided the cash-strapped UN with a state-of-the art communications tool, the system worked primarily to connect the Secretary General and other UN leaders with corporate executives, bypassing the intergovernmental process.[14]

The Secretariat, while signing up for WELCOM, decided to impose a financial charge on NGOs for electronic access to UN documents – a telling coincidence. By this and other moves to restrict the access of NGOs, while widening access for business, Annan and his team made it clear where their priorities lay. The Secretary General's speeches often referred to NGOs as the UN's 'indispensable partners' and the real 'conscience of humanity.' Increasingly, however, the UN leadership referred to 'civil society' – a fuzzy term that embraces business as well as NGOs – when describing its new enthusiasm for non-state partnerships. This helped to impede NGO complaints and access to data.

On 24 June 1997, the UN hosted a high-level luncheon to consider the terms for 'business sector participation in the policy-setting process of the UN' and 'partnering' in UN development assistance funds. In addition to Annan, Maria Livanos Cattaui, Secretary General of the International Chamber of Commerce, attended. The participants included 10 corporate chief executives and 15 powerful government representatives, including three heads of state and US Treasury Under Secretary Larry Summers. General Assembly President Razali Ismail hosted the luncheon with Bjorn Stigson, Executive Director of the World Business Council on Sustainable Development. Millionaire Canadian businessman Maurice Strong, a key figure under several Secretary Generals and a close friend of the White House, is said to have masterminded the initiative. At about the same time, the Secretary General started to promote closer collaboration between the UN and the Bretton Woods Institutions (the World Bank and the IMF), calling for 'greater coherence' at the policy level. Alarmed NGOs asked whether the UN had abandoned its critique of structural adjustment and of neoliberalism in order to please Washington and the ICC. UN leaders insisted that 'coherence' meant real policy change by the Bretton Woods duo, as well as better overall 'teamwork' between Washington and New York.

It soon became clear that officials in the Executive Office of the Secretary General believed that the UN 'must change or die', and that it must reach out to 'new actors' in a globalizing world, beyond the nation-state members. John Ruggie, the Secretary General's Special Advisor, assumed an especially active rôle in preparing the pro-business initiatives, promoting them and developing a rationale to explain them to the many sceptics in the Secretariat, the UN system agencies and the NGO community.[15]

## HOW THE GLOBAL COMPACT COMPLETED THE TAKEOVER OF THE UN

By now numerous UN programmes had become partially privatized or effectively public/private finance enterprises.[16] The Secretary General pressed for a new high-profile programme that would symbolize the new UN–business partnership. The idea for a 'Global Compact' emerged from conversations with business executives in 1997 and 1998, especially with the ICC. After months of preliminary negotiations, the Secretary General formally proposed the idea at the Davos gathering of the WEF on 31 January 1999.

Nine neoliberal principles were put forward by the Compact for corporations in the fields of human rights, labour rights and environmental protection. The principles are worthy but vague. For instance, signatories agree to 'make sure their own corporations are not complicit in human rights abuses.' The UN promises that it will undertake no monitoring. Nor will the companies be under any enforcement procedure or any formal process of scrutiny. Annan's speech says much about his rationale and also about the bargain he was offering to his listeners:

> I propose that you, the business leaders gathered in Davos, and we, the United Nations, initiate a global compact of shared values and principles, which will give a human face to the global market, thus obscuring many of its real purposes.[17]

Annan went on to argue that globalization could only be assured if it was based on broad consensus, and that such consensus would have to be built on efforts to ensure the welfare of all. He called on his audience 'to embrace, support and enact a set of core values' that would define a new era of corporate responsibility.

In retrospect, we can see where all of this led and what it implied. The speech contained all the elements of the thinking that had evolved among Annan and his advisers – partnership with business, 'values' rather than rules, and reminders of the 'threat' that grassroots opposition might pose to globalization. The speech succeeded in its purpose. It drew the attention of many corporate executives and it attracted a good deal of positive comment from the media. Although it was unclear how the proposal would eventually be implemented, at UN headquarters the Secretary General soon made it clear that he intended to develop the idea and give it a highly visible form. He had become a Master Auctioneer.

It was thus easy for corporate executives to support 'values' proposed by the Secretary General, but they were concerned that he might eventually move towards doing something concrete. The UN team, on the other hand, hoped that through this vague commitment they could eventually nudge business into a framework that would become (at least slightly) more concrete. Each party moved forward with caution, as follow-up conversations took place between the UN and the ICC.

However, it was not long before elements of civil society were aroused. NGOs generally were critical or less than enthusiastic. Some agency leaders within the UN system had serious reservations and did not hesitate to say so in public, despite pressures from Annan's Executive Office. UNICEF Executive Director Carol Bellamy, one of the few top UN officials with a substantial background in the private sector, voiced serious doubts. In a speech at the Harvard University International Development Conference on 16 April 1999, she warned that 'It is dangerous to assume that the goals of the private sector are somehow synonymous with those of the United Nations, because they most emphatically are not.'[18]

Nevertheless, the UN continued to rush into business partnerships and neo-liberal concessions at top speed. With UNDP Administrator Gus Speth's term expiring, the Secretary General rejected the candidate from the European Union, the social democratic Danish development minister Paol Nielson, naming instead Mark Malloch Brown, the World Bank's Vice President for External Affairs. Malloch Brown, a former public relations executive, had served as the World Bank's chief apologist. The Europeans were furious and the UNDP staff were shocked. In the months to come, Malloch Brown would reorganize the UNDP and bring in a number of orthodox staff, including World Banker Nancy Birdsall as new head of the Human Development Report. But much worse was to come.

As reported in the daily journal of the Inter Press Services on 8 July 1999, Jayantha Dhanapala, Under-Secretary General for Disarmament Affairs, called for 'creative partnerships' between the UN and arms manufacturing companies in what he described as an effort to control the illicit arms trade.[19] For those who favoured UN controls on all facets of the arms trade, UN partnership with arms manufacturers seemed an outrageous step. In fact, UN guidelines for business partnerships had specifically ruled out links with arms companies. Annan and his team were already testing the limits that they themselves had set. It would be difficult indeed to find a more blatant example of the UN selling out on the UDHR and its other principles.

Then, on 26 June 2000, the Secretary General launched his Global Compact at UN headquarters in the presence of chief executives and other top managers of almost 50 corporations, including such large global companies as Daimler Chrysler, Unilever, Deutsche Bank, BP Amoco, Royal Dutch Shell, Volvo, Credit Suisse, Dupont and Nike, all of whom agreed to sign the Compact and abide by its nine principles. The Secretary General had also invited a small number of sympathetic NGOs, including Amnesty International, the Worldwide Fund for Nature and the International Confederation of Free Trade Unions, but these NGO 'partners' were clearly uneasy at the spectacle. Amnesty International Director

General Pierre Sané said bluntly that he didn't think the Compact was credible in the absence of formal rules. By contrast, the corporate participants made it clear that they wanted no rules – and not even the mildest of monitoring under rules of 'Commercial Confidentiality.'

At the launch meeting in New York, ICC head Cattaui issued the following warning in an article in the *International Herald Tribune*:

> Business would look askance at any suggestion involving external assessment of corporate performance, whether by special interest groups or UN agencies. The Global Compact is a joint commitment to shared values, not a qualification to be met. It must not become a vehicle for governments to burden business with prescriptive regulations.[20]

Alas, there is little evidence that her jeremiad has been heeded!

Protests against the WTO at Seattle in November 1999 had doubtless given the Secretary General's project a boost. 'How prescient he turned out to be', enthused Annan's Senior Advisor John Ruggie, referring to the original Davos speech in January 1999 and the events that followed: 'This was 10 months before Seattle.'[21] In the absence of Seattle, it seems unlikely that 50 corporations would have answered Annan's call, even with UN bluewash on offer.

Kofi Annan decided that the only test of the companies' compliance with the Compact will be a special UN website where they will post information – in the form of 'best practices.' They will control the information flow and the UN will invite the public to examine it and make comments – chat-room democracy. No other test of compliance, much less enforcement, will be available.[22]

Privately, UN spokespeople conceded that corporate scandals could embarrass the organization, and that the UN might have to undertake some limited oversight of the companies just in order to avoid such a pitfall. Licensed use of the UN's logo by corporations (one of the partnership plans) could also lead to UN embarrassment, as special rules for corporate use of this image suggest. Many NGOs from all over the world, led by the Transnational Resource and Action Center, have criticized the Compact in letters, publications and public meetings. They have also released a counter-proposal, namely a Citizens' Compact that calls for a 'legal framework, including monitoring' to govern the practices of the corporations and hold them strictly accountable for their agreements. A number of member states have expressed opposition to Annan's project as well, but the Secretary General has not altered his course. The UN's corporate policy strains the organization's relations with NGOs and many governments. In exchange it will probably produce only the most superficial and cosmetic changes in company behaviour. The UN could lose its public support if it is seen as scarcely distinguishable from business-dominated institutions like the WTO or the IMF. Secretary General Annan was gambling with the UN's most precious heritage – its reputation as an institution that works for the well-being of the world's peoples. We lose that reputation at our peril.

As things stand now, NGOs and their civic society supporters worldwide now have to do two things:

1 We must alert ordinary fellow citizens – who might have decided years ago to shun 'political involvement' – that we are all endangered by the replacement of a trusted transnational arbiter and mediator with the tyranny of market forces.

2 We must organize resistance to it by communicating with our MPs and others who represent our interests, by the way we vote and – perhaps most importantly of all – by discussing the issues in our workplaces, at social gatherings, etc. Ignorance and apathy go well together – and pose a threat to everything we hold dear.

In this respect, the idea of a Citizens' Compact (as suggested by Paul James) could provide a starting point for action. We cannot allow corporations to call the shots. Instead they must be subject to citizen control.

## MARSHALLING NGO OPPOSITION

On 5 May 2006, Catherine Willis published a major literature review for a course she was teaching at the University of Paris and which appeared on the Internet.[23] In it she argues that basically the NGOs have to become both more noisy and more nosy in uncovering the extent to which the policies of the WHO, and of the UN in general, have been infiltrated by neoliberalism. She refers to these interests collectively as 'transnational non-government actions', and argues that some NGOs are well placed to confront them.

The literature that she surveyed presented four main reasons for the emergence of international action by NGOs. The first is the increase in contentious international agreements and organizations at the closing of the century. Schultz[24] and O'Brian and colleagues[25] have observed the all-encompassing effects of the current neoliberal approach of international organizations, and the intense resistance that it has created. This has resulted in increased opposition to both the form and the policies of multilateral economic institutions.[26] Smith argues that one of the reasons for contention is that the positions that governments take in global institutions are subject to little democratic input and are isolated from public view. Transnational Social Movement Organizations (TSMOs) then play a rôle in encouraging global political participation in order to democratize global politics.

Secondly, the increase in power of the international institutions has been accompanied by a decrease in opportunities to influence national governments. Ayres' case study of resistance in Canada to the Free Trade Agreement reveals that the agreement constrained the Canadian government's ability to intervene in the Canadian economy and respond to national demands.[27] NGOs also see new international economic regimes as detrimental to maintaining or raising national standards.

Thirdly, recourse to transnational action or international organizations occurs because it creates more opportunities for influence. This is elaborated upon in the work by Smith on human rights, by Williams with regard to the environmental movement, and by Ayres on the Free Trade Agreement.

Lastly, civil society has gained importance for international institutions because they have been encouraged by governments and international organizations under certain circumstances. International economic institutions (IEIs) have been dealing with NGOs more often, as they are more efficient at delivering services than states are and they are more aware of public opinion. Foreign governments can also use them as a convenient and inexpensive foreign policy tool.

Like states, multinational corporations (MNCs) or business lobbies, NGOs, INGOs (International Non-Government Organisations) and social movements seek policy changes that reflect their interests. Ayres uses the political process model to explain how changes in polity occur. He argues that the fight for power between members and challengers of a polity and the political realities facing the polity gives rise to collective action, and as such a social movement is a political phenomenon. Ayres illustrates through his case study how contention and mobilization changed in relation to the political opportunities available (the same argument is also presented in the work of Stiles[28]). He describes the three factors necessary for the mobilization of collective action. First, a suitable structure of political opportunities must exist. This includes divisions within the elite, major changes in political alignment and the availability of potential partners. His case study reveals that the absence of domestic opportunities resulted in transnational collaboration. Secondly, there must be sufficient organization and resources to take advantage of these opportunities. Leadership, membership and communications networks are key. Thirdly, the solidarity and commitment necessary can be achieved through micromobilization. This includes recruitment meetings, organizational meetings, encounters with allies and opponents, and discussions to share information and experiences. Micromobilization thus has a key role in linking personal preoccupations with collective goals.

The reader can see from this that in many ways the actions of some of the NGOs exploit the same channels as those used by the MNCs, although with more enlightened motives.

Several of the papers reported by Willis illustrate the impacts of transnational action. Desmarais' work illustrates the impact of the Karnataka State Farmers' Association's action on the Indian government's position in WTO negotiations.[29] The association gained public attention which brought India's position in the WTO into public debate, and it managed to educate the public and many government officials on the impacts of trade. Despite the lack of specific policy results, they destabilized the trade negotiations and brought about increased awareness of their issues.

The question must arise as to whether all of this NGO counter-activity actually aggravates or diminishes the lack of transparency. Although it remains difficult to establish the exact influence of NGO action on change, it cannot be questioned that there is an impact. This has brought up a debate about the rôle that NGOs, INGOs or Tribal Security Councils (TSCs) should have in international institutions and in international relations. The participation of NGOs in international institutions has been criticized because they are neither accountable nor representative.[30] However, the same criticism can be brought against the international institutions themselves that they are contesting.

Woods' research identifies several problems in this regard with the IMF and the World Bank, through an analysis of their structures and function. First, representation of members on the board is unequal. As it is based on financial contributions, it does not represent the interest of all members and stakeholders equally. In addition, the heads of these organizations are chosen in a non-transparent process which excludes the participation of many members. Secondly, the board is quite distanced from daily functioning, so staff and management actions are not regularly scrutinized. Lastly, while the rôles of both of these institutions have expanded, their accountability has not: 'IEI (international economic institutes) now make banks responsible for policies that do not lie in the economic domain, which should be the domain of other domestically accountable agencies.' Although it has been argued that countries are not forced to accept IMF policies, its critics have argued differently:

> the political institutions of a country should determine the nation's economic structure and the nature of its institutions. A nation's desperate need for short-term financial help does not give the IMF the moral right to substitute its technical judgments for the outcomes of a national political process.

The legitimacy of transnational activists (and NGOs representing interests other than business) thus comes from the fact that they are addressing a democratic deficit.[31] Some authors argue that they are capable of providing objective expertise due to their apolitical nature. This claim is hard to justify, because defending human rights, for example, is far from neutral. It could be argued instead that their moral principles are their source of legitimacy. Legitimacy can also be claimed from the fact that they do not seek to replace governments, but rather to inform and persuade governments and businesses to modify certain policies or positions. The Zapatista movement in Mexico is an example of this. They did not seek to overthrow to government, but rather to create a more active civil society and democratic government, as Schultz[24] points out. Thus before any question of legitimacy, accountability or representation can be considered, it emerges that such active NGOs promote views and interests that are not catered for by formal agencies. In this way these NGOs effectively become spokespeople for the broader public concerns.

With regard to representation, it is worth noting that international institutions work with and are influenced by NGOs unequally. A few examples of this will be given here. At the WTO Ministerial Conference in Singapore, 65% of the registered NGOs represented business interests. Women's organizations generally have less access to multilateral institutions, because of the loosely structured nature of their organizations. The World Bank tends to fund more technical NGOs than political ones, as they are useful for service delivery. This is problematic in itself, as NGOs then take on responsibilities that should be the domain of the state, and undermine state authority. This illustrates an aspect of complex multilateralism in which the less powerful states are weakened by the participation of non-government actors.

Jan Scholte[32] has put forward a theory to explain the access of civil society actors to international institutions. He categorizes them by the nature of their actions – conformist, reformer or radical. Whereas conformists support the general direction and functioning of international institutions and seek influence, reformers are critical and seek change, and radicals often call for serious overhaul of the institutions or their elimination. With regard to access to institutions, it is the conformists who have the most. This selection represents the interests of the institution more than the representative nature of the organizations. Desmarais[29] comments on this in her work, stating that organizations which accept the basic premise of globalization tend to have greater access than do the grassroots organizations that are highly critical of it. She compares two organizations, namely the IMF and the International Federation of Agricultural Producers, who are pro-liberalization and participate actively in the WTO with Via Campesina. The latter's rights-based perspective on agriculture runs counter to the neoliberal ideologies, and they are excluded from discussion. Scholte's work with the IMF also reveals that various parts of civil society have different degrees of access, academic and business interests being the most important.

Despite this imbalance of represented interests, O'Brian and colleagues[25] argue that the relationships between international economic institutions and government-sponsored mediation (GSM) do nonetheless contribute to a democratization of global governance. Woods has argued that INGOs have increased the accountability of international institutions but have unfortunately undermined the power and relative participation of developing countries and southern NGOs. Despite the difficulties, the collaboration can be worthwhile. Each group has its own set of strengths that can be a powerful tool for change when pooled together – grassroots organizations have good information about policy implications at the ground level, national NGOs have an understanding of government priorities and policies, and INGOs not only have knowledge of global trends, but have a large number of international contacts. They are thus aware of the best targets at which to direct action, as observed by Fox and Brown.[33]

If INGOs and NGOs are key to creating a world polity and to increasing democracy in international institutions, then ensuring their accountability and responsibility is key, at least to their partners within movements and to those they claim to represent. If we understand the objective of NGOs and GSM to be the democratization of international or national policy, it is interesting to ask how developed-world NGOs or INGOs can contribute by increasing the representation of under-represented movements, interests or groups. It is then also important to enquire exactly what developed-world NGOs or INGOs have to lose in this process.

We shall close this chapter with a quote from none other than Joseph E Stiglitz. He was the Nobel Prize Laureate in Economics in 2001, and is now Professor of Economics and Finance at Columbia University in New York. Before that, though, he had been Chairman of President Clinton's Council of Economic Advisers, as well as being the Chief Economist and Senior Vice President of the World Bank! He has obviously thought long and hard about the issues, and his current views on the IMF reflect this. If even he calls for drastic reform, can anyone doubt the credibility of the need for this?

### The IMF Fails Again
(Joseph E Stiglitz)

It is six years since the IMF's fateful meeting in Hong Kong, just before the global financial crisis. I was there. What a peculiar meeting it was. To those paying attention, it was clear that a crisis loomed. Capital market liberalization was the culprit, exposing countries to the vagaries of international capital flows – to both irrational pessimism and optimism, not to mention the manipulation of speculators.

Yet the IMF was still lobbying to change its charter in order to force countries to liberalize their capital markets, ignoring the evidence that this did not lead to enhanced growth or more investment, but only to more instability. The crises that erupted later that year undermined confidence in the IMF and led to discussions about 'reforming the global financial architecture.'

Now, six years later, we can say that those discussions did not lead to much real change. Some suggest that the fancy term 'reforming the global financial architecture' was a dead giveaway. The US Treasury and the IMF knew, or at least hoped, that with the passing of the crisis, global attention would turn elsewhere. While wrong about what to do in the crisis, on this point they were right.

But change has occurred, though sometimes more in rhetoric than reality. Today the IMF is more aware of the impact its programs have on poverty – though it still does not produce a 'poverty and unemployment impact' statement when it presents a program. The Fund has recognized the importance of participation and ownership. No longer are programs simply a matter between the IMF, central bank governors, and finance ministers. The IMF has recognized that there was excessive conditionality, and that these conditions led to a lack of focus.

The IMF has not, however, fully grasped that the conditions were often dangerously misguided, and often dealt with political issues that were beyond its mission. After criticizing the East Asian countries for a lack of transparency, the IMF acknowledged that it, too, was insufficiently transparent, and made reforms – though sometimes it seems that it thinks that a better website is a substitute for real transparency. Unfortunately, it still has not recognized a basic principle underlying modern democracy: citizens' right to know.

After the failure of the Argentina bail-out, the IMF recognized the need for an alternative approach. Earlier, it ignored calls for standstills and bankruptcy, saying that that would entail the abrogation of the debt contract. Finally, the IMF recognized that just as individuals need the right to a fresh start, so do governments. Unfortunately, it did not recognize that as a major creditor it could never be viewed as an impartial judge, and so could not have a pivotal rôle. It never fully grasped the political and economic issues underlying the design of bankruptcy laws.

Under pressure from global civil society, the IMF finally did agree to an enhanced debt forgiveness program for the poorest countries. Regrettably, it set standards and procedures such that few countries achieve the debt relief they need. At least in East Asia, the IMF recognized that excessive fiscal stringency contributed to the downturn, though it still pushed excessive fiscal stringency in Argentina when that country went into crisis, with predictably disastrous results.

It is good news that the IMF has recognized the limits of its policies and positions. But we should expect more of the IMF than just doing less harm than in the past. Even without capital market liberalization, the world will continue to face enormous volatility. Crises will not be things of the past.

Those who expected major reforms in the global financial architecture may well be sorely disappointed by what has happened in the past six years. For any fundamental reforms must address not only the difficult problems posed by the global reserve system and the burdens of risk borne by the developing countries, but also global governance. But there are strong vested interests in upholding the status quo. It is one thing to rearrange the chairs around the table, and quite another to change the table itself or those who have a seat at it.

So it is no surprise that another annual meeting of the IMF passed without any major steps forward in 'reforming the global financial architecture.' Instead, there was much discussion of another one of the symptoms that something is wrong. The issue of the day was whether China's exchange rate is overvalued, and if so, what should be done about it. Developing countries were told, once again, to get their houses in order, to address issues of governance, and to undertake 'painful' structural reforms.

It is, of course, always much easier to encourage others to undertake painful reforms than to look inward. The failed WTO meeting in Cancun of two weeks ago should serve as a warning: something is fundamentally wrong with how the global trading system is managed. So, too, is something fundamentally wrong with the global financial system. How many more meetings of the IMF will pass, how many more crises will occur, before this harsh truth sinks in?[34]

These words from Professor Stiglitz brilliantly exemplify the point that this author has often made in his previous writings, which is that in recognizing that there is an urgent need to move away from neoliberalism because it is an obstacle to global equity, there is no legitimate basis for regarding this as a reason for anti-Americanism. Not only has America's contribution to the philosophical foundations of liberty been seminal in advancing enlightenment values – such as unconstrained debate on intellectual and other issues – throughout the world, but the predicament that the world currently faces requires a strong American input. In fact, this author, while for 12 years an academic in the USA, consistently found that American thinkers and institutions were often their country's most trenchant critics.

In the chapter that follows, we shall consider the details of only a few specific areas in which the auctioning of the UN and the WHO actually undermines the UDHR and the WHO Alma Ata Declaration. However, those few details are enough to substantiate the claims of the present chapter and to give the general thesis of the book as a whole the basis that it needs. That, of course, will leave us with the question of what particular reforms need to be undertaken in order to restore the UN's mandate to its required place of true international authority and respect. Modern warfare, for instance, is completely counter-productive, and for the UN to have become implicated in the arms trade is unimaginable.

More will be said about these issues in the final chapter of the book.

## REFERENCES

1 Annan K. *The United Nations and Civil Society*; www.un.org/issues/civilsociety (accessed 3 August 2007).

2 Third World Network. *TNCs, Global Compact and Dams Face Critical NGOs*; www.twnside.org.sg/title/daros.htm (accessed 3 August 2007).

3 Ibid., p. 2.

4 Paine E. *The Road to Global Compact: corporate power and the battle over global public policy at the United Nations*; www.globalpolicy.org/reforms/papers/2000/road.htm (accessed 3 August 2007).

5 Ibid., p. 13.

6 MacDonald T. *Third World Health: hostage to First World wealth*. Oxford: Radcliffe Publishing; 2005.

7 James P. *The United Nations and Global Social-Economic Policy: Keynesianism for a new era*; www.globalplicy.org/soceocon/un/1996/analysis.htm (accessed 7 August 2007).

8 World Health Organization. *Tobacco Company Strategies to Undermine Tobacco Control Activities at the World Health Organization: Report of the Committee of Experts on Tobacco Industry Documents*. Geneva: World Health Organization; 2000. This story was carried in many leading newspapers. See, for example, Fairclough G. Cigarette firms tried to foil WHO, say investigators. *Wall Street Journal*, 14 August 2000, p. 9.

9 Peekers M. WHO prescribes socialist medicine. *Wall Street Journal*, 14 May 1996, p. 20.

10 Kull S, Destler IM. *Misreading the Public: the myth of a new isolationism*. Washington, DC: Brookings Institution Press; 1999.

11 Paine E. *The Road to Global Compact: corporate power and the battle over global public policy at the United Nations*. Article written for the Global Policy Forum, 5 May 2000.

http://globalpolicy.igc.org/reform/paper/2000/road.htm (accessed 15 December 2007).

12 Ibid.

13 Kennan GF. *Realities of American Foreign Policy.* Princeton, NJ: Princeton University Press; 1954. p. 54.

14 Gertz W. Power brokers' forum wires UN. *Washington Times,* 5 March 1997, p. 3.

15 Ruggie J, Kell G. *Global markets and social legitimacy: the case of the Global Compact.* Paper presented at University of Toronto, Canada, 30 November 1999; www.globalcompact.org (accessed 7 August 2007).

16 Ibid., p. 12.

17 Deutsch C. Unlikely allies join with the UN. *New York Times,* 19 December 1999, p. 2.

18 Bellamy C. *Sharing responsibilities: public, private and civil society.* Speech given at the Harvard International Development Conference, Cambridge, Massachusetts, 16 April 1999; www.bmjjournals.com/reprint/325/374/1240.pdf (accessed 9 August 2007).

19 Deen T. UN calls for new partnership between the UN and the arms industry. *Inter Press Service's Daily Journal,* 9 July 1999, p. 17.

20 Cataui M. Yes to Annan's Global Compact – if it isn't a license to meddle. *International Herald Tribune,* 26 July 2000, p. 1.

21 Ruggie J, Kell G, op. cit., p. 12.

22 James P, op. cit., p. 13.

23 Wilis C. *NGOs, TNGOs, TSMOs: their actions, impacts and concerns* [originally in French]; www.institute-governance.org/en/analyse/richte-analyse-39.htm (accessed 12 December 2007).

24 Schultz M. Collective action across borders: opportunity structures, network capacities, and communicative praxis in the age of advanced globalization. *Sociol Perspectives.* 1998; **41:** 587–616.

25 O'Brian R, Goetz A-M, Scholte JA *et al. Contesting Global Governance: multilateral economic institutions and global social movements.* Cambridge: Cambridge University Press; 2000. pp. 1–66.

26 Smith J. Bridging global divides? Strategic framing and solidarity in transnational social movement organizations. *Int Sociol.* 2002; 17: 505–28.

27 Ayres JM. Studying movements politically. In: *Defying Conventional Wisdom: political movements and popular contention against North America free trade.* Toronto: University of Toronto Press; 1998; pp. 9–20. Ayres JM. NAFTA and the structuring of domestic and transnational protest. In: *Defying Conventional Wisdom: political movements and popular contention against North America free trade.* Toronto: University of Toronto Press; 1998; pp. 117–34. Ayres JM. Political and theoretical implications. In: *Defying Conventional Wisdom: political movements and popular contention against North America free trade.* Toronto: University of Toronto Press; 1998; pp. 143–9.

28 Stiles KW. Grassroots empowerment. States, non-state actors and global policy formulation. In: Higgot RA, Underhill GRD, Bieler A, editors. *Non-State Actors and Authority in the Global System.* London: Routledge; 2000.

29 Desmarais AA. *The WTO . . . will meet somewhere, sometime. And we will be there!* Part of

a series entitled *VOICES: the rise of nongovernmental voices in multilateral organizations.* Ottawa: North-South Institute; 2003.

30 Woods N. Making the IMF and the World Bank more accountable. *Int Affairs.* 2001; 77: 83–100.

31 Price R. Transnational civil society and advocacy in world politics (review article). *World Politics.* 2003; 55: 579–606.

32 Scholte JA. 'In the foothills': relations between the IMF and civil society. In: Higgot RA, Underhill GRD, Bieler A, editors. *Non-State Actors and Authority in the Global System.* London: Routledge; 2000.

33 Willis C. *INGOs and NGOs: Their actions, impacts and concerns.* From the Literature Review, Directed Reading Course, Dominique Caouette; 2005. www.institut-governance.org/fr/analyse/fiche-an (accessed 15 December 2007).

34 Stiglitz J. *The IMF Fails Again;* www.stwr.net/content/view/74/37 (accessed 12 December 2007).

# Chapter 3

# Privatization of water, and the problems of sustainability

## OVERVIEW

Let us begin with a splendid remark made by Kofi Annan[1] within weeks of his becoming Director General of the United Nations:

> There once was a time when water fell freely from the clouds in the sky and bubbled from the springs in the hills . . . when the rivers, streams and lakes were full to the brim . . . When ancient underground aquifers flowed like great veins beneath the continents . . . when water nurtured our people, like babes sustained by their mother's milk.
>
> Today, water has become a scarce resource. Climate change has wreaked havoc with the weather, and the clouds no longer pour their tears of life upon our great forests. Vast agricultural lands suck rivers and streams dry. Our lakes are choked with dead fish which have been suffocated by industrial pollutants. The bowels of the Earth are constantly relieved of their waters, millions of years old.
>
> Experts predict that by the year 2025 our world will be suffering from the dramatic effects of hydrological poverty. There will be great disputes and even wars over water. 'Failure to act could damage the planet irreversibly, unleashing a spiral of increased hunger, deprivation, disease and squalor.'

It would indeed be difficult to find a more coherent statement of the problem. It is all the more surprising, therefore, how quickly Kofi Annan was moved by neoliberal arguments to stop regarding access to safe water as an inviolable human right, and to gradually acquiesce to neoliberal arguments for privatizing it. This event will be dealt with later in this chapter. It is only one of many indications of the extent to which the UN (and the WHO) have been bought out by neoliberal corporate interests.

However, the reader must bear in mind that privatization of water is part and parcel of the link between short-term neoliberal policies, and the whole issue of environmental sustainability generally. As we shall see, those agencies that were set up to protect and defend health and other human rights globally have themselves become increasingly complicit in trading off our long-term requirement for environmental sustainability generally for the short-term financial 'requirements' of neoliberal corporate power. However, we shall begin with the water issue.

One of the most commented upon aspects of what amounts to the privatization of parts of the WHO mandate to promote and defend health rights globally has, for some years now, been the growing practice of privatizing access to water. It is almost impossible to conceive of a more flagrant violation of health as a basic human right, but it has been going on in a big way since 2002, and huge fortunes stand to be made from it. This author discussed the issue in his book *The Global Human Right to Health: Dream or Possibility?*, especially with regard to the situation in Ecuador and in China.[2] The relevant chapters of that book made it clear that when we speak of 'water privatization', we are not only talking about financial barriers that make it impossible for many in the Third World to have ready access to clean and safe water on tap, in (or near) their homes. We are also talking about such major resource implications as the building of dams. Such construction projects are big business indeed, and with immense propensity for the widespread disregard of the rights to shelter, safety and agriculture of millions of displaced people. The profits – and they are handsome – are reaped by a few (usually geographically far removed from the country and people that are immediately affected), while negative impacts on health, especially of infants and children, are felt by many.

By its very constitution, and especially by its supposed commitment to the Alma Ata Declaration[3] of 1979, the WHO (and its parent body, the UN) should be in the front line trying to prevent these assaults on human rights. But instead – as will become clear in this chapter – both of those bodies have allowed themselves to become complicit in these developments. And it is not as if information about this has been lacking. As will be shown in the next section, human rights protagonists – some as non-government organizations (NGOs) and some as individuals – have highlighted the problem in a number of less developed countries since early in this millennium.

However, before dealing with some of these specific cases, let us gain a broader view of the whole problem by briefly considering three aspects of it. These are:
1  varieties of water privatization
2  rationales behind the decision to privatize water
3  how water privatization fits in with neoliberalism.


## VARIETIES OF WATER PRIVATIZATION

People closely associated with the phenomenon tend to recognize two broad categories of water privatization, namely the 'British model' and the 'French model.'[4] The British model involves privatizing both the water supply itself (including the necessary reticulation, sanitation link-ups, treatment plants, etc.) and the operation (management) of all of these facilities. In the French model, however, the assets and their management remain under public control. The British model is largely restricted to the UK itself, except for Scotland and Northern Ireland – where it remains public. However, the reader must appreciate the fact that some British corporations also operate the French model in a variety of Third World countries.

But the situation is not quite as clear-cut as this, because there are three degrees of privatization, all extant in the world today, and referred to as *management contract*, *lease contract* and *concession contract*. Under management contract the private operator is responsible only for running the system at a performance-related fee. Investment in it is generally financed by the government of the country concerned, with everything actually carried out by public finance. The advantage of this approach is that, theoretically, the country concerned can terminate the contract. Under lease contract, the infrastructure is leased to the private contractor, who charges users to make up the costs. Investment and running costs, as with management contract, are funded by the government of the country concerned. The concession contract allows the entire operation to be run privately, and often comes about as a result of the World Trade Organization (WTO) by use of the General Agreement on Trade in Services (GATS). It is much more difficult for a client government to disentangle itself from a concession contract.

Of course, the creation of a water supply system in a country which has never had one is hugely complex, and involves the construction of a wide range of large and expensive infrastructures over and beyond those used directly for water supply. This typically involves what is called a build-operate-transfer (BOT) contract. The BOT contract involves the private firm actually constructing all of the necessary plant, machinery, etc., and then running it for a fixed length of time (often 5 years) before handing it over to public/government control. Such a complex set of arrangements is almost forced to operate as a public/private partnership. Of course, long-term debt at high interest rates is the usual by-product of such systems.

## RATIONALE FOR PRIVATIZING

The most frequent reasons given by desperately poor nations for privatizing are that they must do so as a conditionality for an IMF loan – Structural Adjustment Policies (SAPs). The long-term aims, of course, are to:
- bring about an improvement in water quality
- render it unnecessary to rely on government subsidies
- pay for the infrastructure
- render the system more efficient.

It is instructive to look briefly at the tacit assumption that privatization will automatically result in greater efficiency. This is a view so widely purveyed by most of our media (which, of course, are themselves controlled by corporate interests) that many people take it for granted. However, the World Bank stated in 2007 that 'For utilities, it seems that in general that whether ownership is public or private makes little difference in terms of efficiency.'[5] And remember that the World Bank has not been known as antagonistic to private enterprise. Indeed, one suspects that it may be comparing examples of poorly managed, corruption-ridden public control with examples of more tightly controlled private enterprise!

## WATER PRIVATIZATION AND THE NEOLIBERAL AGENDA

*Masons Water Yearbook*[6] provides a wealth of information on the current situation. From it we learn that, by May 2004, 575 million people (9% of the world's population) were dependent on privatized water supplies. Of particular importance in this provision are three immensely influential multinational corporations:

- Suez, a French corporation with 117.4 million customers
- Veolia Environnement, another French corporation, with 108.2 million customers
- Kemble Water (Thames Water), a German (not British) corporation with 69.5 million customers.

There are other smaller ones, of course, such as:

- Aguas de Barcelona, a Spanish concern, servicing 35.2 million people
- SAUR (a subsidiary of Suez), with 3.5 million customers
- SABESP, a Brazilian state-owned private company with 25.1 million customers
- United Utilities, a French company with 22 million customers.

## OPPOSITION TO WATER PRIVATIZATION

Unsurprisingly, to mount such a blatantly violent assault on the global right to health (which must involve universal and unimpeded access to safe water) as to actually privatize access has attracted high levels of critical publicity and antagonistic commentary. Expressions of this hostility have by no means been confined to petitioning, peaceful demonstrations and academic discussions, but have often involved riots resulting in serious disruption and even death. As will be discussed below, we only have to consider the Cochabamba riots in Bolivia in 2000 and legal actions in various African countries. These will all be discussed in more detail in this chapter.

## IMMINENCE OF THE WATER CRISIS

As oil was the basic cause of wars in the twentieth century, many experts have suggested that water may be the cause of wars in the twenty-first century – and rather sooner than we care to believe. In an excellent paper by Susan Bryce,[7] the issue is discussed in depth. As Bryce points out, relevant opinion was (as far back as 2002) in agreement that a grave water crisis is imminent. Using computerized mathematical models, it was predicted that by 2025 at least 40% of the world population (projected to be 7.2 billion by that time) will be seriously compromised with regard to agriculture, industry and indeed personal basic health. Even such water-rich countries as China and the USA will be affected.[8]

Already 26 countries have more people than their water supplies can adequately support. Tensions are mounting over scarce water in the Middle East, and could ignite during this decade. There is growing competition for water between city dwellers and farmers around Beijing, New Delhi, Phoenix and other water-deficient areas.[9]

All of the evidence suggests that the first quarter of the twenty-first century will be the 'zero hour' for water in some parts of the world. The possibility of a water scarcity has been raised before, but only in the last few years has the language of crisis become all-pervading.

International discussions about the world's water supplies began in 1977 when the UN held the First World Water Conference in Mar del Plata, Argentina. The Conference declared the 1980s to be the 'UN International Drinking Water Supply and Sanitation Decade.' The altruistic goal was to ensure that all people in the world had access to adequate water supplies and sanitation within a decade.

Ten years later, the Brundtland Commission told the world that our approach to development was unsustainable – but it had little to say about water. Then, in 1992, the Rio de Janeiro Conference on Environment and Development, in its 'Agenda for the Twenty-First Century (Agenda 21)', considered the issue of availability of fresh water.

## GROWTH OF NEOLIBERAL CONTROL OF WATER

Concern about universal and unimpeded access to water as a fundamental human right has been increasingly preoccupying the WHO since the mid-1990s, and led to the first World Summit on Sustainable Development. The first of these 'Earth Summits' was held in Rio de Janeiro in 1992, and the Johannesburg Conference that was held in 2002 was therefore also referred to as 'Rio +10.' The original idea, as the reader will see in the next section, was more of a 'holding operation' on the part of the WHO and of the UN as a whole to create a 'balanced' approach to the problems, rather than accepting that such a problem should not exist and should be rectified immediately. A sense of 'fairness' was promoted by allowing the meetings to be discussion forums for business interests and people's groups. At the meeting in September 2002, corporative interests became obvious, especially with regard to fresh water. The reader should bear in mind that, even at this stage, the main issue was with regard to domestic supply. Looming large, though, and only latterly systematically addressed, was the issue of dam construction. This is so crucial an issue – and one that has been very much the concern of (often expatriate) corporate interests rather than of the communities immediately affected – that the author devotes an entire section to it below. For now, though, let us focus on domestic supply and use of fresh water.

The September 2002 meeting has been well described by Maude Barlow and Tony Clarke, and much of what follows is derived from their paper.[10] The setting of the summit paints the picture, one in which gross discrepancies in wealth, power and health are virtually flawed as 'inevitable', and where financial poverty and poverty of the imagination come face to face. This has given rise, in South Africa itself, to a particularly strong grassroots reaction. For instance, in Johannesburg itself (where Rio +10 was taking place), we have two adjacent townships – one wealthy and one poverty stricken.

Throughout South Africa, 'people's' conferences sprang up where activist and oppositional voices were also heard at various parallel meetings. One of the main ones took place in Alexandra Township, one of the poorest communities in South Africa. By and large, the people involved were not opulent, high-profile academics and apologists for big business, but were intimately familiar with life at the edge of economic ruin, where human rights were not discussed over cocktails and canapés. In Alexandra Township, water services (including sanitation) and electricity had already been privatized. In addition, many of these people had already experienced the harsh face of capitalism by having these vital services discontinued because they had not paid their bills.

As Barlow and Clarke point out, poverty-stricken and degraded Alexandra Township is separated by a fairly narrow river from the much more opulent town of Sandton. However, the river is so polluted that the people of Sandton do not use it for their supplies of drinking water, whereas those from Alexandra Township do. Local government demonstrated its concern about this situation by placing notices on the Alexandra side warning people that the water which they were compelled to use was a source of cholera!

In fact, South Africa – with its obscene difference between consumer-driven opulence and degrading poverty, the one living cheek-by-jowl with the other (especially in its large cities) – could hardly have been a more apt setting for Rio + 10. Not unnaturally, that country has given rise to the most articulate expressions of outrage at the idea of approaching these inequities by 'discussion' rather than by active remediation. This counter-movement stems from nothing less than a fight for survival, for we live in a world that is literally running out of fresh water. As this author pointed out in 2005,[11] while millions of babies die unnecessarily of gastric diseases caused by drinking polluted water, gallons of good-quality fresh water are wasted on golf courses for a small wealthy elite.

As Barlow and Clarke point out in the paper cited above, people are polluting, diverting and otherwise removing fresh water from circulation at an alarming rate. Day by day the levels of demand for fresh water increasingly exceed easily accessible supply. This puts more and more people at serious risk. By the turn of the millennium, the phenomenon of conflicts arising over water availability was becoming widely recognized as a destabilizing influence. Certainly within the next two decades almost two-thirds of the world's population will be faced with acute shortages of fresh water. The health implications are enormous.

However, this problem has only become widely appreciated recently, as if it had crept up on us unawares. It didn't, of course, because it has been well known by powerful corporate interests for years, but a compliant media has said little. For instance, until the turn of the millennium, analysis of the fresh-water disaster had remained sequestered among specialized groups of limnologists, hydraulic engineers, meteorologists, town planners, etc., and the ordinary consumer remained blissfully ignorant. Those who were aware of the desperately sad issue of babies in the Third World perishing in their millions, due to lack of access to safe water, tended to think of this as a highly localized issue with no impact on themselves, and to link it exclusively to personal poverty, along with endemic corruption, injustice, etc.

But now the message is getting through – finally – that our worldwide sources of fresh water are definitely finite and of comparatively low volume. We have allowed our precious aquifers to be prodigiously exploited, leaving us little on which to fall back. Put even more starkly – of the total water supply available on the planet, less than 0.5% is fresh water. Furthermore, the world's population is increasing by almost a billion people a year and, as education spreads, per capita water use is growing. At present it is doubling every 20 years. Even as things stand now – towards the end of the first decade of the twenty-first century – we cannot, without dramatic changes in both technology and political will, meet the needs of all of our people.

As was mentioned above, the problem is exacerbated by our propensity for building dams – to say nothing of the intense usage of fresh-water sources in factory farming, dumping of toxic wastes, destruction of rainforests, drainage of swamps, etc. In fact, the legacy of our poor stewardship has so severely compromised the Earth's surface water that we are now using up aquifer water reserves far faster than we can possibly replace them. Areas in which this has already happened are referred to as 'hot stains', and include parts of Spain, Morocco and France, huge tracts of the Middle East, Northern China (where most of that country's wheat is produced), Mexico, California and much of Sub-Saharan Africa.

It was said that, in 2000, one billion people lacked access to clean water.[12] Out of the entire panoply of environmental crisis that we now face, this acute shortage of ways to access even enough fresh water to meet basic needs is by far the most catastrophic. Yet few discussions about environmental issues give it the high profile that it urgently needs. The question might well arise as to why this should be so and (a closely related question) why the World Health Organization has not been more pro-active. To address these issues, we shall now consider the relevant history of the above-mentioned World Summit(s) on Sustainable Development, and then consider more closely the link between neoliberalism and those agencies (such as the WHO) which should long ago have visited it as part of their mandate.

## POLITICAL USE OF THE EARTH SUMMITS

Rio + 10, to which some reference has already been made, took place in Johannesburg, South Africa, from 26 August to 2 September 2002. It was a UN project – the UN World Summit on Sustainable Development (WSSD) and the entire history of those summits already illustrate the impact of corporate financial interests on their proceedings and recommendations.[13]

Consider the principles of the Earth Summit idea, as of 2002, as summarized in the Johannesburg Declaration. The following is a quote of items 16 to 37 of the Declaration accepted by the UN Department of Economic and Social Affairs Division (Division of Sustainable Development), and agreed to as UN policy at the September 2002 Earth Summit. The Declaration was called 'From our origins to our future.'[14]

16. We are determined to ensure that our rich diversity, which is our collective strength, will be used for constructive partnership for change and for the achievement of the common goal of sustainable development.

17. Recognizing the importance of building human solidarity, we urge the promotion of dialogue and cooperation among the world's civilizations and peoples, irrespective of race, disabilities, religion, language, culture and tradition.

18. We welcome the Johannesburg Summit focus on the indivisibility of human dignity, and are resolved through decisions on targets, timetables and partnerships to speedily increase access to basic requirements such as clean water, sanitation, adequate shelter, energy, healthcare, food security and the protection of bio-diversity. At the same time, we will work together to assist one another to have access to financial resources, benefit from the opening of markets, ensure capacity building, use modern technology to bring about development, and make sure that there is technology transfer, human resource development, education and training to banish forever underdevelopment.

19. We reaffirm our pledge to place particular focus on, and give priority attention to, the fight against the worldwide conditions that pose severe threats to the sustainable development of our people. Among these conditions are: chronic hunger; malnutrition; foreign occupation; armed conflicts; illicit drug problems; organized crime; corruption; natural disasters; illicit arms trafficking; trafficking in persons; terrorism; intolerance and incitement to racial, ethnic, religious and other hatreds; xenophobia; and endemic, communicable and chronic diseases, in particular HIV/AIDS, malaria and tuberculosis.

20. We are committed to ensure that women's empowerment and emancipation, and gender equality are integrated in all activities encompassed within Agenda 21, the Millennium Development Goals and the Johannesburg Plan of Implementation.

21. We recognize the reality that global society has the means and is endowed with the resources to address the challenges of poverty eradication and sustainable development confronting all humanity. Together we will take extra steps to ensure that these available resources are used to the benefit of humanity.

22. In this regard, to contribute to the achievement of our development goals and targets, we urge developed countries that have not done so to make concrete efforts towards the internationally agreed levels of Official Development Assistance.

23. We welcome and support the emergence of stronger regional groupings and alliances, such as the New Partnership for Africa's Development (NEPAD), to promote regional cooperation, improved international co-operation and promote sustainable development.

24. We shall continue to pay special attention to the developmental needs of Small Island Developing States and the Least Developed Countries.

25. We reaffirm the vital röle of the indigenous peoples in sustainable development.

26. We recognize sustainable development requires a long-term perspective and broad-based participation in policy formulation, decision-making and implementation at all levels. As social partners we will continue to work for stable partnerships with all major groups respecting the independent, important rôles of each of these.

27. We agree that in pursuit of their legitimate activities the private sector, both large and small companies, have a duty to contribute to the evolution of equitable and sustainable communities and societies.

28. We also agree to provide assistance to increase income-generating employment opportunities, taking into account the International Labour Organization (ILO) Declaration of Fundamental Principles and Rights at Work.

29. We agree that there is a need for private-sector corporations to enforce corporate accountability. This should take place within a transparent and stable regulatory environment.

30. We undertake to strengthen and improve governance at all levels, for the effective implementation of Agenda 21, the Millennium Development Goals and the Johannesburg Plan of Implementation.

31. To achieve our goals of sustainable development, we need more effective, democratic and accountable international and multilateral institutions.

32. We reaffirm our commitment to the principles and purposes of the UN Charter and international law, as well as the strengthening of multilateralism. We support the leadership rôle of the United Nations as the most universal and representative organization in the world, which is best placed to promote sustainable development.

33. We further commit ourselves to monitor progress at regular intervals towards the achievement of our sustainable development goals and objectives.

34. We are in agreement that this must be an inclusive process, involving all the major groups and governments that participated in the historic Johannesburg Summit.
35. We commit ourselves to act together, united by a common determination to save our planet, promote human development and achieve universal prosperity and peace.
36. We commit ourselves to the Johannesburg Plan of Implementation and to expedite the achievement of the time-bound, socio-economic and environmental targets contained therein.
37. From the African continent, the Cradle of Humankind, we solemnly pledge to the peoples of the world, and the generations that will surely inherit this earth, that we are determined to ensure that our collective hope for sustainable development is realized.

All of the above became UN policy as of 4 September 2002. And it illustrates, if one reads it carefully, how far acquiescence to neoliberal interests had gone even by that time. Thus the original declaration indicated – by subheadings – this gradual move from guaranteed human rights to how their objectives would be financed. In the section quoted above, paragraphs 16–30 were subheaded 'Our Commitment to Sustainable Development', paragraphs 31–33 were subheaded 'Multilateralism is the Future', and paragraphs 34–37 were subheaded 'Making it Happen.'

The reference to multilateralism should arouse suspicion in the minds of anyone familiar with WTO jargon. The reference in paragraph 31 to 'more effective, democratic and accountable . . . multilateral institutions' refers to the 'need' to privatize certain activities with regard to achieving the goals in paragraphs 16–30. Once the UN has agreed to this, it not only restricts the rôle of the WHO in promoting and defending its commitment to global human rights, but also in effect renders those rights realizable on the basis of business/marketing criteria rather than inviolable in all circumstances. 'Making it Happen' (paragraphs 34–37) confirms this in their emphasis on the need for public-private 'cooperation' and – as we shall see – despite Kofi Annan's statement at the beginning of this chapter, he became a strong proponent of this acquiescence to market forces, during his last five years in office.

Even so, the forces of neoliberalism were not completely satisfied. President George W Bush stayed away from the Summit and, accordingly, the USA did not feel bound by those UN commitments. Colin Powell, the US Secretary of State, did make a cursory appearance at the Summit – not to listen, but to briefly address the other delegates on the USA's expectations for just a few minutes before flying home. The US government refused to send a delegation as such, and back in the USA this snub earned President Bush praise from a number of corporate leaders.

As implied in Barlow and Clarke's paper,[10] many protagonists of people's right to water, and to environmentally sustainable policies in general, regarded the World Summit of 2002 as having been welcome. Earth Summit 2002 delegates were criticized for their hypocrisy in providing expensive catered food and drink for dignitaries while a few miles away there were starving South Africans. The Summit organizers were also criticized by others for excluding a variety of organizations and individuals, particularly those early founders who were instrumental in the nation's conservation and green history. The Summit also excluded critics in the movement who believe that the 'sustainable development' mantra is being misused in order to greenwash economic development at the expense of long-term environmental goals. However, had such critics been evenly marginally aware of the history and background of these 'Earth Summits', they would not have been surprised. The influence of corporate interests was there from the start.[15]

## A BRIEF HISTORY OF THE SUMMIT

A number of accounts of this are easily accessible in the literature. For instance, the Wikipedia report is adequate.[16] Bear in mind that it was a UN project from the start.

The United Nations Conference on the Human Environment was first held in Stockholm, Sweden, in June 1972, and marked the emergence of international environmental law. The Declaration on the Human Environment, also known as the Stockholm Declaration, set out the principles for various international environmental issues, including human rights, natural resource management, pollution prevention and the relationship between the environment and development. The conference also led to the creation of the United Nations Environment Programme.

The Brundtland Commission set up by Gro Harlem Brundtland, the pioneer of sustainable development, provided the momentum for the first Earth Summit in 1992 – the United Nations Conference on Environmental Development (UNCED). It was also headed by Maurice Strong, who had been a prominent member of the Brundtland Commission – and of Agenda 21. As readers may be aware, Gro Harlem Brundtland was the fifth Director General of the WHO (from 1997 to 2003).

South Africa's first National Conference on Environment and Development, entitled 'Ecologise Politics, Politicise Ecology', was held at the University of the Western Cape in conjunction with the Cape Town Ecology Group and the Western Cape Branch of the World Conference on Religion and Peace in 1991. Prominent individuals involved in this conference included Ebrahim Rasool, Cheryl Carolus, Faried Esack and Julia Martin.

What quickly becomes evident upon analysing this background, however, is that the principles of monetarism (as initially developed by Milton Friedman, the eminent American economist, and 1976 winner of the Nobel Prize in that field) became enthusiastically endorsed by powerful right-wing governments. Paramount in this respect were the US government under President Ronald Reagan and the UK government under Prime Minister Margaret Thatcher. In this context, and from its origins, the Earth Summits were dominated by monetarist thinking – also widely referred to as the 'Washington Consensus.' The Washington Consensus derives from the tacit assumption that neoliberalism is the only logical way forward for global finance. This has had the effect of discouraging nations from concerning themselves with environmental issues, and instead privatizing their maintenance of ecological protection. Everything has to be administered in terms of market forces rather than basic moral principles – and this has to include such services (and their supporting structure) as education and healthcare. Environmental sustainability was no longer seen as a 'social right' but as a bargainable financial proposition. It was therefore easy for governments to have no qualms about handing over water supply, and the care of freshwater resources generally, to those bent on making a profit out of this.[17]

Therefore, faced with the suddenly well-documented freshwater crisis, governments and international institutions are advocating a Washington Consensus solution – the privatization and commodification of water. Price water, they chorus – put it up for sale and let the market determine its future. For them, the debate is closed. Water, say the World Bank and the UN, is a 'human need', not a 'human right.' These are not semantics – the difference in interpretation is crucial. A human need can be supplied in many ways, especially for those with money. No one can sell a human right.

So a handful of transnational corporations, backed by the World Bank and the IMF, are aggressively taking over the management of public water services in countries around the world, dramatically raising the price of water for the local residents, and profiting especially from the Third World's desperate search for solutions to its water crisis. Some are startlingly open about this – the decline in freshwater supplies and standards has created a wonderful venture opportunity for water corporations and their investors, they boast. The agenda is clear – water should be treated like any other tradable good, with its use determined by the principles of profit.

It should come as no surprise that the private sector knew before most of the world about the looming water crisis, and has set out to take advantage of what it considers to be 'blue gold.' According to Barlow and Clarke,[18] the annual profits of the water industry now amount to about 40% of those of the oil sector, and by 2002 were even higher than those of all of the pharmaceutical corporations combined – close to US$1 trillion (1000 billion). However, only about 5% of the global water supply is privately owned. Just think, therefore, of the even larger profits to be made as the shortage of water becomes more acute. In the USA alone, 1999 saw in excess of US$15 billion worth of water acquisitions.[19] In fact, all of the major water companies are currently listed on the Stock Exchange.

We have to ask ourselves the following questions. Do basic human rights belong on the Stock Exchange? Are they commodities? If 'rights' become marketable commodities, how can we call for them to be 'global'? If the UN acquiesces to this, is it meeting its basic commitment to the UDHR?

## WHO ARE THE OWNERS OF WATER?

As already mentioned earlier in this chapter, there are three main providers of privatized water (which together dominate most of the market), and a number of smaller ones. The top ten of these corporations provided private water for more than 200 million people in 150 countries as far back as 2002. However, in recent years – as already noted – a number of countries have terminated their contracts because of quality/quantity problems. The British firm, Biwater, even took legal action against the desperately poor country of Tanzania[20] in an effort to force it to pay for a private water contract which it had to terminate because of complaints from its users – to say nothing of the violent street riots by thousands of people with no access to safe water because they couldn't afford to pay for the privatized supply. Where was the WHO which was supposedly protecting public health?

The answer is that the UN (and hence the WHO) have been sold out to the highest bidders by the IMF's SAPs and by the WTO enforcing GATS as part of loan and development conditionalities. Private water companies from the First World are actually assisted by the IMF and the World Bank, which through various WTO mechanisms, especially GATT and GATS, are forcing Third World countries to abandon their public water delivery systems and contract with the water giants in order to be eligible for debt relief. The performance of these companies in Europe and the developing world has been well documented – huge profits, higher prices for water, cutting off the supply to customers who cannot pay, no transparency in their dealings, reduced water quality, bribery and corruption.

The catalogue of such abuses by corporate agencies under the IMF and the World Bank affects not only tap water to people's homes, but also even the provision of a high standard of unpolluted bottled waters. In fact the bottled water industry is virtually unregulated, yet it is growing by leaps and bounds in many poor townships. Globally it is galloping ahead at an annual growth rate of more than 20%. In 2001, nearly 90 billion litres of bottled water were sold around the world – most of it in non-reusable plastic containers, bringing in profits of US$22 billion to this highly polluting industry. Bottled-water companies such as Nestlé, Coca-Cola and Pepsi are engaged in a constant search for new water supplies to feed the insatiable appetite of this business. In rural communities all over the world, corporate interests are buying up farmlands, indigenous lands, wilderness tracts and whole water systems, and then moving on when these sources are depleted. Fierce disputes are being waged in many places over these 'water takings', especially in the Third World. As one company explains, water is now 'a rationed necessity that may be taken by force.'[21]

The private water industry has a large and varied infrastructure. Corporations are now involved in the construction of massive pipelines to carry fresh water long distances for commercial sale, while others are constructing supertankers and giant sealed water bags to transport vast volumes of water by ocean-going vessels to reach more inaccessible areas. If a profit can be made from this (which clearly it can), why can't such transnational agencies as the UN do it more cheaply because they don't have to pay dividends to stockholders? The World Bank is even quoted[22] as stating that 'One way or another, water will soon be moved around the world like oil is now.' Even omitting the more obvious human rights implications, think of the carbon footprint that such activity would leave.

This author has already considered the social implications of huge commercial projects like this[23] when discussing the Three Gorges Dam in China, and some of those in South America. It is also known that some proposed projects would even reverse the flow of the Athabasca and other large rivers in Canada. The environmental implications of such an event would exceed even those of the Three Gorges project in China.

With regard to China's escalating problems with water, that country is increasingly having to turn to large-scale desalination of sea water, as it has already so heavily compromised even its aquifer sources of fresh water. A report published in the *London Evening Standard*[24] announced that China is in the process of constructing one of the largest desalination plants in the world in Zheiziang, near Shanghai. As the article points out, China has over 20% of the world's population, but only has access to 7% of the world's fresh water. In order to secure IMF loans for the project, it will have to undertake not to devote public funding to it, but to engage private contractors.

As we have implied, the World Bank and the IMF have been particularly active in what amounts to opening UN contracts to private contractors. The author will consider this issue in greater detail later, but before doing so, it would be instructive to consider specific case histories of water privatization as they have impacted on different countries. Although most of the egregiously bad instances are drawn from Third World countries, it must not be imagined that neoliberalism is particularly 'loyal' to its own countries! Keeping this in mind, let us first consider privatization of water in Argentina, Bolivia, China and several African countries, and then move on to consider the situation in Australia, Canada, France, the UK and the USA.

## SOME NATIONAL CASE HISTORIES
### Argentina

In theory, water supply is not privatized because it is operated by a state-owned company, Obras Sanitarias de la Nacion (National Sanitation Works), but it is not supported by taxation, nor is it universal. Supply of water from Obras calls for payments from individual customers. Those who cannot afford to pay have to obtain their water from sources such as polluted rivers. Then, in 2001, the state sold the business to the French privatized water firm Suez Lyonnaise. The new owners expanded the network to include 600 000 more customers. The service in the big cities is apparently adequate (if expensive), but with many households not provided for. However, in rural areas – even where services *are* provided – the water is even more expensive and the service is poor. The firm (referred to as 'Aguas Argentinas' rather than being called by its French name, to make people think that there is some state control involved) promised to cut prices by 27% and to invest US$4 billion to improve the service by 2032. The World Bank (through a South American private intermediary making a profit of 4% on grants under the name 'International Finance Corporation') gave the firm a grant of US$172 million as far back as 1994.

Under the WHO's mandate, safe potable water is supposed to be provided universally at low cost. It never was the idea that intermediary corporations should make a handsome profit out of it. And neither the WHO nor the UN gains any of that profit, nor does the Argentinean Government or its citizens. It goes straight into the pockets (and Swiss bank accounts) of the corporate owners, who themselves are not even resident in the country. In effect this means that, once again, the UN has had its activities farmed out to make a profit for big business.

Worse still, Aguas Argentinas has been called to account on several occasions by state health agencies for malfeasance in not providing an adequate standard of service. Outside of the capital, Buenos Aires, many customers complain that the water supply is often cut off for hours.

## Bolivia

The situation here is even more grim than it is in Argentina. In 1998, the water reticulation system in Bolivia's third largest city, Cochabamba, had become so decrepit that the government applied to the World Bank for a loan so that it could carry out the necessary repairs. The World Bank is, after all, a UN agency. However, the World Bank stated that it would *only* lend the money if Bolivia stopped supporting the project with public funds. They were forced to privatize. Naturally, Cochabamba's City Council had no choice, and they were forced to recover the extra money (required for a private corporation profit margin and for the dividends to stockholders) by raising the rates for individual customers. At this point, many urban customers were reluctantly forced to give up using the service. To privatize the service, as the loan conditions required, the state had to sell the entire water service to the highest bidder.

Only one bid reached the table, and that was from Bechtel. The author has shown in a previous book[25] that Bechtel had been implicated in the disastrous Three Gorges Dam in China, which caused the eviction of nearly 1.5 million people and the loss of their livelihood. As Susan Bryce[26] points out, 'in January 1999, before it had even hung up its shingle, the company announced a doubling of water prices.' The effect of this, for the majority of the people affected, was that water costs would now exceed those for food! For the poorly paid (about 55% of the people), water would now cost half their total income. The privatizing hand of the UN was once more visible in this, because the World Bank granted monopolies to all the private companies involved and announced, moreover, that the water pricing would need to be met fully by customer charges, and this cost of water was pegged to the US dollar. This now applied to all sources of water – people required paid permits to use even previously established community wells. Indeed, even peasants collecting rainwater for their needs were charged.

Riots broke out on 10 April 2000, when close to half a million people marched to Cochabamba City Hall, smashed up government vehicles and even forced entry into offices. The government quickly responded by kicking Bechtel out of the country. The people had won – even though their enemy was basically the UN, which was supposed to promote and defend their human rights.

## China

This author has alluded to China several times in previous publications, especially with regard to its prolific dam-building enterprises, such as the now infamous Three Gorges Dam mentioned above. However, it is widely assumed that since China classifies itself as communist, privatization of domestic water supplies for corporate commercial gain would not be a problem. In fact, though, despite Chinese insistence on its 'communism', many of its social policies out-capitalize capitalism! With regard to access to safe drinking water, the Chinese commentators Au Loong Yu and Liu Danqing,[27] writing in 2006, are very clear on this matter.

They point out that during the days of Mao Tse-Tung, and even as late as 1979, water supply was organized by the state. Since water supply was regarded ideologically as a public good, water rates charged to individual consumers were kept as low as possible, with water-processing and piping facilities being subsidised by the government. However, problems soon arose, especially under the twin pressures of increasing urban development and increases in population generally. Water quality gradually dropped to substandard levels as the need for greater financial investment in the infrastructure became more evident.

As with so many business-related activities in modern China, neoliberal approaches soon made themselves felt. By 1995, the Chinese government had decided that the solution was to commercialize and privatize water supply. It is often claimed that one of the underlying factors in the shortage of fresh water is that people have no concept of how to conserve water. Therefore the imposition of a water fee or rate became seen as the core reform in the supply of water – not only to force people to save water, but also to generate funding for additional investment. After 15 years of neoliberal policy on water supply, today it is clear that the only success is the massive increase in market penetration and the high profits earned by water companies, at the expense of the poor.

Thus China in many ways finds itself in a catch-22 situation. If it assumes that access to clean water is a fundamental human right, then supply of it has to be undertaken as efficiently as possible. Yet state authorities had shown that they could not adequately meet these needs with government finance alone, especially when the government was also bent on maintaining China's very high rate of economic growth as a worldwide trading partner at the same time.

With regard to fresh water, China is resource poor, the availability of fresh water per capita being only 25% of the world's average. The pollution of rivers and groundwater, as a result of the onslaught of industrialization and urbanization on a vast scale, has further exacerbated the problem. Today two-thirds of Chinese cities have an inadequate supply of fresh water, and in 110 of them the freshwater supply is critically inadequate. Meanwhile, the use of water per capita in China has fallen by 1.7% in the past 7 years.

The water supply infrastructure suffers from both a lack of investment and mismanagement. The problem is more acute in poorer areas of China – some areas have pipelines dating back to the 1940s. This means that the poor have to drink poor-quality water. Because of the chronic lack of investment in rural areas, 360 million peasants do not have piped water. Among them are households who suffer from a severe shortage of fresh water because they lack the money to dig deep wells. In many places the water table has fallen and deeper wells are needed in order to obtain a water supply from the wells.

Solutions based on privatization have been shown to create enormous profits for the few owners and stockholders. However, privatization of the water supply market has resulted in vast increases in water rates. A recent survey has shown that average water rates in 35 cities increased from 0.14 RMB per ton in 1988 to 1.26 RMB in 2003, an eightfold increase in 15 years. In Beijing the hike has been even more dramatic. Between 1989 and 2003 water rates were raised nine times, from 0.12 RMB to 2.9 RMB, a 23-fold increase. RMB means 'Renminbi', the Chinese unit of currency, and 1.8 RMB (as of 2007) is equivalent to one US dollar. In 2005, the average paid by consumers was 2.29 RMB per grade per month. The 'grades' refer to the household's income ranking, of which there are five, namely low income, lower-middle income, middle income, middle-higher income and higher income. Each grade represents 20% of the population. Thus some element of socialism still prevails in this marketplace system at present. However, in this author's view, even that will be sacrificed to growth.[28]

According to a study conducted in 1985 by Dong Fuxiang, water bills account for 2.5% of the monthly household income, and water is deemed to be unaffordable –hence the need to conserve water. In 2000, researchers surveyed five provinces and found that among the poorest 20% of households, water bills far exceed 2.5% of monthly income (*see* Table 3.1).

**TABLE 3.1** Households water bill and electricity bill as percentage of monthly income

| Households | Water bill as percentage of monthly income (%) | Electricity bill as percentage of monthly income (%) |
|---|---|---|
| 1/5 of low-income households | 4.19 | 11.62 |
| 1/5 of lower- to middle-income households | 1.87 | 5.05 |
| 1/5 of middle-income Households | 1.26 | 3.55 |
| 1/5 of middle- to higher-income households | 1.20 | 2.69 |
| 1/5 of higher-income households | 1.40 | 2.37 |

Table 3.1 shows that in 2006, among low-income households, water and electricity bills accounted for 15.8% of their average monthly income, a severe burden on these households. A book entitled *The Consciousness of Saving Water* recounts

strategies adopted by low-income households in order to save money on water bills. These range from barely opening taps so that the water meter might not record any water flow, to the use of water in public toilets, with huge crowds flocking to the toilets at the end of the day to wash clothes, vegetables, etc.[29]

But what of the corporations that are thus raking in huge profits from exploiting access to what the UN's own UDHR, and the WHO's Alma Ata Declaration, both define as a basic human right? Where did the corporations concerned, who have condemned thousands to death in infancy from enteric disorders, obtain the original capital to get the enterprises under way? The answer is from the IMF usually, and under conditions that compelled the government to privatize rather than to use state subsidization.

Such IMF loans, and these conditionalities, greatly enhance the power of the corporations because, as water rates increase, more and more private entrepreneurs crowd in to reap the profits. In this case, the now well-known French corporation, Suez, has moved into China in a big way. In fact, Suez, together with a Chinese/French Corporation 'New World Development' from Hong Kong, have undertaken to build 15 water-processing plants across China.[30]

Before leaving Asia, about which much more could be said, we shall briefly consider water privatization, its impacts and its UN support in Indonesia.


## INDONESIA'S EXPERIENCE WITH WATER PRIVATIZATION

In 1999, when the Indonesian government sought a World Bank loan to improve its water supply, it was advised that, as a condition for such a loan, it must become much more proactive in calling in private water firms to assess and then meet its needs. The companies that were specifically recommended to the government were Suez and Thames Water. Once the necessary contracts had been signed and the projects had been undertaken, complaints from aggrieved communities began to flood into the government. Rising prices and poor service led thousands to forsake the companies and dig their own wells.

However, as will be seen in a subsequent chapter, Indonesia has suffered massively – and continues to do so – at the hands of neoliberal forces applied through such UN agencies as the WHO (with regard to flu vaccine virus sources), the WTO, etc.


## AFRICA'S EXPERIENCES WITH WATER PRIVATIZATION

Many countries in Africa have unwittingly served as guinea pigs for the water privatization business, and have also served as a means for the WTO to test out various approaches to GATS. The case of Ghana has been dealt with in some detail by this author.[31] However, at least Ghana's government fought back. Much worse befell South Africa, as has been described by Barry Manson and Chris Talbot.[32] A very detailed study of water privatization in Africa was undertaken by UK researchers from the Public Services International Research Unit (PSIRU), and their report was presented at Witswatersrand University in early 2002.

When considering South Africa, Manson and Talbot commented that only a small number of the areas mentioned in the PSIRU report have had full privatization inflicted on them. The fact is that the ANC government has been persuaded by various UN agencies, and not only the IMF, that unless they become more energetically committed to moving towards full privatization, they will be disadvantaged with regard to access to development loans. However, when they started to implement this conditionality, they met with widespread and violent opposition, especially from poor communities.

As a result of this increase in implementation of full privatization, the worst outbreak of cholera in South Africa's history began in late 2000, and by February 2001 the death toll had reached at least 260. South Africa's Water and Forestry Minister, Ronnie Kasrils, agreed that the outbreak – and those deaths – had been caused by the lack of free access to safe and potable water.

Further analysis showed that although residents of the Empangeni district did have access to government-provided water schemes, many of them were too poor to pay the R51 ($4.80) registration fee charged by the local water board. Although the district municipality had a reserve of R98 million at the time, and was offering tax concessions to businesses to invest in the area, it demanded that communities should pay cost-recovery for water.

We have already referred to Alexandra Township earlier in this chapter. In the Johannesburg suburb of Alexandra, four people who were protesting against water privatization were recently injured in clashes with the police.[33] The area has been identified as a cholera danger zone. Residents believed that they were to be provided with clean water and sanitation, but the newly privatized water company run by Suez had refused to install taps in the area. Moreover, there were no sewers, and people had to use chemical toilets. Efforts to investigate what the company is contracted to provide have been blocked, but the project was financed by the IMF.

Biwater's activities, also discussed earlier in this chapter, showed up here, too. Other experiences of South African water privatization that were detailed in the PSIRU report include the British firm Biwater operating in Nelspruit, capital of Mpumalanga Province, and the French-owned SAUR, in a public-private partnership operating in the Dolphin Coast resorts of Kwazulu-Natal. That company experienced financial problems in 2001, with the result that water prices rose by 15%, with more increases likely to follow. A local investigation has revealed that enlargement of the project 'faced difficulties' because of the 'higher charges it makes for water provision to the poor.'

Biwater's project had likewise faced strong local opposition. An investigation indicated that:

> Biwater has not extended services and water infrastructure over the past three years – it stood at only one tap for every 10 households' and 'the [local protest] organizations say that residents were paying a flat rate of R70 a month

before Biwater took over in 1999, but were paying in 2002 between R400 and R500. Where residents have stopped paying, their water supply was cut off . . . Residents who are in arrears now risk being sued by the council, which has just hired a legal firm to track down defaulters.

One could select a number of African countries for analysis in this context, and others will feature later on in this chapter, but for now we shall restrict our discussion to the situation in Guinea, and more hopeful developments arising from the privatization fiasco in Tanzania. An excellent insight into Guinea's problems can be found in a report from the Integrated Regional Information Network (IRIN), a UN sub-agency on Africa.[34]

Although it was not published until 2007, the original report was written in Conakry (the capital of Guinea) on 13 October 2005, during the rainy season there. The report reminds us that Guinea is so well endowed with fresh water that it has been nicknamed 'the water tower of West Africa.' Yet by 2005 the taps in many of its towns had run dry. Frequent breakdown in the national water company's treatment centres and reticulation system have left many towns without running water for weeks at a time. Indeed, N'zerekone, a town near the Liberian border, has been without running water since 2001!

To put this in context, Guinea is a country that is enormously rich in resources (bauxite, gold and diamonds), but where the majority of the people live on under US$1.00 per day. Even in Conakry, many residents have to go foraging for water from polluted sources.

'It's been two years since we had drinkable water in our neighbourhood', Thiany Yansane, a local councillor, told IRIN. 'That's why I always keep jerry-cans in my car in order to fill them up with water at the office.'

Mohammed Dangoura, a Red Cross official in Conakry, says that there are two reasons, both linked to the country's poverty, for people's inability to gain access to proper drinking water. First, the vast majority simply do not have the money to pay for the service. And secondly, the national water company cannot afford to provide it.

In a report released in June, the international think tank Crisis Group warned that Guinea was on the verge of becoming West Africa's next failed state.

Lansana Conte, Guinea's president since coming to power in a 1984 coup, is seriously ill and lacks a clear successor, while the opposition has yet to provide a strong alternative. This combination leaves the future uncertain and the present increasingly difficult as the state breaks down.

'This [water issue] is not out of character with the problems that Guineans are living with in every aspect of their lives', said Mike McGovern, the West Africa project director at Crisis Group, adding that similar difficulties exist in other areas, including transportation, health and education.

'There's no real excuse for the current problems', McGovern told IRIN. 'The bottom line is it's a very rich country that should have the ability to provide things for its people, and it's not doing it.'

'Although water cuts are not uncommon in Guinea, the present shortages are especially difficult for this mostly Islamic country, as last week marked the beginning of Ramadan, a period in which many Muslims go without food and drink during daylight hours. As evening falls and the fast is broken, people require access to water for replenishment, a fact which the government readily admits.'

'We have called together officials from the interior of the country to ensure that everybody has access to water during the holy month of Ramadan', Fatoumata Binta Diallo, Guinea's energy minister, told IRIN.

But one week into this year's fasting period, the problem had not been solved, and the government decided on Monday to replace the heads of the troubled water and electric companies.

The utility's ex-director, Acheick Mouctar Youla, speaking to IRIN shortly before the high-level reshuffle, admitted to some supply problems, which he blamed on poor maintenance and the soaring cost of fuel necessary to keep the treatment centres running. He said that the 24 facilities in the country's interior require 10 000 litres per month, leaving the company with a tab of close to US$9000.

However, if we look a little closer, we see that the problems cannot be blamed on oil price rises – which occurred after the water problem became acute – but originate in the water privatization programme, taken on as a condition for an IMF loan to the country. As the IRIN report[34] shows, widespread complaints about the inadequacies of the water supply led the country's government to terminate the contracts, and resulted in the re-nationalization of the water system in 2000. However, matters have only got worse, due less to malfeasance than to lack of technical know-how. It is here that the UN could have played a crucial rôle, but their aim seemed to be to promote privatization. The Government caved in by renegotiating with the private water corporations!

The French companies SAUR and Electricité de France (EDF) and the Canadian company Hydro-Québec agreed to waive 70% of the debt that they claimed to be owed by the government, leaving a total of 3 million euros (US$3.6 million) to be repaid over the next 36 months.

In recent years, corruption and the lack of democracy have made foreign donors increasingly reluctant to lend money to Guinea, but EDF representative André Jaujay said that this new deal could help to change all that.

'With foreign loans serving as a foundation, our companies will be happy to be serious partners in Guinea', he said, speaking on behalf of the three multinationals at the signing of the accord.

But still there is no water.

Let us now turn to Tanzania's stormy experiences with IMF-impelled water privatization. The intention was to show the less developed countries of the world just how brilliantly effective an idea water privatization could be, but it failed dismally. The private water company concerned was Biwater, and it was contracted in 2003 to make sure that the citizens of Tanzania's capital, Dar es Salaam, at least had ready access to clean and safe tap water. The contract was also supposed to provide service to 'surrounding areas', although these were not clearly defined – all within 5 years.[35]

As indicated above, the World Bank funded the plan as part of an IMF loan conditionality at a cost of US$140 million. In undertaking this arrangement, Tanzania and Biwater were strongly supported by the UK government under Prime Minister Tony Blair. Altogether it was one of the most involved and ambitious such plans in all of Africa. However, it failed badly to deliver water reliably, even in Dar es Salaam itself. The supply was frequently cut off, and the water was often dirty and smelled so bad that people rioted in the streets in protest. And within 2 years, the Tanzanian government terminated the contract unilaterally. They made a number of specific complaints, namely that no new domestic pipework had been installed, that water quality had actually declined, and that revenue had decreased because many customers stopped paying for what they weren't getting.

Although Biwater had the contract, it had been subcontracted to City Water, one of its subsidiaries. The British Chief Executive of City Water denied the claims and even filed a court suit against the Tanzanian government for breach of contract! The news of a wealthy First World country (the UK) actually suing a poor Third World country did not exactly enhance the humanitarian reputation of Britain! However, the Chief Executive went on to say that he accepted that the project was behind schedule and that no pipes had been installed, but he claimed that water quality and quantity had improved and that 10 000 new customers had been signed up in the last 2 months.

He said 'We have been trying to renegotiate the terms with a view to continuing', and claimed that the Tanzanian government had given the company wrong data about water supplies, and that the delays were not of City Water's making.

'We accept there is a serious problem, but we proposed on May 9 that we put in a further US$5 million over the next year and borrow a further US$6 million. We said "Let's talk about it", but the government announced to the press that the contract had terminated.' He said that the Tanzanian government owed the company US$3 million.

The privatization scheme was facilitated by British aid money. The Department for International Development had paid Adam Smith International, sister organization of the Adam Smith Institute, a free-market UK think tank, more than £500 000 to provide advice to the Tanzanian government. More than £250 000 of that sum was spent by Adam Smith International on a video which included the words 'Our old industries are dry like crops, and privatization brings the rain.' However, according to the World Development Movement (WDM) in London, Tanzania was forced to privatize its water as a condition of international debt forgiveness. 'The International Monetary Fund forced water privatization on one of the poorest countries in the world in order to benefit western water companies', said Dave Timms of the WDM.

Naturally, the collapse of the contract throws into question other water privatizations planned around the world, and the UK government's involvement in them has also been questioned. Resentment of private water monopolies is growing, and there have been demonstrations in South America, Africa, the Caribbean and Asia. Many western companies are accused of profiting from the poor and raising prices above what they can afford.

However, City Water claimed that it stood to make little money out of the scheme. We have since witnessed a rather undignified squabble among the capitalists themselves. 'Our declared profit was to be just 10%. There is no way we can make super-profits in Dar es Salaam', said a spokesperson for the firm. 'We have been losing money. Profits always come at the end of a contract. The plan was to use this as a model for other projects and recoup money later on.' The Department for International Development has said that it has paid more than £36 million in the past 7 years to Adam Smith International and PricewaterhouseCoopers to advise countries on privatizing utilities.

Accusations and counter-accusations still continue, with ActionAid (an NGO that promotes the rights of less developed nations) roundly condemning the World Bank and other associated agencies of the UN. However, a spokesman for the UK's Department for International Development tried desperately to defend this country's honour by putting the blame on Tanzania itself, stating that:

> It is for the government of Tanzania to set its own policies and priorities. It was their decision to introduce private sector participation in the water sector in Dar es Salaam, so it is not appropriate for us to comment on contractual issues.

Surely this was said with tongue in cheek, for he would have realized only too well that Tanzania had been forced to privatize its water system as an IMF Structural Adjustment Policy.

All in all, the Tanzania experience has succeeded in being a model for other Third World countries – but not in quite the way that was intended by the rich and powerful who stood to gain from it!

## WATER PRIVATIZATION IN THE USA

Water privatization in the USA has a long and complex history because each state draws up its own regulations. And even within some states there is sometimes freedom for different counties to exercise choice as to how and under what auspices their water is to be privatized. However, since 1995, water privatization has grown exponentially. The main corporations involved are Consumers Water Company, Domingues Services, Southwest Water, Connecticut Water and E'Town Corporation, and they have seen their profits soar, increasing by more than 20%.

US Water News Online reported a major paradigm shift[36] involving overt cooperation between elected politicians and the water corporations. Their collective aim – a truly breathtaking expression of monetarist philosophy – is to reduce each component of nature (most of which have been taken for granted as 'free' or 'God-given') to the status of a commodity, which can be bought and sold subject to the rules of the marketplace. Is this a foretaste of the *reductio ad absurdum* of neoliberalism? And if so, what are the purposes of the UN, the WHO and many of their other agencies?

To give substance to these rhetorical questions, many examples from the world's most highly developed nations can be cited. However, we shall content ourselves with just one, namely Atlanta, Georgia.

## LESSONS LEARNED IN ATLANTA, GEORGIA

One would think that the citizens of the USA, especially the municipal officials of its larger cities, would be pretty much immune to the blandishments of water privatization companies. Yet Atlanta, Georgia – one of the largest cities in the USA – fell for it hook, line and sinker. However, unlike some of the other victims of water privatization, Atlanta managed to disengage itself when things went wrong for the consumers. Let us go back to the beginning of the interaction.

In 1999, Atlanta's city fathers were persuaded to hand over the management of the municipal water system to United Water which, as we have seen, is really a subsidiary of Suez. The initial contract cost US$420 million. The engagement lasted for only 4 years, and the Mayoress of Atlanta, Shirley Franklin, ended the contract on 2 January 2003.[37] In her public announcement to the citizenry – many of whom had been complaining about United Water's failings – she is reported to have said that 'Atlanta will once again run its own water system, and I want to reassure all citizens of Atlanta that your water supply is in good hands.'

It is interesting to see how easily the original takeover was managed, even in a sophisticated American city. Lee Morris, who had trained as both a lawyer and an accountant, sat on the panel that made the original decision, and he described the transaction as follows:

> I personally agreed with the concept of turning it over to a private operator because the former municipal water department had been a poster child for government inefficiency, where politicians would dump their friends and relatives when they needed a job. It was not a well-run department, and it was a very costly department.

Now, with the deal cancelled, it's hard to find anyone in Atlanta who thinks that privatizing the water system was a good idea. And many people, like Morris, just shake their heads in disbelief that so much has gone wrong. As Morris stated:

> It's a cautionary tale because quality has been jeopardized. In my old councillor district particularly there have been a dozen or more instances where people had brown water running through their faucets and advisories to boil it before you drink it. In a large world-class city like Atlanta, that just should not happen. It might happen in Third World countries, but it should not happen in Atlanta.

How did the citizens at the grassroots level regard the privatization? As Frank

Koller of the Canadian Broadcasting Corporation (CBC) described it, he couldn't find anyone who supported the privatization! He cited several examples, one being that of the single mother Lamar Miller. She had three children living at home, and consequently was a heavy consumer of water, as her washing machine was on almost daily. She was described as 'comfortably middle class', yet she found the water rates exorbitant.

Over the years she had had water problems from time to time, but nothing like the summer of 2001:

> When you turn on the water, you expect to have water come out of your faucet. That summer we had, multiple times, when you would turn on the faucet and nothing would happen, sometimes for a couple hours, sometimes for a couple days. And then when the water comes back, it looks like dirty creek water. It clogs up all the filters in your refrigerator, it destroys your laundry, and there's no warning when you're going to get these discolorations.

One day, she loaded more than a dozen of her husband's white dress shirts into the washing machine. Thirty minutes later they weren't white. She added:

> During the summer, when the water pressure was going down, we were getting a lot, so you could actually see it coming out of the faucet.

Then consider Walda Lavroff's comments. In the summer of 2002, a severe drought forced the people of Atlanta to follow strict water rationing. However, when a fire hydrant at the foot of Walda Lavroff's driveway broke a leak like a gusher, Lavroff says it took 10 days of constant phone calls to United Water to get it fixed. By then, the pavement was eroding away.

On other occasions, Lavroff received notices from United Water to boil her water, days after breaks in water lines had created health concerns. She pointed out that she didn't have these problems when the City ran the water system, and went on to state:

> When water pipes and valves had broken in this neighbourhood, there was a boil advisory out for water and we didn't get the advisory until a day or two later ... [This] is serious business because if the water is not safe to use as they said for baby formula or for elderly, ill people and so on, we should be notified at once, not a day or two later. The City cannot wash its hands of the responsibility of supplying water.

Despite repeated complaints, United Water would not talk to the CBC reporter when I was in Atlanta just before the City ended the water contract. The company had said publicly that the City of Atlanta hid the true state of the pipes from contract bidders. The company complained that it only realized after winning the deal how bad things were when brown water started to flow.

Howard Shook, an Atlanta City Councillor, says that he was drowning in complaints:

> I spend way too much of my time acting as a grief counsellor for bereaved United Water customers. We have raised property taxes 50%, and we have done all sorts of things poorly that have aggravated the citizens, but I have never run into anything that has aggravated my constituents more than the inability to provide clean tap water every time they reach out and turn that tap.

Atlanta's city government was also disappointed with United Water because the company failed to deliver on promises to save the city money. A recent audit of United Water's performance, ordered by the mayor, revealed uncollected bills, demands for even more money from the City, and delayed repairs.

Clair Muller, who chairs the City's Utility Commission, says that those problems were all supposed to end when the private company took over the system:

> It was said at the time that we would save $20 million per year of the 20 years. Even people who believed in this privatization buzz word were calling me saying even the city can't be doing that bad a job that you'd save $20 million. And indeed they were right, we've saved about eight.

When it was decided to privatize its water system, the world's water management companies flocked to Georgia. This was the largest water privatization deal yet in the USA. Winning it was regarded as getting a toehold in a huge untapped market. Competition was fierce.

Five major bidders spent millions on public relations campaigns, lobbyists and lawyers courting City politicians. In the end, United Water, owned by Paris-based Suez, won with the lowest bid.

Lee Morris, then chair of the Utilities Commission, said he and his other elected colleagues knew that the Atlanta contract was a highly valued prize:

> We certainly heard that it was important to all of these large companies, that this was going to be the first one, the toehold if you will, and it was important for them to land it even if it meant they did not necessarily make a lot of money or maybe even any money. So certainly it took deep pockets.

One thing is certain about Atlanta's experiment with water privatization. City Councillors Howard Shook and Claire Muller say that they have learned a tough lesson. As Howard Shook commented:

> My inner conservative no longer worships at the altar of privatization as I might once have done. That is for sure. Sometimes it is the best answer, but I now know that it is not always the answer, and we have to be very careful about it.

Claire Muller expressed the following view:

> Water is something very important to everybody, and I do think that we got a
> little carried away four years ago with the hype of this being the silver bullet that
> was going to solve all our problems. We went down the wrong path.

One could cite many more examples from the USA, but most of them have ended
in the same way, and with the same bitter lessons learned. But how much more
serious it is for less developed nations, especially under UN pressure, to make the
same mistake.

## EARLY EVIDENCE OF THE NEOLIBERAL TAKEOVER

In fact, participants at the Rio + 10 meeting in Johannesburg recall that, among
the stalls run by publishing companies and academic institutions, were dozens
run by private water companies. Their aim, clearly, was to get poverty-stricken
less developed nations to 'do the right thing' on IMF conditions by signing up for
privatized deals for water and sewage infrastructures. This author has mentioned
in a previous book that the eight Millennium Development Goals (MDGs) were
designed to put the world back on the path laid out by the Alma Ata Declaration.
One of these MDGs was to halve the number of people (2 billion) lacking access
to safe and potable water by 2015 and, almost cynically, these private operators
flaunted their services as helping poor countries to meet that target. Yet, as
Manson and Talbot[32] make so clear, such advertisements represented empty
rhetoric, with no commitment from Western governments. However, the fact that
this was one of the few areas in which the USA and the European Union were
not at loggerheads reflects the almost universal agreement in the West to step up
the pressure on the developing world – including some of the poorest countries
– to sell off their water provision to big business. Despite Kofi Annan's words, the
Third World's experiences with private corporations in other areas (e.g. breast
milk substitutes and tobacco products) has made it abundantly clear that their
first objective must be (under neoliberal competition) nothing more than profits
and sufficiently high dividends to hold on to their stockholders. Why should a
corporation be committed to 'working with' Kofi Annan to bring about equity?
The very notion of equity gives no legitimacy whatsoever to competition and thus
to neoliberalism.

The appalling conditions that result from lack of clean water and sanitation
were described in a report by two British charities, namely Tearfund and WaterAid.
Inadequate sanitation results in an environment in which debilitating and life-
threatening diseases can flourish. The consequence is that 2 million children a year
(one every 15 seconds) are dying from wholly preventable diseases. In developing
countries, waterborne disease is the second commonest cause of death, with half
of all visits to a clinic due to diarrhoeal disease from waterborne pathogens such
as cholera, *E. coli* and *Shigella*, which causes dysentery.

However, as was mentioned earlier, it is not only the poor and underdeveloped countries that are victims of water privatization. Anywhere where a profit can be made from water will attract such corporations. Let us therefore consider a few wealthy countries whose less well off citizens have become victims of such neoliberalism.

## AUSTRALIA AND UNESCO

One UN agency that has so far not been implicated in the auctioning off of human rights is UNICEF. However, that agency certainly featured in Australia's involvement with water privatization, as reflected in Susan Bryce's research.[26]

A report entitled *A Vision for Australia's Water Resources 2025* was prepared for the World Water Forum 2000 by Integrated Resource Management Ltd under contract from UNESCO. The Australian report recommends water pricing related to volume and timing, as well as the elimination of subsidies.[38]

Australia has already undertaken a programme of far-reaching changes in the way in which the water sector is organized and managed, with an increasing rôle for the private sector. In 1994, the Council of Australian Governments (COAG) declared that 'business as usual' in the rural water industry was not a viable option for irrigators – or for the environment.[39] They are now implementing changes which will affect pricing, water allocation, institutional arrangements and environmental management. These reforms are to be implemented together, as a package, this year (2007).

The reform package included an agreement to introduce full-cost recovery pricing in rural areas. Hence, prices paid for water increased dramatically after that. But even prior to that, prices had started to increase already. Many local governments in Australia have made rainwater tanks and recycling of 'grey water' illegal, because these would interfere with corporate profits.

## THE UK

The idea of privatizing household water supplies had not been considered in Britain since 1945, and many people thought that it would remain as a government service. However, when Margaret Thatcher became Prime Minister, the philosophy of monetarism was applied widely. A number of sacred cows were sold off, and there was a widespread rush to buy shares. Water was no exception, and thus water supply and services were privatized.

It all turned out to be the most total and expensive water privatization programme carried out to date. The UK's 10 regional water authorities (RWAs) were sold off as private profit-making enterprises. They were sold at visibly low prices and on 25-year concessions through the issue of stock-market shares. The Government wrote off all the existing debts of the water companies – at a cost of US$8 billion! The media were freely used to encourage ordinary people of all social classes to become stockholders. The only parts of the UK which did not become involved were Northern Ireland and Scotland.

To make the project more attractive, government subsidies were employed to render the venture even more certain of bringing in huge profits. Of course, payment for these inducements became part of the general tax burden. Another inducement was the fact that private companies were given a start-up fund of US$2.6 billion. Moreover, the companies were exempted from taxes on their profits.

Within a very short time, customers started to realize that they had been 'had.' Prices rose by more than 5% in the first 4 years. Over the first 9 years – adjusted for inflation – there were price increases of 46%.[40] Popular anger was increased still further when the media, especially the tabloid press, informed the public of the fact that, as their water rates rose, the managers of the companies were raking in obscenely large salaries and enormous bonuses. It turned out that the real value of the fees, salaries and bonuses paid to the directors increased by between 50% and 200% in most of the water companies. The profits of the 10 water companies rose by 147% between 1990 and 1997. Profit margins in the UK are typically three or even four times as high as those of water companies in France, Spain, Sweden or Hungary. This could explain why most of the 10 UK companies were quickly purchased (after the 5-year 'protection' period) by the big corporate water multinationals – including Suez, Vivendi and RWE.[41]

As might be expected, the increase in water prices for customers was followed by an increased rate of household disconnections due to non-payment. The disconnection rate tripled in the first 5 years, with 18 636 households disconnected in 1994. Again, there was a wide public outcry arguing that cutting off the water supply endangered public health. A 1994 study showed rates of dysentery rising in most major urban areas. When disconnections for non-payment became more controversial, the water companies started to use 'pre-payment meters' for customers who were unable to pay their bills. These meters only supplied water when customers had paid money charged on a plastic card. When the account was empty, the meter cut off the water supply. The companies called these 'self-disconnections.' By 1996, over 16 000 pre-payment meters had been installed. Public outrage continued to grow until Parliament passed a new public water law called the Water Industry Act of 1999, which outlawed both disconnections for non-payment and the use of pre-payment meters.[42]

There have been serious transgressions in the environmental performance of the UK companies, such as lack of basic conservation measures, sewer back-flow, waterway pollution, and poor drinking water quality. In 1998, the major water companies in the UK were ranked as the second, third and fourth worst polluters. The UK's Environmental Agency regularly prosecutes the water companies for pollution offences. The 10 water companies were prosecuted a total of 260 times between 1989 and 1997. However, paying the fines was simpler than making the necessary investment in rehabilitation of infrastructure and treatment plants. Since 1998, the situation has improved somewhat, and the water companies have been prosecuted for a total of 22 water pollution offences. Lack of attention to maintaining the water and sewerage system has contributed to wastage from leaks, and to poor drinking water quality. The Drinking Water Inspectorate (DWI) identified lack of compliance with regard to key parameters (excessive amounts of nitrite, iron, lead and other pesticides) in more than 20% of water zones.[43]

The 10 UK water companies have little incentive to make capital investments to rehabilitate and improve the water and sewer infrastructure. In fact, capital expenditure started to accelerate before privatization, peaked in 1991–92, and then began to fall in the post-privatization period. It appears to be common practice for the companies to budget large capital expenditure needs (which are then used to calculate the allowed price rises). However, rather than making the budgeted infrastructure improvements, the companies use the shortfall in expenditure to boost their profits. For example, Southern Water submitted plans for a series of new sewage treatment plants that were never built. Yorkshire Water 'saved' on its capital expenditure budget by getting a promise from government to redefine coastal waters as sea waters instead of estuary waters – permitting the company to dump raw sewage instead of expanding treatment plants.

The widely read *Daily Mail* ran a scathing article[44] in the mid-summer of 1994 – when many were feeling the worst effects of water control bans. It contained the following quote:

> The water industry has become the biggest rip-off in Britain. Water bills, both to households and industry, have soared. And the directors and shareholders of Britain's top ten water companies have been able to use their position as monopoly suppliers to pull off the greatest act of licensed robbery in our history.

## CANADA

As a country, Canada has always been bountifully supplied with water. Hydroelectric power was (and still is) a widely used source of energy, and even a decade ago few Canadians regarded water rates as anything other than one of their more trivial expenses. But now neoliberalism has well and truly taken over, and water is becoming a commodity to be traded and sold. Pressures within Canada to privatize control of municipal water services and treat water resources as an export commodity are increasing. French and British companies are vying with American firms to control Canada's water services.

Many municipalities have entered into 'partnerships' with private organizations. For example, Moncton in New Brunswick has entered into a 20-year agreement that will see the city's water filtration plant maintained and operated privately. The company concerned, US Filter, will build the plant and sell it to the city upon completion, in exchange for a guarantee that it will have exclusive rights to sell Moncton its drinking water. The company has sought status as a municipality for tax purposes, arguing that it should be exempt from Goods and Services Tax.[45]

## FRANCE

In France the situation with regard to water privatization has been made worse not so much by bad management, as by what might be called 'sharp practice' even within the government itself. In fact, in France, private companies have been prosecuted for providing water that is polluted and unfit to drink. A French Government report revealed that more than 5.2 million citizens received 'bacterially unacceptable' water. Corruption is also rampant, with water-related bribery schemes resulting in convictions of municipal officials and water company board members under investigation. French cities with private water charge 30% more than cities with public water. In France, as well as in Germany and the Czech Republic, municipalities guarantee payments to companies if consumption or prices are not sufficient to ensure a profit.[46]

## HAS WATER PRIVATIZATION FULFILLED ITS PROMISE?

Whenever this author reads the rhetoric – from WHO agencies and others who should know better – about the advantages to the poor of privatization, he is reminded of a splendidly apt comment attributed (uncertainly) to the renowned British economic theorist, John Maynard Keynes:

> Capitalism is the extraordinary belief that the nastiest of people, for the nastiest of motives, will somehow work for the benefit of all.[47]

As we have already seen, enthusiastic claims were made by WHO-based proponents of water privatization that it would contribute to achieving the Millennium Development Goals by 2015! To what extent, however, has water privatization really been beneficial? Is it really true that the private sector is so much more efficient than the public sector that, even when the need for profits and dividends is taken into account, the needs of masses of people are met more cheaply, swiftly and to a higher standard than could be expected of government-run agencies? From everything that has been said so far in this chapter, privatization can only spell disaster for the MDGs – and for any hope of realizing the targets of the Alma Ata Declaration.

In 2004, the Global Policy Forum[48] asserted that the Structural Adjustment Policies of the IMF and the World Bank have grossly undermined health in much of the Third World. With their energetic support for water privatization, they have created unemployment and food scarcity, and left millions of people without access to water. In doing this, these UN agencies are effectively, and with ghastly efficiency, undermining the WHO's commitment to basic human rights. Thus the UN, instead of defending and promoting the UDHR, has been serving the interests of private water companies – and the corporate sector generally – through its loan programmes to governments of less developed countries.

Kofi Annan, despite the impression given by his quote which headed this chapter, increasingly throughout his post as Director General of the UN stressed the need to achieve the MDGs by closer cooperation with the private sector. As long ago as 2002, he was quoted as saying:[49]

> Lasting and effective answers can only be found if business joins in partnership and works with public agencies. We can only make significant progress if we mobilize the corporate sector.

One can only wonder at his naivety, so well characterized by the above quote attributed to Keynes, especially when one considers the vast number of well-known cases in which the corporate dedication to a 'profit-first' policy trumps any more altruistic concerns.

As far as water supply is concerned, the eagerness with which UN agencies have jumped into bed with the private sector has been amply documented above. Indeed, the corporations are only too ready to forsake any commitment to public service if their profits become threatened, whatever the prevailing need of the people. Maude Barlow and Tony Clarke give some startling accounts.[10,18]

In July 2002, Suez terminated its World Bank-backed 30-year contract to provide water and sewerage services to the city of Buenos Aires, when the financial meltdown of Argentina's economy meant that the company would not be able to maintain its profit margins. To make matters worse, the company also left a mess behind it. During the first 8 years of the contract, weak regulatory practices and contract renegotiations that eliminated corporate risk enabled the Suez subsidiary, Aguas Argentinas S.A., to earn a 19% profit rate on its average net worth. Water rates, which the company said would be reduced by 27%, actually rose by 20%. In total, 50% of the employees were laid off, and Aguas Argentinas reneged on its contractual obligations to build a new sewage treatment plant. As a result, over 95% of the city's sewage is now dumped directly into the Rio del Plata River.

SAUR, whose activities have been discussed above, distributes the water on a for-profit basis for all of Senegal. In 1996, the company was awarded the contract with a US$96 million loan from the World Bank. The deal explicitly states that its aim is 'cost recovery' – meaning profit for investors – and stipulates the need to charge for the cost of water, even to poor households. As a result, as in many other countries in Africa, many Senegalese citizens are forced to turn to untreated water sources for their water needs. For instance, the government of South Africa has cut off water supplies to over 10 million people in the last 2 years because they could not afford to pay for the newly privatized service – despite a constitutional guarantee of access to water for all!

In an effort to attract World Bank funds, President Vicente Fox of Mexico has established a national programme called PROMAGUA. Now operating in 27 of the country's 30 states, PROMAGUA actively promotes the privatization of water services in cities with a population of over 100 000 people. Largely financed by a World Bank grant of US$250 million, PROMAGUA encourages cities to open up their public water systems to private water corporations by signing concessions that last for between 5 and 50 years. As a result, the two water giants, Suez and Vivendi, together with United Utilities and Aquas de Barcelona, have developed joint ventures with Mexican companies to take over the running of public water systems on a for-profit basis. Close to 20% of municipal water systems in Mexico are now privatized. Furthermore, there are numerous instances where these private water companies have jacked up water rates and cut-off services to those who can't pay the bills, while reducing water quality and refusing to make investments for the improvement of infrastructure such as leaky pipes.

As we have already seen in this chapter, these shenanigans have lent strength and coherence to much of the growing grassroots opposition to water privatization. Various individuals and organizations have become increasingly vocal in attacking the WTO, and other agencies of the UN, for their complicity. Much of this opposition has been based on analysis of the implications of GATS as a cause of ill health and degradation.

However, despite all of this, less developed countries in particular are still being put under great pressure by the World Bank, the IMF and the WTO to privatize their water supplies. The International Institute for Environment and Development (IIED) published a paper in June 2007,[50] from which the following information is drawn.

Research from the IIED warns that privatization is unlikely to contribute to achieving the MDG of halving the number of people without access to water and sanitation by 2015. Despite its prominence in current debates, only around 5% of the world's population is served by the formal private sector. Water privatization in developing countries is concentrated in wealthier states, cities and neighbourhoods where companies know that users can afford to pay for new or improved services. Areas on the outskirts of cities, smaller urban centres and rural areas (home to some 80% of the estimated 1.1 billion people who lack access to improved drinking water supplies) are often excluded from private contracts.

As we have already seen, over 80% of the private water and sewage market is controlled by four multinational companies. Local operators in developing countries have often found it difficult to get into the market because they cannot raise sufficient finance. Contrary to the hopes of market reformers, privatization has not eliminated political involvement or corruption. Bidding processes have not always promoted competition, as some companies have underbid competitors with a view to subsequently raising charges, or colluded with rival companies to win follow-on contracts.

However, despite ongoing encouragement from development institutions, the rate of privatization is slowing down. After underestimating risks and overestimating potential profits, companies are becoming more wary of getting involved. Several large contracts have been terminated prematurely. Companies have failed to mobilize substantial private finance, and most investment has come from development loans, government funding and user charges.

## GROWING OPPOSITION TO WATER PRIVATIZATION

Fortunately, popular opposition to these activities is funded by the very international agencies to which the neediest people would ordinarily have looked for protection, and the people of poorer countries are beginning to oppose their government's involvement in such scams. If nothing else, this has been a lesson in empowerment at the community level! Consider recent events in South Africa.

On 29 May 1994, as South Africa was gearing itself up to celebrate the anniversary of its first democratic elections, riots began to break out. These disturbances were not led from above, but broke out almost spontaneously from grassroots discontent over the recently privatized water supply, and in particular from the way that the corporate owners were cutting off the supply due to non-payment of bills. To add to the growing resentment, electricity supplies were suffering the same fate. Street riots broke out, and when police tried to quell them many officers were injured by showers of stones and bottles. Even government offices and other facilities were destroyed. In fact, the number of such disturbances exceeded by five times the number of anti-apartheid riots only a few years before.[51]

The ANC government, at one time the people's champion, immediately launched a campaign to identify the organizers, and referred officially to such people as 'a conspiracy against order, and a dark force.'[52] However, spokespeople for the protesters pointed out that the 'dark forces' were the conditions under which the people were being forced to live.[53] As was stated by Kerry Chance,[54] there was no way that these events could be swept under the carpet, and they even received embarrassingly huge coverage in the media worldwide. Such events were not confined to South Africa, and have become increasingly common in many other countries, as we shall see.

In the Philippines such resistance began to make itself felt as far back as 2002. In December 2002, after 5 years of controversy, Maynilad Water (co-owned by Suez and a wealthy Filipino family) threatened to terminate their water contract in Manila. Maynilad Water was unable to pressure the regulator to approve its requested rate increase. Approval had been granted for six previous rate increases, and countless other contractual obligations had been re-negotiated away since the contract was signed. Debt ridden and unable to raise more capital, Maynilad Water's creditworthiness was at stake. The company's operating expenses were more than 40% higher than projected, although major investment and performance targets were never met. In the aftermath of the Asian financial crisis, the company repeatedly demanded coverage of its foreign exchange losses. Although many of Maynilad's demands were granted, eventually the regulator started to refuse them, and Maynilad Water, assessing their rates of return to be inadequate, began to threaten to pull out.[55]

Can the hand of UN agencies be traced in all of this? Indeed it can. The International Finance Corporation (IFC) had advised Manila to privatize its water services on a 'user pays' basis as the only feasible way of meeting the people's needs. However, the IFC is a private lending sub-agency of the World Bank. In

1994, it sought to privatize Manila's publicly owned Metropolitan Waterworks and Sewer System (MWSS). Suez was given those rights, through a World Bank loan, in 1997. That company had promised to provide water for 7.5 million households, at a rate of 4.96 pesos (about US$1) a week. It also claimed that Manila City Council would save US$4 billion over 25 years!

However, within a year things were turning out badly. The water company sought to increase the water charges, and by 2000 the price had gone up to 15.46 pesos (US$3.40).

In a Christmas 2000 press release the Asian Labor Network stated:

> The additional cost of water will ensure a bountiful New Year to Maynilad and Manila Water. But an ordinary Filipino family will now have to forego an additional 87 to 147 pesos a month. In effect, Maynilad and Manila Water with the full blessing of MWSS have deprived the Filipino family of three full meals or three kilos of rice. The ordinary vendor will now have to surrender one full day of income to pay for the cost of water. To poor families who can only afford instant noodles the water increase might mean they cannot eat for two days.[56]

Despite all of this, the water company Maynilad tried to re-negotiate the contract that it had so egregiously broken, and the World Bank still backed it. Rate increases continued, and it kept deferring obligations with regard to infrastructure that had been part of the original contract. Technically, this constituted grave and persistent breach of contract, and should have forced the company to forfeit its performance bond. However, the company, backed by WTO lawyers, fought the government in the local courts. This allowed Suez to use its well-versed corporate lawyers and supplies, while also billing customers for losses caused by the gradual devaluation of the peso! Not only is the company seeking US$303 million as compensation, but MWSS will now have to cover US$530 million in loan repayments. Ultimately it is taxpayers in Manila who will end up shouldering this burden. They have learned the hard way not to trust UN agencies to protect their human rights under the UDHR.

One could go on listing similar accounts as country after country comes to realize that neoliberalism rules the UN and most of its agencies. However, enough has been said to persuade the reader that the entire system of mediation of human rights globally needs to be re-addressed. Therefore, rather than presenting more details of particular cases, let us set all of these particulars within the broader context of international trade. When we do so, we gain an insight into the real degree to which the UN and its agencies have become complicit in promoting the interests of global neoliberalism.

## INTERNATIONAL TRADE AND NEOLIBERALISM

As we have seen from the foregoing account, governments have since the 1990s been signing away their control over their nations' water supply. This has not only been happening in individual cases with individual private water companies, but is also steered globally through such WTO arrangements as multilateral trade agreements – for example, GATT and GATS. Global instrumentalities like these have led to transnational corporations having almost total access to freshwater sources worldwide. As we have seen, some corporations have even gone so far as to sue governments for terminating unsatisfactory contracts.

This means that what most thinking people, until recently, regarded as unquestionable rights have become commodities instead. As Maude Barlow and Tony Clarke have pointed out,[57] the North America Free Trade Association (NAFTA) and the Free Trade Area of the Americas (FTAA), along with the WTO itself, exert enormous power on behalf of neoliberalism globally.

Water is listed as a 'good' by the WTO and NAFTA, and as an 'investment' by NAFTA. It is to be included as a 'service' in the upcoming WTO services negotiations (the General Agreement on Trade in Services) and in the FTAA. Under the 'National Treatment' provisions of NAFTA and the GATS, signatory governments that privatize municipal water services will be obliged to permit competitive bids from transnational water-service corporations. Similarly, once a permit is granted to a domestic company to export water for commercial purposes, foreign corporations will have the right to set up operations in the host country.

NAFTA contains a provision that requires 'proportional sharing' of energy resources that are now being traded between the signatory countries. This means that the oil and gas resources no longer belong to the country of extraction, but are a shared resource of the continent. For example, under NAFTA, Canada now exports 57% of its natural gas to the USA and is not allowed to cut back on these supplies, even in order to cut fossil fuel production under the Kyoto Agreement. Under this same provision, if Canada started to sell its water to the USA – something President Bush has already stated he considers to be part of the USA's continental energy programme – the State Department would consider it to be a trade violation if Canada tried to turn off the tap. And under NAFTA's 'investor state' Chapter 11 provision, American corporate investors would be allowed to sue Canada for financial losses.[58] Already a California company is suing the Canadian government for US$10.5 billion because the province of British Columbia banned the commercial export of bulk water.

The WTO also opens the door to the commercial export of water by prohibiting the use of export controls for any 'good' for any purpose. This means that quotas or bans on the export of water imposed for environmental reasons could be challenged as a form of protectionism. At the December 2001 Qatar Ministerial meeting of the WTO, a provision was added to the so-called Doha Text, which requires governments to give up 'tariff' and 'non-tariff' barriers – such as environmental regulations – to environmental services, which include water.

## CAN WE IMPROVE ON THIS?

It might well be asked whether there is any hope, given the present ubiquity of neoliberalism. This author believes that there is still plenty of realistic scope for effective opposition to 'The Empire.' However, in order to develop a coherent opposition to it, let us be clear as to what exactly is wrong with the prevailing model. First of all we do have the technical know-how – vastly under-utilized at present – to reclaim 'grey' and otherwise jettisoned water. For instance, widely used and monstrously wasteful systems of flood irrigation can easily be replaced by drip irrigation and repair programmes for existing reticulation systems. We referred earlier to China's plans for a massive desalination plant, and such plants are held out by some as a rational response to the growing shortage of fresh water. However, what is not generally realized is just how environmentally destructive such plants are. They produce massive carbon footprints, as well as impacting negatively on the surrounding marine environment, interfering with fish populations, etc. As the situation stands even now, the developed nations could – without having to set up desalination plants – supply all of water-deprived China (and the rest of the world) with good-quality fresh water.

However, in order to do this, we would have to enter into hugely cooperative and well-run programmes of international action. If the UN had not become so enmeshed in the short-term gains of corporate private profit, it could provide the necessary global mediation to accomplish this. Thus we are talking about nothing more technologically demanding than a change of global politics! For a start we could *really* cancel the Third World debt, *actually* meet the G8 promises for foreign aid and *realistically* tax the privatizing corporations.

In other words, we have to bring water supply under internationally administered law. However, our window of opportunity for doing anything so rational and morally responsible is perilously narrow, and closing all the while, the longer we persist in the insanity of treating fresh water as a market commodity. Thus a new international ethic is called for, and one critical tenet of this new ethic has to be 'Thou shalt not commodify vital natural resources.'

The Earth and its myriad resources must sustain us all, and not only the temporarily privileged, if even we are to survive. At the practical level – and on an international basis mediated by a reformed UN – we must set about defining which natural occurring resources are of universal necessity to life.

Existing national governments – backed as they are in competition in a neoliberal matrix – are unlikely to unilaterally set about creating such legislation. The lead must come from a redirected UN, and be supervised by a similarly redirected WHO. We are already on the cusp of such reforms becoming feasible. As Barlow and Clarke[51] have pointed out, a useful lay common front already exists. Public sector workers, human rights organizations, medical teams and a whole range of social classes – from peasants to professors – are determined to bring about a water-secure future for all.

They have already done much along these lines – coordinating strategy at the World Social Forum at Porto Alegre, Brazil, in January 2000. And they were actively vocal at the Rio + 10 talks in Johannesburg, South Africa in 2001. Likewise, they made their presence felt in Kyoto in 2002 at the Summit on Sustainable

Development, and in 2003, when the UN and the World Bank convened over 8000 people at the Third World Water Forum. They have stood – and still do – with local people fighting World Bank-sponsored water-privatizing enterprises in Bolivia and dam construction in India. They have led an inspiring opposition in the developed countries as well, such as attacks on the obscene profits made by Perrier in Michigan. All of these local struggles must be reaffirmed as part of a global movement with a common political agenda.

Steps needed for a water-secure future include:

❏ the adoption of a 'Treaty Initiative to Share and Protect the Global Water Commons'

❏ a guaranteed 'water lifeline' – free clean water every day for every person as an inalienable political and social right

❏ national water protection acts to reclaim and preserve freshwater systems

❏ exemptions for water from international trade and investment regimes

❏ an end to World Bank and IMF-enforced water privatizations

❏ a Global Water Convention that would create an international body of law to protect the world's water heritage based on the twin cornerstones of conservation and equity.

A tough challenge indeed, but – given the stakes involved – we had better be up to it.[59]

## REFERENCES

1 United Nations. Press release, 23 June 1997, at a Special Session of the UN convened to implement 'Agenda 21' – the programme of action adopted in Rio de Janeiro in 1992 by the UN Conference of Environment and Development. In making the cited comment, Kofi Annan was discussing what would happen if 'Agenda 21' was not realised.

2 MacDonald T. *The Global Human Right to Health: dream or possibility?* Oxford: Radcliffe Publishing; 2007. pp. 43–4, 87–8, 96–8.

3 MacDonald T. *Health, Human Rights and the United Nations.* Oxford: Radcliffe Publishing; 2007. pp. 232–5.

4 Wikipedia Encyclopaedia. *Water Privatization*; http://en.Wikipedia.org/wiki/water_privatization (accessed 16 June 2007).

5 Ibid., p. 1.

6 Holland A. *The Water Business: corruption vs. people.* London: Zed Books; 2005. pp. 64–6.

7 Bryce S. Privatization of water. *Mexus Magazine.* 2001; **8:** 61–74.

8 Gleick PH. Making every drop count. *Sci Am.* 2001; **February issue:** 29–33.

9 Postel S. *Last Oasis: facing water scarcity.* Worldwatch Environmental Alert Series. New York: WW Norton and Company; 1997. pp. 21–30.

10 Barlow M, Clarke J. *Who Owns Water?*; www.thenation.com/docprint.mintrol?I=20020902=Barlow (accessed 17 June 2007).

11 MacDonald T. *Third World Health: hostage to First World wealth*. Oxford: Radcliffe Publishing; 2005. pp. 12–21.

12 Barlow M, Clarke J, op. cit., p. 3.

13 Wikipedia Encyclopaedia. *Earth Summit 2002*; http://en.Wikipedia.org/wiki/world_summit_on_sustainable_devel (accessed 16 June 2007).

14 United Nations. *From Our Origins to Our Future*. First published in 2002, and adopted as a United Nations Policy Document at the 17th Plenary Meeting of the World Summit on Sustainable Development, 16 September 2007.

15 MacDonald T. *The Global Human Right to Health: dream or possibility?* Oxford: Radcliffe Publishing; 2007. pp. 16–31.

16 Wikipedia Encyclopaedia. *Water Privatization*; http://en.Wikipedia.org/wiki/water_privatization (accessed 16 June 2007).

17 Barlow M, Clarke J, op. cit., p. 3.

18 Barlow M, Clarke T. *Blue Gold: the fight to stop the corporate theft of the world's water.* London: Earthscan; 2002. pp. 42–7.

19 Barlow M, Clarke J, op. cit., p. 4.

20 MacDonald T. *The Global Human Right to Health: dream or possibility?* Oxford: Radcliffe Publishing; 2007. pp. 44–6.

21 Barlow M, Clarke J, op. cit., p. 5.

22 Barlow M, Clarke J, op. cit., p. 5.

23 MacDonald T. *The Global Human Right to Health: dream or possibility?* Oxford: Radcliffe Publishing; 2007. pp. 40–48.

24 China to build desalination plant. *London Evening Standard*, 14 June 2007, p. 24.

25 MacDonald T. *The Global Human Right to Health: dream or possibility?* Oxford: Radcliffe Publishing; 2007. pp. 40–44.

26 Bryce S. The privatisation of water. *Nexus Magazine*. 2002; 8: 9.

27 Au Loong Y, Liu D. *The Privatisation of Water Supply in China*; www.tri.org/books/waterchina.pdf (accessed 16 June 2007).

28 Li T. China water shares are very profitable. *Wanbao Weekly*. 2006; **January issue:** 3.

29 Ibid., p. 5.

30 Wang Y. *Behind the 3.3 Billion RMB Water Business*; www.people.com.en/GB/huanbao.html (accessed 17 June 2007).

31 MacDonald T. *The Global Human Right to Health: dream or possibility?* Oxford: Radcliffe Publishing; 2007. pp. 44–6.

32 Manson B, Talbot C. *What Water Privatisation Means for Africa*; www.wsws.org/articles/2002/sept.2002/water-s07.shtml (accessed 17 June 2007).

33 Ibid., pp. 2–3.

34 Integrated Regional Information Network. *Guinea: water, water everywhere but not a drop to drink*; www.irinnew.org/report.aspx?reportid=56708 (accessed 18 June 2007).

35 Vidl J. Flagship water privatisation fails in Tanzania. *Guardian*, 25 May 2005.

36 US Water News Online; www.uswaternews.com/homepage.html (accessed 18 June 2007).

37 Koller F. *No silver bullet: water privatisation in Atlanta, Georgia – a cautionary tale*. CBC Radio, broadcast 1 February 2003; www.cbc.ca/news/features/water/Atlanta.html (accessed 18 June 2007).

38 UNESCO. *A Vision for Australia's Water Resources 2025. Final Report.* Brisbane: Integrated Resource Management Research, Pty. Ltd; 1999. p. 13.

39 Council of Australian Governments Communiqué. Hobart, Tasmania, 25 February 1997; www.dist.gov.au/science/pmsec/14meet/inwaterr/app3form.html (accessed 18 June 2007).

40 OFWAT (Office of Water Services). *OFWAT Memorandum,* 18 March 1998. House of Commons Research Paper.

41 Ibid., p. 2.

42 Alberni Environmental Coalition. *Annual Report on Privatisation*; www.portaec.net/library/ocean/water/profiting_from_water.html (accessed 18 June 2007).

43 Ibid., p. 11.

44 The rip-off of water rates. *Daily Mail,* 11 July 1994, p. 4.

45 Keasy K, Thompson S, Wright M. *Corporate Governance, Economic Management and Financial Issues.* Oxford: Oxford University Press; 2001. pp. 31–9.

46 Ibid., pp. 9–10.

47 This is very uncertainly an attribution distributed by Leeds Postcards (www.leedspostcards.com), who claim that they cannot find the source for it.

48 Global Policy Forum. *New Humanitarian Empire?*; www.globalpolicy.org/empire/humanist/2004/01newhumanitarianism.htm (accessed 18 June 2007).

49 Annan K. Press comment on his award of the Nobel Prize on 12 October 2001; www.un.org/news/press/docs/2001/sgsn7992.com (accessed 18 June 2007).

50 International Institute for Environment and Development (IIED). *Privatisation and the Provision of Urban Water and Sanitation in Africa, Asia and Latin America.* London: IIED; 2007. pp. 20–42.

51 Barlow M, Clarke T. *Blue Gold: the fight to stop the corporate theft of the world's water.* London: Earthscan; 2002. p. 7.

52 NIA launches probe into riots. *Sunday Times,* 29 May 2006, p. 3.

53 Ibid., p. 3.

54 Chance K. *The Cut-Off: electricity and water politics in the 'new' South Africa*; http://humanrights.uchicago.edu/workshoppapers/kerrychancepaper.pdf (accessed 20 June 2007).

55 International Consortium for Investigative Journalism. *Loaves, Fishes and Dirty Dishes: Manila's privatised water utility can't stand the pressure*; www.wateractivist.org (accessed 18 June 2007).

56 Statement from the Asian Labor Network (a sub-agency of the International Labor Organisation) in its Philippines Chapter Newsletter, December 2000; www.wateractivist.org (accessed 18 June 2007).

57 Greider W. *The Right and US Trade Law: invalidating the 20th century*; www.thenation.com/doc/20011015/greider-37k (accessed 20 June 2007).

58 Ibid., p. 46.

59 Ibid., p. 51.

# Chapter 4

# Dams and dambusters

## ANOTHER FACE TO WATER PRIVATIZATION

In our discussion of UN involvement in water privatization, so far we have largely concentrated on user-pay schemes for domestic water supplies. However, equally threatening to human rights has been the widespread and forceful application of neoliberal principles by the UN, and its agencies, in imposing dam construction on various countries and river systems. Indeed, in general one can say that the infrastructure implications of dam construction are even more destructive globally to environmental sustainability and to human rights than is the idea of privatized supply of good-quality water for domestic use. Dam building also involves a much greater capital outlay and provides much greater scope for corporations in the First World to literally (and figuratively!) make a killing in the Third World. On top of this, and unlike discrepancies in local domestic water supply, dam building has immense potential for environmental damage far beyond the localities in which the dams are constructed.

This chapter will deal with recent examples of the long-term harm that is often done by such enterprises, and will also discuss various levels of local and international opposition to dam building.

Many people have already remarked on what might appear to be similarities between oil and water, with regard to the importance of making money out of ways of accessing it. However, the analogy is superficial – as we shall see – and Jean-Michel Cousteau, of worldwide fame for his underwater photography of fish and other less understood life forms, commented that 'Water cannot really be thought of as the next gold or oil.' He made that observation at the World Water Forum in Kyoto in March 2003.[1]

In this chapter we shall concern ourselves primarily with dams and with what the author calls the 'mega-effects' of ordinary domestic exploitation of water. Out of both, of course, private enterprise – with the ready help of the World Bank and allied UN agencies – generates millions of pounds. However, before considering specific dams, it is worth providing an overview of the environmental impact of dams. It has even been said, for instance, that the huge number of dams built in Asia since 1990 has actually altered the tilt of the Earth on its axis.[2]

## FATE OF THE ARAL SEA

Damming on a smaller scale is regularly carried out for 'industrial agriculture' purposes. Consider the Aral Sea (actually a lake) in the former Soviet Union. Until only four decades ago, it was the fourth largest inland body of water on Earth, and the largest inland body of salt water. It was obviously of huge ecological significance, and also supported thriving communities of trawlermen. Some of the boats used were enormous, of a size normally used for open ocean fishing. When this author first saw the Aral Sea in 1960, he was impressed with its vastness (one couldn't see across it) and great depth. It seemed absolutely indestructible. It was 36 260 square kilometres in area – as permanent a geographical fixture as one could hope to find. However, within 30 years it has effectively vanished, leaving only a series of moist slimy patches on which today one can walk out to rotting ships beached in the mud and far from any open water. How could such transformation happen, and so quickly?

The death of the Aral Sea came about through a barrage of environmentally unsustainable assaults on the two main river systems feeding it. These two rivers are the Amu Darya and the Syr Darya. As will be seen, damming these rivers and diverting much of their water flow for irrigation had catastrophic consequences. Details of the stages by which the Aral Sea was destroyed, those who provided the capital necessary to fund this monumental degradation, and those who profited from it are all highly instructive lines of enquiry.

The impacts of this decline will be described at some length because it so clearly demonstrates the dangers of allowing large-scale infrastructure on the landscape, guided by neoliberal considerations, to proceed without first routinely carrying out some check, such as International Health Impact Assessments (IHIAs). This issue has been discussed by the author in a previous book.[3] Of course, such precautionary checks are often discouraged and/or ignored by UN agencies that are determined to promote development under privatization.

A number of accounts of catastrophes attendant upon such neglect are available from various Internet sources, the *Environmental Times* being especially informative.[4] From such sources we learn that the Aral Sea has in previous millennia undergone expansions and contractions with dramatic climate change. However, it was only when vast farming operations started in the 1960s and 1970s in the surrounding region for producing cotton on a large commercial scale that really big problems arose. Creating the necessary field irrigation networks involved the partial damming of the two key rivers, and diversion of their waters. This was accompanied by industrial-level extraction of enormous volumes of water to irrigate the huge cotton plantations. The enterprise was funded by the World Bank, with Structural Adjustment Policies and other loan conditionalities – the issue of human rights barely being considered. Moreover, IMF regulations required that the entire enterprise be privatized.

Today the Aral Sea and surrounding territories are world famous for ecological disasters attributed mainly to man-made factors. As a result of the increase in water consumption connected to cultivation of new irrigated territories, where mainly cotton and rice are grown, together with the increase in the population working in agriculture, the flow of water to the sea from the two major river systems – the Amu Darya and Syr Darya – stopped altogether. Despite intensive glacier melting which should have led to an increase in the territory of the Aral Sea, during the last 25 years a disastrous reduction in the area of the largest inland water body has taken place.

Because the Aral Sea is situated in the Central Asian deserts, and at an altitude of only 53 metres above sea level, it functions as a gigantic evaporator. Approximately 60 km$^3$ of water evaporate annually. In this way the 'sea' contributed to hydrothermal regime improvement, modifying the water supply to desert flora, creation of pastureland and creation of artesian wells. Up until at least 1960, this all served to maintain a stable ecological balance.

Eventually, though, due to irreplaceable loss of water from the rivers largely as a result of damming, the ecological balance suddenly began to collapse. Over only a decade the Aral Sea was deprived of about 50% of its river water supply. Thus the established altitude above sea level of 53 metres could no longer be sustained. Along with all of this, the pace of economic development in the cotton plantations led to an expansion of irrigated areas and thus further irrecoverable loss of increasing volumes of river water. The delta areas of both rivers gradually began to dry out. Since 1961 the sea level has dropped at an increasing rate, from 20 cm per year in 1965 to 85 cm per year in 2005.[5]

Between 1960 and 2000, the Aral Sea received less than 1000 km$^3$ of river water, resulting in a drop in water level of 17 metres and a volume loss of 75%. Even in 1998 (when the author visited it), the area was already constantly beset by 'dust storms' – in which salt granules were a major component of the windblown dust.

As a result of the complete cessation of the Amu Darya and Syr Darya runoff and the expansion of irrigated territories without any control of the Aral Sea and environmental needs, seriously complex ecological, social and economic problems developed in the Aral area. These problems, as we shall see, have had an international character. The sea has lost its fishery and transport importance. It was divided into two parts, the Bolshoi and the Maly (Northern) Aral, and has moved 100–150 km away from the original shore.

Up to 100 million tons of salty dust flew out from the exposed salty beds annually. Suspended solids in the form of aerosols with agricultural pesticides, fertilizers and other harmful components of industrial and municipal waters were major constituents of these winds.

Table 4.1 gives an idea of the full ecological horror of all these effects.

**TABLE 4.1** Development of the ecological crisis in the basin of the Aral Sea from 1966 to 1996[6]

| | Units of measurement | 1966 | 1976 | 1996 | 2000 |
|---|---|---|---|---|---|
| Territory of 'new' salty desert appeared as a result of the sea drying off | km² | No | 130 200 | 38 000 | 42 000 |
| Physical mass of salt, dust and wastes within salty desert | million tons | No | 500 | 2300 | 3300 |
| Territory of salt and dust spread | 1000 km² | No (in fact, mitigation and favourable impact of the Aral Sea on territory 68 900 km²) | 100–150 | 250–300 | 400–450 |
| Growth of withdrawal and fallout of salts and dust | kg/hectare | No | 100–200 | 500–700 | 700–1100 |
| Population in the zone of ecological crisis | 1000 people | No | 500–600 | 3000–3500 | 3500–7000 |

Because of this steady reduction in both the area and the volume of the Aral Sea, along with the increasing rates of evaporation and drainage, the salinity of collected water increased dramatically, from 9.9 g/litre in 1996 to 15 g/litre in 2000. And it has increased greatly since then.

All of this has not only caused a local violation of human rights and a loss of fisheries, but has also had global impacts, particularly by precipitating climate change and accelerating the rate of desertification. Let us briefly consider each of these issues.

## EFFECTS ON CLIMATE

During the last 5 to 10 years the drying off of the Aral Sea has brought about noticeable changes in climate conditions. In the past the Aral Sea was considered to be a regulator, mitigating cold winds from Siberia and reducing the summer heat. Climate changes have led to a dryer and shorter summer in the region, and longer and colder winters. The vegetative season has been reduced to 170 days. Pasture productivity has decreased by 50%, and destruction of meadow vegetation has decreased meadow productivity by 10-fold. On the shores of the Aral Sea, precipitation has been reduced several-fold. The average precipitation is 150–200 mm, with considerable seasonal non-uniformity.

There are high evaporation rates (up to 1700 mm per year), while air moisture is reduced by 10%. Air temperature during the winter have fallen, and summer temperatures have increased by 2–3 °C, including observations of 49 °C.

Frequent long dust storms and ground winds are now a characteristic feature of the Aral area climate. Strong winds often blow in the region. They are the most intensive on the western coast – with perhaps more than 50 days of storms per year. The maximum wind velocity reaches 20–25 m/s.

These climatic conditions mean that agriculture without irrigation is impossible. The result is intensive accumulation of salt in the soil, leading to greater volumes of water being used for watering plants and washing off lands.

Can anyone really believe that such severe localized climate changes will not have a wider impact? Indeed, we know that taking local barometric changes only into account, the global configuration of wind velocities and directions is changed. And this does not take into consideration the effects of increased air-borne salt particles. In turn, these changes have implications for soil structure and global agriculture and trade.

## LOCAL DESERTIFICATION AND ITS WIDER IMPLICATIONS

As we have seen, much of the Aral area soil is light and easily shifted about by changes in wind direction and velocity. In fact, the huge loss of water from the Aral Sea has resulted in two different types of desertification. The recently dried out Aral Sea, together with what can only be called 'anthropogenious' (caused by people) water-logging of irrigated land, has created a new desert. This has been called Aralkum. It appeared in the middle of the great 'dry soil' desert.

This distinction perhaps needs some explanation. A 'desert' is not necessarily either hot or dry. The word 'desert' refers only to annual rainfall levels. Areas that receive less than 25 cm (about 10 inches) of rain a year are technically desert. They obviously don't have to be hot, because much of the Arctic is desert, nor does that definition exclude areas that are already waterlogged.

In much the same way, the Aral Sea bed, formerly referred to as a 'fresh water maker' – a huge water-collecting basin –has now become analogous to an anthropogenious volcano, hurling great masses of salt and dust into the atmosphere. This pollution is exacerbated by the fact that the Aral Sea lies along the same axis as a powerful air stream running from west to east over its length. This has already contributed to aerosol transference into the upper layers of the Earth's atmosphere. Thus it has a truly global impact. Indeed, traces of pesticides from the cotton fields of the Aral region have been found in the blood of Antarctic penguins. Such traces have also been found on glaciers in Greenland and in Norwegian fjords – that is, in areas thousands of kilometres away from the source of the pesticide.

Both of these factors have significantly reduced the total area of the Earth's surface which can be described as fit for habitation – at a time when the very size of the world's total population is posing such concern about environmental sustainability. In other words, the issue can no longer be regarded as local, meteorological or economic – it is political, and globally political at that. It calls for a UN committed to long-term goals, with human rights paramount, rather than one committed to short-term goals, with corporate profits paramount.

## ARAL SEA DESPOLIATION AND THE GLOBAL INHABITATION AREA

The links between Aral Sea despoliation and its consequent jeopardizing of ecological sustainability are not hard to find. Field withdrawal from dry parts of what was once the Aral Sea bed ranges from about 400 000 tons to 20 to 30 million tons annually. Above that sea bed rise clouds of dust which are then whipped all over locally at lower levels, but internationally carried by winds in the upper reaches of the atmosphere. The composition of these menacing clouds includes suspended solids in the form of aerosols, agricultural pesticides, nitrogenous fertilizers and a host of other harmful components. Even fine powders consisting of industrial and domestic sewage are present. Salt accounts for about 0.5% to 1.5% of the total content. The effect on soils is that multi-layer herbage tends to be replaced by a single layer, which depletes the quality of useful fodder plants and grazing herbage. In fact, the study cited above estimated that at least 2 million hectares of fertile land vanished because of over-watering and the rising level of already polluted ground water.

A natural consequence of this is that the condition of irrigated soil throughout Eastern Asia – whether for commercial crops or for grazing – is impaired, fed as it is on an increasing intake of collective-drainage water that has been saturated with pesticides. It is discharged as run-off into any available depressions in the local landscape. These then constitute poisonous reservoirs, with disastrous consequences for the surrounding fields. It is by no means rare for secondary pollution to occur when the poison-saturated beds dry out and themselves give rise to clouds of poisonous dust that are scattered by the wind.

As the above-mentioned Aral Sea study[7] goes on to show, the extent of harm caused by this totally unnecessary pollution is vast. The most widely spread pollutants in the Aral Sea are oil hydrocarbons, phenols, synthetic surface-active substances (SSAS), chlororganic pesticides (COP), heavy metals and minerals. The large-scale use of pesticides with strong physiological effects (e.g. B-58, metaphos, corotan, butiphos, hexachloran, lindan, DDT, etc.) poses a tremendous threat to living organisms. Reservoirs carrying water containing undecayed compounds of heavy metals and chlororganic pesticides have led to the destruction of fisheries, the appearance of cancerogenic diseases, and changes in cytogenetic indices.

## BAD NEWS OF BIODIVERSITY

One of the major concerns of those committed to environmental sustainability is that biodiversity – which is widely threatened by more common types of pollution – should be maintained and even increased. However, the fate of the Aral Sea gravely threatens global biodiversity. This is particularly tragic in view of the fact that, before 1960, the Aral Sea had been contributing uniquely to biodiversity. But what has happened since then? Prior to the demise of the Aral Sea (what is termed the 'Pre-Aral' times), the region exemplified such a wealth of biodiversity that it was often compared with the continent of Africa. The Pre-Aral area possessed fully half of the biological species extant in the whole of the former Soviet Union. For example, there were 500 species of bird, 200 species of mammal, 100 species of fish, and thousands of species of invertebrate, such as insects. The change since 1960 has been dramatic.

Prior to 1960 the river deltas were home to over 70 kinds of mammal and 319 species of bird. At present only 32 kinds of mammal and 160 species of bird remain. In low streams of the Syr Darya River, more than 100 000 hectares of alluvial soils became salt marsh, and more than 500 000 hectares of swamp and meadow-swamp soil became dry. This resulted in the transformation and destruction of five to seven kinds of herbs needed for fodder for sheep, horses, camels and goats. Diseases and death of cattle began, muskrat cultivation stopped, and sheep livestock decreased sharply.

The study cited above ends with the following details of an ecological disaster with global implications. As readers consider this catalogue of calamity, they should remember the rôle played in it by the UN agencies, and the extent to which such acquiescence to the dictates of neoliberalism violates the Universal Declaration of Human Rights – the UN's most definitive document on what its function should really be.

> Before 1960, the regional flora was impressive and included 1200 flowers, and 560 types of tugai forests, of which 29 were endemic to Central Asia. The flora of the Aral Sea coast included 423 kinds of plants of 44 families and 180 genera. The highest diversity of sand vegetation was concentrated on the former islands of the western coast. The dry strip of the Aral was characterized by lower diversity in comparison with the coast. Among them were 30 species which are valuable fodder plants, 31 kinds of weeds, and more than 60 kinds of local flora were potential phytomeliorants for dried coasts. Changes in water balance caused mineralization of the water in the Aral Sea basin, and this led to the loss of unique biocenosis and a number of endemic species of animals.
>
> Inflow reduction into the Aral Sea caused irreversible changes of hydrological and hydrochemical sea regimes and hydrosystems. Salt-balance changes increased the sea salinity three times, transforming it into a desert. The formerly flourishing sea ecosystem supported 24 species of fish that are now disappearing. These include carp, perch, sturgeon, salmon, sheat-fish and spike. There were 20 kinds of fish in it, but the commercial fishery was based mainly on bream, sazan and aral roach (vobla). Barbel and white-eye fish were caught in the Aral Sea.

Early evidence of the negative impact of salinization on fish life in the Aral Sea appeared in the mid-1960s, when salinity reached 12–14%. In shallow water the salinity of water increased faster than in the open parts of the sea, negatively affecting spawning sites. By 1971 the average salinity exceeded 15% and resulted in the destruction of fish spawn. Since then the average salinity reached 12% in the open part of the sea, and the first signs of a negative impact on fish appeared. Some kinds of fish slowed their growth, and the number of fish was sharply reduced. By the mid-1970s the average salinity of the sea exceeded 14%, and the natural reproduction of the Aral fishery was completely destroyed. In the late 1970s several species of fish did not reproduce at all, and by 1980 the salinity exceeded 18%.

Now the Aral Sea has lost its fishery completely. Of the fish life of the Aral Sea, only aboriginal species – pricles and acclimatizers – bullheads and sprats are left. In the estuaries of the Syr Darya and Amu Darya, adult fishes were caught occasionally. The researchers of the Aral Department of the Kazakh Research Institute of Fishery in the 1970s collected eurigaline and salt-loving kinds of fish. They conducted experiments with Caspian sturgeons, Kurine salmon, Asov and Black sea plaice-glossa and plaice-kalkan. The most promising were the experiments with plaice-glossa which, having ecological plasticity, spawned at the sites with 17–60% salinity. At present its catch accounts for 30% of the total. Plaice quality is very high, and Dutch research showed that there are no traces of pesticides and heavy metals in these fish.

## THE COMMERCIAL CONTEXT OF DAMMING

Dam construction, as well as having such an immense environmental, climatic and social impact, requires a financial outlay that puts the GNPs of many nations to shame. In the next section, we shall consider the political and economic impact in terms of human rights, but let us first address the question of where such enormous amounts of money come from. We have indicated the degree to which the UN is complicit in making funds available, but the World Bank and the IMF themselves do not have ready funds for such projects. We shall start, then, with one of the largest dam projects ever undertaken – the Three Gorges Dam in China – and analyse its financial backing.

In June 2005, after 18 months of meticulous accountancy research, Probe International drew up a list of nations and institutions which were the source of most of the funding.[8] None of these countries or institutions were Chinese. They include Brazil, Canada, France, Germany, Italy, Japan, Norway, Sweden, Switzerland, the UK, the USA, the World Bank, and various export credit agencies and financiers. Of course, this is not to say that China was not in any way financially involved. However, the extent of its involvement was much less, as Chinese state agencies – rather than private contractors – coordinated the allocation of incoming finance, pouring much of it into a number of auxiliary state-owned enterprises producing supporting infrastructure, as we shall see. Two questions immediately arise. First, what was in it for them, since they were so remote from any hydroelectric advantage that could be gained? And secondly, since China classifies itself as a communist country and is ideologically opposed to capitalism, why did it place such a project that was so pivotal to its own national development in the hands of its natural enemies?

Isolating the nations (and the agencies) involved gives little away and – as we shall see – the hand of the UN is pretty well concealed, even if we look at the complexities of financial involvement within some of the nations concerned. This information is provided in full in the Probe International document.[8] The partial breakdown is as follows.

Sae Vigese, a Brazilian manufacturer of power generation turbines, produced some of the apparatus for General Electric in Canada, which was supplying the turbines for the project. The Brazilian government found this outlay to represent a social investment, as finance for it came from the World Bank, from which a comfortable project margin was harvested, even after the debt was paid off to the World Bank. In Canada, once her involvement became known, there was considerable public opposition to the way in which the transaction was handled, with so many middlemen making profits at each stage in its execution.

The main private company in Canada was Aeres International in Toronto. However, it was only one of five Canadian firms which together formed a consortium called the 'Canadian International Project Managers Yangtze Joint Venture' (CYJV), in order to carry out a US$14 million feasibility study on the project for China. On completion of the study they did approve the project – but only on the basis of technical geological criteria. They did not interview any of the hundreds of thousands of people who stood to lose everything – including their homes and livelihoods. Nevertheless, the Canadian International Development Agency (CIDA) agreed to finance the project.

Probe International used the Canadian Access to Information Act to obtain the feasibility study, and then had it evaluated by independent experts at various Canadian universities. They were horrified by its ecological implications and by the fact that many of its conclusions were not even substantiated by the evidence offered. As described by Margaret Barker and Grámine Ryder,[9] CIDA with some embarrassment was forced to withdraw from the Three Gorges Project after it attracted multi-party comment in the Canadian House of Commons.

'This is not engineering and science, merely an expert prostitution, paid for by Canadian taxpayers', said Professor Vaclav of the University of Manitoba, an expert on Chinese energy and environment issues. 'It would never get approval in Canada', he added.

Based on the independent experts' findings, Probe International filed complaints against the Canadian engineers who conducted the feasibility study, accusing them of professional negligence, incompetence and professional misconduct.

Canada had many other fingers in the financial pie initially, but several withdrew over widespread objections on humanitarian and ecological grounds. Hydro-Québec International was one of the firms so involved. It is a subsidiary of Hydro-Québec, which mediates the Province of Québec's domestic and industrial electrical supply needs. However, Hydro-Québec International signed a US$2.85 million contract in June 1999 with China's Power Grid Development Company to supervise installation of a 900-kilometre transmission line from the Three Gorges Dam to Changzhou, 80 kilometres northwest of Shanghai.

Hydro-Québec International is also a member of the CYJV consortium that conducted the now discredited feasibility study for the dam. In 1993, Hydro-Québec Vice President Pierre Senecal, one of the authors of the feasibility study, stated at a 1993 conference in Shanghai that due to population increases and a lack of available land in the Three Gorges area, 'the study's recommendation that resettlement is feasible is not valid anymore' – a complete and sudden change of mind.

China's own involvement is interestingly peripheral, linking with large international corporations. It also generates foreign finance by raising the tax rate on foreign-held enterprise, so it did rather well out of capitalist neoliberalism – and got many of the dams built. But at what cost to human rights? In terms of financial gains to be made from the enterprise, just consider one state-owned enterprise, namely Yangtze Power. It was able to report a fourfold increase in its first-half earnings for 2004, and was able to buy two generating units from the parent company. The government meanwhile increased its yearly tax by 37%. At that point, the Gezhouba Dam Hydro project, the main stockholder in Yangtze Power, was sold Yangtze Power by the state at a low valuation. This generated so much money internally that it was reported by Reuters News Agency, and the project attracted more speculation from the developed countries. The *South China Morning Post*, a government newspaper, ran the story:[10]

> Yangtze Power, Shanghai-listed operator of Three Gorges dam hydro project, reported a net profit of US$286.2 million in the first 9 months of 2004. The strong profit mainly came from high power demand in Central, East and South China, and from a sharp increase in the company's power generation due to its acquisition of a 2.8-million-kW installation capacity of the Three Gorges Dam project and favourable water levels on the Yangtze River, according to the company.
>
> Yangtze Power will spend 9.8 million yuan (US$1.2 billion) – most of its loans from 12 institutions – to buy two 700-MW hydropower generators from its parent company – China Yangtze Three Gorges Development Corp – increasing the company's generation capacity to 6915 MW from 5515 MW. According to the A-share company's filing to Shanghai Stock Exchange, the acquisition is part of the company's listing promise to gradually buy the 22 generating units that it does not already own from the parent firm by 2015. It will finance the acquisition with 9.5 billion yuan of bank loans from 12 institutions, which have provided five-year loans at a 5.26% interest rate.[11]

China Construction Bank, one of Yangtze Power's biggest creditor banks and China's top property lender, launched an initial public offering by 2005, estimated to raise as much as US$10 billion, making it the largest ever Chinese profit.

China Development Bank (CDB) registered a US$500 million bond sold by US-based Morgan Stanley with the US Securities and Exchange Commission (SEC) on 30 July 2004. Goldman Sachs, Merrill Lynch and Morgan Stanley will lead the sale of US$500 million worth of bonds to US dollar investors, while BNP Paribas, HSBC and UBS manage a separate 500 million euro (HK$4.79 billion) offering. Standard & Poor's estimate that 40% of the loans on the books of state banks are non-performing reports. This deal was carried with the blessing of the UN.

China Development Bank and another eight Chinese banks are providing a total loan of US$5.86 billion to finance the South-North Water Diversion (SNWD) Project. This project includes three water diversion routes connecting the Yangtze River, the Huai River, the Yellow River and the Hai River, bringing water to drought-hit regions such as Shandong Province, the municipality of Tianjin, and Beijing. China Development Bank will provide US$2.4 billion. The first phase of the eastern and central routes will require an investment of almost US$15 billion. As of 2007 the third and most challenging phase involves a 750-mile canal connecting the upper reaches of the Yangtze and the Yellow Rivers and dissecting the Qinghai-Tibet Plateau.

The financial details are of lasting interest, and although there is not space here to provide further accounts from individual countries, the reader may well find it worthwhile to consult the Probe International report[8] for further insights. However, it is worth considering the rôle of the USA in the enterprise. In doing so, we see once more America's capacity for internal opposition to much that its corporate interests do. This is not only reassuring in itself, but illustrates a point often made by this author in previous publications – that few things are more unhelpful to the human rights debate than the sort of 'reflex anti-Americanism' that characterizes much of the critique of neoliberalism.

In 1999, Atkinson Construction of New York succeeded in contracting to provide 'consultation services' in overseeing purchases of large-scale equipment for the Three Gorges Dam Project. This represented a change entirely brought about by humanitarian considerations, for from 1986 to 1999 Bechtel (another American corporation) had held that contract. However, in 1997 Joe Ferrigno, Bechtel's Managing Director for their involvement with the project, was quoted as saying that Bechtel 'could not possibly continue with the Three Gorges Project because the dam is extremely controversial from an ecological perspective.'[12] At the same time as he was independently taking this stance – despite encouragement and grants from the IMF – Caterpillar Tractor Ltd, a construction company in Illinois, sold US$15 million worth of equipment to the Yangtze Three Gorges Project Development Corporation in 1996, and in the same year this was turned down. The scenario unfolded as follows, and is one that this author often uses to illustrate the point that, to whatever extent the USA may currently dominate the operation of global neoliberalism, it is often prevented from its worst excesses by the sheer genius of its emphasis on the importance of the individual conscience.

Caterpillar, Rotec Industries and US Voith Hydro had applied for loans from the US Export-Import Bank to support their bids for Three Gorges contracts, but they were turned down in 1996. Following an intensive campaign led by Probe International and US environmental groups, the US Export-Import Bank announced in May 1996 that it could not support US companies seeking contracts to build the dam, because 'the information received, though voluminous, fails to establish the project's consistency with the bank's environmental guidelines.' The Three Gorges Dam became the first serious test of the bank's new guidelines, introduced by Congress in 1992, which required the bank to conduct environmental reviews of foreign projects that sought its backing. The US Export-Import Bank asked the National Security Council to convene a panel to consider the merits of US participation. In September 1995, the National Security Council delivered its recommendation that the US government should not 'align itself with a project that raises environmental and human rights concerns on the scale of the Three Gorges.' Martin Kamarck, President and Chairman of the US Export-Import Bank, toned its decision down, noting only that there was not enough information, and that for the bank to reconsider its decision it 'would need further evidence that these issues will be adequately addressed, resolved and/or mitigated by the project's sponsors.' Kamarck noted at the time that several US companies had sold US$60–100 million worth of equipment and services to the project without US Export-Import Bank support.[13]

Of course, there were plenty of US corporations unaffected by such matters of conscience and human rights. For instance, consider ITT Industries who, under GATS and IMF Structural Adjustment Policies, took advantage of the requirement that China should throw open the supply of pumps to competitive bidding. ITT Industries, one of the world's largest pump manufacturing groups, announced on 8 November 2000 that its Chinese subsidiary, Nanjing Goulds Pump Co., received a contract worth US$604 595 to provide 48 deep-well pumps for the five permanent ship locks to be built in the Yichang section of the Yangtze River in Hubei.

Then again, consider the complex involvement of the United States Bureau of Reclamation (USBR), a large construction engineering corporation with a long history of organizing major infrastructure projects, under IMF Structural Adjustment Policies in developing countries as part of 'development plans.' In fact the USBR not only has direct links with the World Bank, but is also a federal building agency for the US government. Since 1990 it had been involved with the government of China in initial feasibility studies of such a dam, along with the US Army Corps of Engineers. The company has been a member of the Three Gorges Working Group ever since.

The USBR went on a World Bank-sponsored trip to the Three Gorges area. Upon returning, they and other experts submitted a report to the Chinese and US governments, expressing many doubts and concerns with regard to geology, sedimentation, flood control, navigation, hydraulic engineering and construction, electric systems, economic analysis and environmental issues. A senior analyst, who was also a member of the World Bank's panel of experts, reviewed the Canadian feasibility study for the dam in 1988. In 1992, the US Bureau of Reclamation signed a second agreement with China's Ministry of Water Resources to provide technical assistance to the Three Gorges Project, related to data management, computer software, drill-hole survey technology and dam-safety monitoring.

But again, in June 1993, the Bureau officially terminated its Three Gorges contract. A Bureau of Reclamation press release stated that 'further involvement in this project is not consistent with Reclamation's mission. Reclamation's current priorities are water resource management and environmental restoration, not large dam projects.' Bureau of Reclamation spokesperson Lisa Guide explained:

> It is now generally known that large-scale water retention dam projects are not environmentally or economically feasible. We wouldn't support such a project in the US now, so it would be incongruous for us to support such a project like this in another country.

The Bureau's decision to withdraw came in mid-September 1993. This was to a large extent because seven US environmental groups filed a lawsuit against the Bureau, arguing that the government agency was violating the US Endangered Species Act, because the Three Gorges dam 'will threaten the continued existence of several species that the US lists as endangered.'

Is it not mordantly instructive that, while the World Bank was so determined to follow the process through, individual consciences of 'ordinary' people led them away from it?

## THE WORLD BANK

As mentioned above, the World Bank has been one of the major financial supporters of the Three Gorges Dam. Its credentials as a multilateral lending institution have confronted it with much commentary from various human rights groups – not all of it supportive by any means. Therefore it is only appropriate that we examine in some detail its involvement with a project that has involved such a vast catalogue of human rights violations. Initially the World Bank approved a US$200 million loan to Chongqing Municipality Bank in June 1960 for a project costing US$500 million, scheduled for completion six and a half years later, at the end of 2006. It was to include wastewater treatment facilities and solid waste collection services in areas affected by the Three Gorges Dam.

Chongqing, itself an industrial centre, is located at the Three Gorges Dam reservoir's upper end, and dumps almost all of its industrial wastewater and sewage untreated into the Yangtze River. Almost all urban wastewater flows untreated in the Yangtze and its tributaries through 200 open discharge points, mixing untreated sewage and industrial wastes with drinking water supplies. This immediately violates the most elementary health rights of millions of people, and should therefore be of imperative interest to the World Health Organization. It would certainly have been forestalled by any kind of International Health Impact Assessment, as advocated in the past by this author and by many other public health specialists. The 2006 deadline was not met, but for a project of this magnitude, that is not entirely surprising.

However, a crucial question surely is what its overall health impact will be once it has been completed and is functioning. In this regard, even World Bank estimates[14,15] are not exactly reassuring – and even more alarming, these assessments were made prior to their agreement to make the loan! If the Three Gorges Dam is completed, scientists predict that it will slow the Yangtze River's flow, backing up water and concentrating sewage and other pollutants in its 600-kilometre-long reservoir. The Canadian proponents of the Three Gorges Dam left the cost of controlling increased pollution in the dam reservoir and of providing water supply services to resettled communities out of the official project budget.

The project includes providing new water supply and treatment facilities for new towns associated with the Three Gorges Project in the Fuling area, and replacing existing water supply infrastructure that will be flooded by the Three Gorges Dam reservoir in areas including Wanzhou, 320 kilometres downstream of Chongqing. However, the World Bank's involvement started with its support for the Canadian International Development Agency (CIDA), which made an initial loan – which in turn depended for its notification on an initial feasibility project financed by the CIDA.[16]

The World Bank was part of a steering committee formed in 1986 to supervise the CIDA-financed feasibility study, which included CIDA and China's Ministry of Water Resources and Electric Power. The World Bank also set up an international panel of experts whose rôle, according to panel member and US sediment expert John Kennedy, was 'to evaluate the study and to ensure that it met very high standards of international practice for these kinds of studies.' On resettlement, the World Bank's panel concluded that 'feasibility is not yet clearly demonstrated. Unresolved issues pertaining to land availability, job creation and host population, and other issues need further clarification.'

However, even that didn't seem to alert the relevant UN human rights agencies. We can learn a little more by going behind this 'expatriate' (outside of China) involvement, to consider what China's internal strategy had been to initially secure CIDA and World Bank finance It is necessary here to point out that the CIDA only sponsors UN-approved projects and, of course, the World Bank is already an agency of the UN.

China's State Development Bank (SDB) made its first commitment to the Three Gorges Project in 1996, with a 10-year $3.6 billion loan, making the dam the SDB's number one debtor. According to *China Daily* of 7 April 1998:

> Huge amounts of loan money (from the SDB) have propped up the development of the country's key electric power projects. Since its establishment in 1994, the bank has injected about $15 billion into the construction of hydroelectric, nuclear, and thermal power stations, including the Three Gorges Project, the World Bank-financed Ertan Dam, and the Qinshan Nuclear Power Plant. SDB continues to favour large power plants, making it one of the most important sources of funds for China's power industry.[17]

The SDB receives its capital and funding from the government. It also issues debentures to domestic financial institutions, construction bonds in China, and bonds in international capital markets – and it borrows money from foreign governments, international financial institutions, and foreign commercial banks. Sovereign guarantees make these debt instruments relatively risk free.

The promise of sovereign guarantees was the inducement that the private sector in the industrialized countries needed to invest in the Three Gorges Project. In 1996, the SDB launched its first international bond, offering ¥30 billion ($269 million) underwritten by Nomura Securities and IBJ Securities of Japan. When a Japanese critic of the Three Gorges Dam discovered that the bond issue violated Japanese security laws because it failed to provide clear information on the use and risks of the bonds, Nomura Securities cancelled a second bond issue for 1998.

And it is here that the merry-go-round of private financiers really begins a matrix of borrowings and futures trading that would cause the head of any non-corporate banker to spin. However, the thing to remember is that at each juncture in the proceedings, huge profits are made for shareholders and bonuses for CEOs, while the lack of provision for adequate human rights protection has been suspended entirely by financial considerations – with the UN's World Bank looking on in splendid isolation. It is also interesting to note that the Power Technology report, cited above, assumes that – even if no unforeseen circumstances arise – the project will be at least 3 years late, with 2009 being accepted as the earliest possible completion date!

However, we shall close this section with just a brief overview of the high points of the inter-agency horse trading that lies behind the project. Very little of it is Chinese, although the SDB set the chain off. We can establish that the SDB issued its second bond in January 1997. This time US$330 million in bonds were underwritten by Lehman Brothers, Credit Suisse, First Boston, Smith Barney Inc., J.P. Morgan & Co., Morgan Stanley & Co. Incorporated, and BancAmerica Securities Inc. On 17 December 1997, BancAmerica Securities announced that it would not invest in the Three Gorges Project in future, in response to public pressure from environmental and human rights groups.[18]

In May 1999, the SDB (now called the China Development Bank) issued a US$500 million bond. Merrill Lynch & Co. (a subsidiary of Citigroup) and Chase Manhattan Bank were the lead managers for the bond issue, each responsible for underwriting US$225 million. Chase Securities, J.P. Morgan & Co. and Morgan Stanley Dean Witter contributed US$6.25 million each, while Credit Suisse First Boston and Goldman Sachs each contributed US$1.25 million.

Morgan Stanley helped to underwrite a total of US$830 million in bonds to the China Development Bank, the single largest funding arm for the dam, in 1997 and 1999. The firm's continued involvement with the dam is through their joint venture with the China International Capital Corporation (CICC), the lead adviser on raising overseas capital for the Three Gorges Project Corporation. CICC is managed and 35% owned by Morgan Stanley.[19] And that same report points out that a wide group of people – Chinese, Tibetan and Indonesian among them – were all adversely affected. They lost their homes, their security and their livelihoods – and were then left destitute to fend for themselves. As the next section makes clear, the Three Gorges Dam has not been the World Bank's only collusion in big dam construction to have deprived millions of their human rights.

## OTHER WORLD BANK-SPONSORED DAM PROJECTS

The World Bank Group[20] published a list of some of the dams financed by the World Bank and the IMF which have been 'successful' primarily as a source of income for private corporations. In fact, they point out that the World Bank is the largest single source for such projects, and had – as of 1992 – provided US$50 billion for construction of more than 500 large dams in 92 countries. The World Bank has been 'directly or indirectly associated' with around 10% of large dams in developing countries (excluding China, where it had funded only eight dams up to 1994). The importance of the World Bank in major dam schemes is illustrated by the fact that it has directly funded four of the five highest dams in developing countries outside China, three of the five largest reservoirs in these countries, and three of the five largest hydroplants.

According to the Manibeli Declaration, these large dams have had 'extensive negative environmental impacts; destroying forests, wetlands, fisheries, habitat for threatened and endangered species, and increasing the spread of waterborne diseases.' In addition, the World Bank has 'tolerated and thus contributed to gross violations of human rights by governments in the process of implementing Bank-funded large dams, including arbitrary arrests, beatings, rapes, and shootings of peaceful demonstrators.' The Manibeli Declaration[21] called for a moratorium on World Bank funding of large dams as far back as September 1994. The full document is well worth reading, and a section on it follows this brief survey of such World Bank-funded projects.

In Latin America, the World Bank's activities in this regard have been discussed in some detail in a previous book by the author.[22] Here, though, let us consider Argentina (which was not mentioned in the cited reference).

The World Bank is one of the major funders of the 67-kilometre-long Yacyreta Dam, which joins the Argentine and Paraguayan sides of the Parana River. So far, more than 5000 people have been forced to move from the flooded banks of the Parana River because of the dam construction. Most of them were not properly compensated for their losses, and many were moved to resettlement colonies that had begun to crumble even before they were completed. Workers struggled to get to their jobs, and children often failed to get to their schools. Diseases flourished because there were no working sewers and few healthcare facilities. New nature reserves, set up to compensate for the loss of unique habitats, include one which contains a military base, an international highway, a large refuse dump and the quarry from which the stone for the dam was taken. That quarry is now a source of danger and disease for the poverty-stricken children who swim in it.

Much further north of this, in Central America, the World Bank has also been active, especially in Guatemala, where it financed the Chixoy Dam. Construction of the dam displaced about 75 000 of the Maya Achì indigenous people who have lived there for hundreds of years. An intimidation campaign against the Maya Achì Indians began in 1980, following the community's refusal to move to the new settlements provided by the government. Prior to dam completion and the resettlement of local residents, between February and September 1982, the death squads and the army killed about 400 men, women and children from Rio Negro, during both massive and individual massacres.

The dam has also turned out to be a financial disaster. The final cost of the project has not yet been clearly defined. Evaluations range from US$1.2 billion (521% higher than predicted) to US$2.5 billion. Nor does the dam meet the country's energy needs. Guatemala still spends US$150 million a year on producing electricity. Every year a minimum of US$8 million are spent on structural maintenance costs of the Chixoy Project, and only when fully operating will it cover about 50–60% of the country's needs. Energy costs supported by the population have steadily increased during the last few years, but still only 30% of the population benefit from electric power.

There are other examples that could be cited from Latin America, but let us now consider one World Bank-funded dam in Lesotho, an already desperately poor country, which was until recently part of South Africa. The World Bank is funding the Lesotho Highlands Water Project (LHWP), Africa's largest infrastructure project, which involves five dams (of which one is built and a second is under construction), miles of tunnels through the Lesotho mountains, and a small hydropower component. The project delivers Lesotho's water to Gauteng Province, South Africa's industrial heartland and the site of metropolitan Johannesburg, in the suburbs of which many of the country's wealthiest citizens have made their homes amid plush lawns and swimming pools. Most of the poor in South Africa's townships, who suffer from water inequity dating back to apartheid, will be unable to afford the project's expensive water.

The project's social impacts in Lesotho have been especially hard on the rural highlands communities, who have lost fields, grazing lands and access to water sources due to the project. Despite decade-old promises, their livelihoods have not been re-established, and poor people have been pushed further to the edge in their struggle for survival. Furthermore, a dozen major international dam-building companies involved in the LHWP were recently caught lavishly bribing at least one top official on the project, and have allegedly given nearly US$2 million in bribes over 10 years.

In addition, in Africa the International Finance Corporation (IFC), backed by the World Bank as one of its private-sector sub-agencies, is engaged in negotiations to finance the largest single independent power producer in the world, a US corporation (AES), to construct a dam near Bujagali Falls on the Nile, at a cost of US$520 million. The dam would create a socially and environmentally destructive reservoir, would worsen downstream impacts (as it would be the third dam in the upper Nile), and would drown the spectacular Bujagali Falls. This dam will permanently displace 820 people, and will affect an additional 6000 by submerging communal lands, burial sites or portions of their land. Replacement land for those who would lose homes or crops is practically non-existent in the area. In addition, the reservoir is expected to increase serious waterborne diseases such as malaria and schistosomiasis. Stagnant pools of water are breeding grounds for malaria-carrying mosquitoes and schistosomiasis-spreading vector snails. Malaria is already the leading cause of death in Uganda.

The World Bank is also not unknown for dam financing in India. It has provided loans for the Sardar Sarovar Dam on the Narmada River. This dam has a proposed height of 136.5 metres, to irrigate more than 1.8 million hectares and quench the thirst of the drought-prone areas of Kutch and Saurashtra in Gujarat. The opponents of the dam counter that these benefits are grossly exaggerated and would never accrue to the extent suggested by the government. Instead the project would displace more than 320 000 people, and would affect the livelihood of thousands of others. Overall, due to related displacements by the canal system and other allied projects, at least 1 million people are expected to be affected if the project is completed. After an independent review was extremely critical of the plans for the dam, the World Bank bowed out of the project.

Shortly after the World Bank withdrew from the Sardar Sarovar Dam Project, it also pulled out of the US$1 billion Arun III hydroelectric project in eastern Nepal, after local groups exposed the Bank's faulty project planning and appraisal process. However, neither the UN nor its agencies have been immune from active opposition to their activities in the dam construction business. One of the most articulate of these opponents has been the Manibeli opposition group.

## THE MANIBELI DECLARATION

Set up initially by an NGO – River Net – in 1994, the Manibeli group has since become one of the best known and best informed of opposition groups to large dam building generally. The World Bank itself has long claimed that it only provides loans for locally approved projects in the countries to be effected, but this is loosely defined. River Net speaks for the European Rivers Network, and the following relevant information is drawn from the Manibeli Declaration.

Since 1948, the World Bank has financed large dam projects which have forcibly displaced around 10 million people from their homes and land. The World Bank's own 1994 'Resettlement and Development' review admits that the vast majority of women, men and children evicted by Bank-funded projects never regained their former incomes or received any direct benefits from the dams for which they were forced to sacrifice their homes and land. The World Bank has consistently failed to implement and enforce its own policy on forced resettlement, first established in 1980, and despite several policy reviews the Bank has no plans to fundamentally change its approach to forced resettlement.

Over the next 3 years the World Bank is planning to fund 18 large dam projects which will forcibly displace another 450 000 people, without any credible guarantee that its policy on resettlement will be enforced. Meanwhile the Bank has no plans to properly compensate and rehabilitate the millions displaced by past Bank-funded dam projects, including populations displaced since 1980 in violation of the Bank's policy. Large dams funded by the World Bank have had an extensive negative environmental impact, destroying forests, wetlands and fisheries, and habitat for threatened and endangered species, and increasing the spread of waterborne diseases.

The World Bank has tolerated and thus contributed to gross violations of human rights by governments in the process of implementing Bank-funded large dams, including arbitrary arrests, beatings, rape and shootings of peaceful demonstrators. Many large dam projects funded by the World Bank cannot be implemented without gross violations of human rights, because affected communities inevitably resist the imposition of projects that are so harmful to their interests. The World Bank plans, designs, funds and monitors the construction of large dams in a secretive and unaccountable manner, imposing projects without meaningful consultation or participation by the communities affected, often denying access to information even to local governments in the areas affected.

The World Bank has consistently ignored cost-effective and environmentally and socially sound alternatives to large dams, including wind, solar and biomass energy sources, energy demand management, irrigation rehabilitation, efficiency improvements and rainwater harvesting, and non-structural flood management. The Bank has even persuaded governments to accept loans for large dams when more cost-effective and less destructive alternative plans existed, as may be the case again with the Arun III Project in Nepal.

The economic analyses on which the World Bank bases its decisions to fund large dams fail to apply the lessons learned from the poor record of past Bank-funded dams, underestimating the potential for delays and cost overruns. Project appraisals are typically based on unrealistically optimistic assumptions about project performance, and fail to account for the direct and indirect costs of negative environmental and social impacts. The Bank's own 1992 portfolio review admits that project appraisals are treated as 'marketing devices which fail to establish that projects are in the public interest.'

The primary beneficiaries of procurement contracts for large dams funded by the World Bank have been consultants, manufacturers and contractors based in the donor countries, who profit while citizens of the borrowing countries are burdened by debt and the destructive economic, environmental and social impacts of the large dams themselves. The World Bank has consistently failed to build up local capacity and expertise, promoting dependency instead. Large dams funded by the World Bank have flooded cultural monuments, religious and sacred sites, and national parks and other wildlife sanctuaries.

In its lending for large dams, the World Bank has tolerated and even condoned theft of funds supplied by the Bank, often by corrupt military and undemocratic regimes, and has often made additional loans to cover cost overruns brought about by what the Bank refers to as 'rent-seeking behaviour.' Examples of this include Yacyretá Dam in Argentina and Chixoy Dam in Guatemala.

The World Bank has consistently violated its policy on environmental assessment, and has allowed environmental assessments to be produced by project promoters and used to justify prior decisions to proceed with destructive large dam projects.

It has never addressed in policy, research or project planning documents the decommissioning of large dams after their useful lifetime has expired due to reservoir sedimentation and physical deterioration.

Furthermore, it has never properly assessed its record of funding large dams, and it has no mechanism for measuring the actual long-term costs and benefits of the large dams that it funds.

Throughout its involvement in the Sardar Sarovar Dam in the Narmada Valley, a worldwide symbol of destructive development, the World Bank has consistently ignored its own policy guidelines with regard to resettlement and environmental assessment, and has attempted to cover up the conclusions even of its own financed and severely critical official independent review, namely the Morse Report. With the ongoing forcible evictions and flooding of tribal lands, the World Bank bears direct legal and moral responsibility for the human rights abuses that are taking place in the Narmada Valley.

The above information, drawn from the Manibeli Declaration, strongly supports this author's thesis that the UN – through one of its agencies, namely the World Bank – has in effect allowed itself to become involved in projects which violate its own UDHR. To underline this point, let us briefly consider some further details relating to the Three Gorges Dam. The Power Technology report[17] provides us with the following information about the ecological concerns raised by the project.

The long-term ecological effect of the dam has been described as possibly catastrophic. The dam will disrupt heavy silt flows in the river. It could cause rapid silt build-up in the reservoir, creating an imbalance upstream, and depriving agricultural land and fish downstream of essential nutrients. Since these problems would also hit the plant's turbines and millions of farmers and fishermen, considering ecology is common sense.

Environmentalist and political opposition to the Three Gorges Dam has been intense. The most emotive issue has been the forced relocation of between 1.2 and 1.9 million people. China points to detailed plans to actually improve the lives of those affected, but independent reports suggest that residents are privately convinced that their compensation is miserly. The farmland which will be flooded is more fertile than higher ground, and around 1600 factories will be submerged.

Opponents of the Three Gorges Dam have had more success outside China. The World Bank, stung by vicious critiques of other hydro projects that it had sponsored, decided not to fund the project. The US Export-Import Bank also bowed to pressure. The Bank hoped to gain further environmental information from the Chinese that would allow a positive decision – it is not against the project in principle. Moreover, its stance did not prevent US groups from bidding for contracts, or US commercial banks from financing their operations.

## BUT ALL OF HUMANKIND LIVES DOWNSTREAM!

One of Canada's leading scholars in the field of public health and health promotion, Ron Labonté, is also known for his capacity to draw people's attention to crucial issues through the use of parables. One of these runs as follows.[23]

A community living by a fast-flowing river had to make do with a rather flimsy bridge. On wet or icy days, it was not uncommon for people to slip off the bridge, fall into the river and be carried downstream. Not far downstream lived another community made up of people who could swim. They were always rescuing people who had fallen in upstream, some of whom had already died. When the lucky ones had recovered, they returned home, where sooner or later they would fall in again, and again be pulled out – either dead or alive. The moral of the parable, of course, is that if the people upstream had been 'empowered' by knowing how to swim, the 'healthcare system' (swimming out and rescuing people) would have been much more efficient.

In a sense, then, we all live downstream. People already affected by dam construction can – at great cost and loss to their own communities – be rescued. More worthwhile, however, would be to empower people (which the WHO, and the UN generally, are intended to do) so that they can prevent such adverse dam construction, or moderate its impact if they decide to allow it. The casual and uncritical acceptance of a philosophy of neoliberalism has made it possible for financial gain for a few to trump the human rights of the many, but we can change that.

Despite the spirit of the age – untrammelled greed, casual cruelty, unabashed corruption and fatal short-sightedness – we still find people who want to redeem the time, to make a difference. Fortunately for humankind, these people have encouraged conservation of natural resources for the last 50 years.

For example, the Tree People, a California-based ecological group, have shifted their focus from planting trees to renewing the watershed that nurtures the trees. In Pacoima and Westchester schoolgrounds they have mounted demonstration projects using landscaping and underground cisterns to retain rainwater. If parks and schools spent a little more on cooling trees and underground watering systems, they would save money on water and energy while preventing pollution and erosion from pavement runoff.

The many proponents of organic farming want us to stop growing water-intensive crops in the desert with scarce irrigation water and government subsidies, as the industrial agriculturists are doing all over the world. Drought-resistant plants grown on pesticide-free small plots prevent pollution and conserve water. We have learned from the water privateers how important definitions are. Water defined as a right rather than as a commodity can be protected from predators.

Dianne Wassenich is taking the definition a step farther. In the USA, the western states have traditionally granted water rights on the basis of 'beneficial needs.' Beneficial needs have included mining, building and agriculture, but not conservation. Therefore Wassenich has applied for a permit to allow the water flowing through her property to continue on its course to the Gulf of Mexico, and she has set up a one-person foundation that is part of an emerging movement to redefine beneficial use.

One seasoned warrior in the water wars is Rajendra Singh, who makes rivers flow in the desert. Using traditional methods, his organization has rejuvenated land in India's driest area. A seasonal campaigner in his own country (India), he is now known worldwide for his advocacy of water rights for all of humanity.[24]

When asked how he rejuvenated the dry land without large injections of money, infrastructural intrusion, etc., Rajendra Singh replied:

> The farmers taught me. How you harvest water depends on your objective, the geography, topography, catchment area, pond area and soil type and costing between 100 000 and 500 000 rupees ($2000 to $10 000), depending on the size. The first one was built with my efforts. Today, the local contribution is up to 90 per cent. Rajasthan has had drought for the past five consecutive years. But there is no migration from the region around the Ruparel and Arvari rivers. The water that had flowed away in flash floods is now accumulating underground. Farmers' crops are growing and there is fodder for their cattle.

His low-tech procedure involves the use of fairly small tanks or basins (referred to locally as 'johads') for conserving water that would otherwise be lost. He explained how the 'powerful forces' (rich landowners, banks, etc.) opposed his techniques:

> In the beginning the power brokers and moneylenders – those who mistakenly think that economic empowerment of the poor means loss of their riches – were against me. And the government engineers felt illiterate villagers had no right to enter their domain of construction.
>
> When we built our first johad, the state irrigation department issued warrants for its removal under the Irrigation and Drainage Act of 1954. I told them we cannot stop rain falling on our land. Last year the people of Lava ka Baas village built a pond to collect run-off water. The area became green and farmers started growing vegetables. But the act forbids stopping the flow of water. The state irrigation department sent earth-movers to demolish the water-harvesting structure. How can the government come between nature and people like that?

When asked if the government owned the water, he said:

> No king in history has claimed to rule over water. They only had rights in water management. Government alone cannot own water. Civil society has a right in water management, but even it does not own water. Nature owns water. Before they lost their rights over common land and forests, these communities had a

rich tradition of building johads and other rainwater-harvesting structures. With government centralisation, the johads were neglected and allowed to die.

You know, Jaisalmer in the west of Rajasthan – the last town before the border with Pakistan – is in one of the driest areas in the world. Yet 100 years ago it was India's major trading centre. It had twice the population it has today, and 15 times more camels. It survived on a traditional water-harvesting system. But now society has become indifferent as it thinks that water is the responsibility of the government that collects taxes. Only when a community realizes that it owns water will it treat it with care and stop misusing it.

Communities should manage their water resources and the government should help them. In a democracy, it is the duty of the government to make sure every person has drinking water. If the government is unable to provide it, it should take help from communities. They can work together. The government should have declared water a common natural resource.

With regard to any possible rôle for the private sector, he commented:

Government has failed in water management. So it is handing over to the private sector. Fine. But what private sector? Communities or multinational corporations? If multinationals gain control of water, they will squash the rights of the poor. The National Water Policy implies water privatisation. That would spell doom for society. But the government has favoured big dams because big projects mean more money and more scope for corruption.

I am not against private schemes because of their size. It is not a question of big or small structures. Small projects are not automatically sustainable either. Sustainability comes with a sense of community ownership and participation. Big dams displace a lot of people and raise issues of equity. You have to think hard, and go for such projects only if there is no other option.

It is the modern engineers who destroyed the traditional water-harvesting systems. The new technocrats and scientists have not concerned themselves with nature and ecology. They are intellectual giants, experts in calculations and research. But more problems arise when you seek solutions without understanding the underlying circumstances. Consider massive, centralised schemes like the Indira Gandhi Canal. Is this wise in a desert state like Rajasthan? There are problems with increasing soil alkalinity and rises in malaria due to waterlogging and waterborne diseases like diarrhoea. No local would have advised such a canal here.

Traditional knowledge is often dismissed as unscientific. But what's really unscientific is not trying to understand local agro-ecology-climate dynamics, local culture and needs, and soil characteristics. Our scientists think problems should be solved by any means necessary. But they looked only at the benefits of their schemes, not the harm. You should not dismiss everything emanating from illiterate villagers as unscientific.

May the wisdom of Rajendra Singh prevail. Think globally and act locally.

That last comment is a well-known mantra for the philosophy of 'empowerment', basic to the ideas of health promotion. It can easily be applied to the way in which we use agencies like the WHO, and even the World Bank. The UN is for all of us, and it belongs to all of us, but its powers are soon exploited by forces which are hostile to the basic human rights that it was founded to defend. It is up to ordinary people – perhaps sometimes doing extraordinary things – to make proper and frequent use of such agencies and yet to prevent them from being exploited for private gain.

## REFERENCES

1 Cousteau M. Quoted by Michelle Mairesse in her paper *The Global Water Crisis* (p. 4); www.hermes.press.com.htm (accessed 15 June 2007).
2 Piquepaille R. NASA looks at the Great Wall of China. In: *Dam Construction*; www.blogs.znet.com/energingtech/index.php?cat-z (accessed 15 June 2007).
3 MacDonald T. *The Global Human Right to Health: dream or possibility?* Oxford: Radcliffe Publishing; 2006. p. 209.
4 United Nations Environment Programme (UNEP). *The Disappearing Aral Sea*. Oslo: UNEP; 2002; www.environmentaltimes.net/article.cfm?pageID=7 (accessed 15 June 2007).
5 *The Aral Sea*; www.evrin.grida.na/arel/aralsea/english/arsea/arsea.htm (accessed 15 June 2007).
6 Ibid., p. 6.
7 Ibid., p. 8.
8 Probe International. *List of Financiers and Companies Involved in the Three Gorges Project*; www.threegorgesprobe.org/pi/documents/three_gorges/who.htm (accessed 15 June 2007).
9 Barker M, Ryder G. *Damming the Three Gorges: what dam builders don't want you to know*. London: Earthscan Publications; 1993. pp. 14–17.
10 Lee Kwok Chang. Yangtze power in bank ploy. *South China Morning Post*, 29 July 2004, p. 11.
11 Ibid., p. 11.
12 Probe International, op. cit., pp. 26–7.
13 Probe International, op. cit., p. 13.
14 World Bank. *China: Chongqing Urban Environment Project. Volume 12*. Washington, DC: World Bank; 2000.
15 World Bank. *China: Chongqing Urban Environment Project. Volume 14*. Washington, DC: World Bank; 2002.
16 Canadian International Development Agency (CIDA). *Three Gorges Water Control Project Feasibility Study*. Ottawa, Canada: CIDA; 1989.
17 Power Technology. *Three Gorges Dam Hydroelectric Power Plant, China*; www.power-technology.com/projects/gorges (accessed 15 June 2007).
18 Probe International, op. cit., p. 20.

19 Rogue Traders. *Disastrous Impacts on the Human Rights of millions of Asian People*; www.foe.co.uk/resource/reports/roguetraders.pdf (accessed 15 June 2007).

20 World Bank. *Dams and the World Bank*; www.worldbank.org/environment.dams.html (accessed 15 June 2007).

21 Manibeli Declaration. *Calling for a Moratorium on World Bank Funding of Large Dams*; www.rivernet.org/manibeli.htm (accessed 15 June 2007).

22 Piquepaille, op. cit., pp. 46–7.

23 MacDonald T. *Rethinking Health Promotion*. London: Routledge Publishers; 1998. pp. 4, 70–72.

24 Maiesse M. *The Global Water Crisis*; www.hermes-press.com/water.htm (accessed 15 June 2007).

# Chapter 5

# WHO: accessory after the fact?

## AUCTIONING YOUR VIRUSES!

Some of the worst examples of the degree to which the UN and its agencies have become ready accessories to neoliberalism involve the collection of viruses and bacteria for use in elaborating vaccines for disease which could become pandemic. In this chapter we shall deal in some detail with such procedures as a preliminary step to developing vaccines for diseases like smallpox, poliomyelitis and avian flu. At its simplest level, let us assume that country A is beset with an outbreak of, say, a highly contagious viral disease X. Such a situation is tailor-made for the intervention of the WHO.

The standard procedure would be for country A to provide the WHO with samples of virus X active in that country. The viruses can of course vary slightly from one geographical area to another. If a vaccine against X(A) (X as found in country A) is to be elaborated, it can only be done on the basis of a genetic analysis of X from country A. It is here that problems arise, for two reasons:

1  Only in the last two decades or so has such detailed DNA sequencing been possible.[1]
2  It is only since 1995 that TRIPS (Trade Related Intellectual Property Rights) have allowed for the possibility of people or organizations actually patenting such sequences.

TRIPS has made it increasingly difficult for the WHO to abide by the Alma Ata Declaration, because patent protection invariably involves patient costs, whether paid directly by the patient or by some other agency – a further acquiescence to neoliberalism – and a huge stratification in access to health. Indeed, according to Alma Ata and the UDHR, health is a 'human right', whereas neoliberalism has turned it into a 'commodity.' This is so vastly at odds with both UN and WHO mandates that, in the author's view, the very concept of TRIPS, or of patenting access to health in any way, should be absolute anathema to the UN. It violates the very core of the UDHR. However, since 1988, the WHO has been increasingly dominated by neoliberal approaches to business. In this chapter we shall concern ourselves with the issue of how neoliberal approaches under TRIPS are serving to deny the right to protective vaccines against dangerous pandemic diseases.

A particularly active proponent of health rights in the less developed countries is the Third World Network (TWN), and much of the detail in this chapter is derived from their excellent reports. Indeed, the TWN is one of the principal NGOs in the People's Health Movement (PHM), and the latter regards the growing privatization of the UN and of the WHO with the same degree of alarm as does this author.

Let us begin this account with the smallpox (a viral infection, also called variola) issue. In many ways it is a source of great pride to the WHO, because the latter systematically set out to eliminate it, and by 1977 had succeeded in doing so. This was achieved by a systematic and global campaign of vaccination. Until this campaign had been completed, smallpox regularly killed and disfigured many, especially in the Third World. The disfigurement is caused – especially on the face – by the pustules which eventually erupt, leaving unsightly pockmarks. Its eradication represented a great step forward, but was not as straightforward as many people think, for some smallpox still existed after that 1977 'victory' date.

This is because, although the WHO called on all countries to destroy any remaining stocks of the virus by 1999, neither the USA nor the former Soviet Union (the former two superpowers) wished to comply. Each was afraid of it being used as a biological weapon. Because smallpox (variola major) is so highly contagious, it is dangerous to have any stocks in hand. Once released and allowed to spread, it can kill 25% of its victims. Thus it is not a matter to be taken lightly. Just as the collapse of the former Soviet Union suddenly flooded the world with stolen supplies of weapons-grade uranium, we have no guarantee that the remaining stocks of smallpox will not fall into the wrong hands.

Could the WHO have prevented this potential calamity from arising? To answer this question, we go back to analogy of virus from country A. The WHO had requested virus samples initially from each country in which smallpox had occurred, but itself had no facilities for developing a vaccine. Instead, it gave samples to the Centre for Disease Control in Atlanta, Georgia, and to St Jude's Children's Research Hospital (Immunization Centre) and a similar institution in the former Soviet Union for the necessary scientific work to be undertaken. Such ancillary institutions used by the WHO are referred to (by the WHO) as Collaborating Centres. However, as subsequent events have shown, the WHO had not placed any prior restraints on these institutions about how they would handle the virus. They were free, once they had succeeded in elaborating the vaccine, to share it with other laboratories, and those laboratories were free to patent it. Under TRIPS, any country wishing to buy the vaccine would therefore have to pay for the privilege. Moreover, they would not have to pay the WHO, but whatever institution had received the original virus from the WHO. A more rational approach, surely, and one in keeping with the WHO's mandate, and with the UN's own UDHR, would have been for the WHO to have been able to designate certain medical research centres in state-run universities to do the work and give the resulting findings to the WHO. It would then be up to the WHO to ensure that the vaccine would definitely be made freely available to meet the needs of the country that had provided the original sample, and at cost price only to other countries that needed it. Monies required for this could be billed to various UN member states according to their ability to pay.

As mentioned earlier, the danger of 'leakage' from stores of the smallpox virus cannot be underestimated. And because of these residual supplies in the USA and in what is now the Russian Federation, the world is not yet secure from the threat of a smallpox epidemic.


## VICTORY OVER SMALLPOX

What we know about the history of smallpox over several centuries does not exactly inspire confidence that the present sequestration of the virus is safe! Let us briefly consider that history. In the twentieth century alone, about 300 million people died of the disease. As the reader probably knows, it was Edward Jenner who first discovered a safe method of protection from catching smallpox, but not a cure for people afflicted with the disease. What Jenner confirmed, about two centuries ago, was that inoculating people with cowpox conferred immunity to smallpox. Cowpox is much more benign, usually only causing minor skin irritation in humans, and although it affects cattle more severely, even among them it is rarely serious. Of course, it is the rôle of the cow in the process from which the term 'vaccination' is derived. Even within Jenner's lifetime, though, cowpox inoculations were replaced with an even milder relative of the smallpox virus.

However, even vaccination was not widely used, and as late as the 1960s smallpox was still accounting for 2 million deaths a year. As already stated, the disease was eliminated by WHO-led global public health surveillance, which has since then constituted a model for epidemiologists. The WHO mass-vaccination campaign began in 1976. The victory proceeded relentlessly, with smallpox being eliminated from Asia in 1975. In 1977, there was a localized smallpox epidemic in Somalia. In 1978 the last reported case occurred at the University of Birmingham in England. That case was particularly tragic, and it illustrated clearly the unbelievable difficulty of keeping samples of the disease safely locked away in laboratories.

It started when a medical photographer working above a laboratory where smallpox virus was being studied contracted the disease from a laboratory leak. Before the photographer died, her mother became infected with the disease. Although the mother survived, the photographer's father died of a heart attack after visiting his daughter in hospital. The head of the laboratory from which the leak occurred came under intense criticism, and committed suicide. It was a tragic episode that should humble researchers to this day; but it has frequently been downplayed, even by well-known virologists specializing in the most dangerous diseases.[2]

The above account should remind us that although there have been no cases of smallpox under natural conditions for more than three decades, we cannot claim that it has been eradicated – not so long as any laboratory in the world houses the virus. WHO officials, very much aware of such dangers, convened a global commission to certify that smallpox was no longer being transmitted under natural conditions. Then, in December 1979, the World Health Assembly (WHA) adopted that commission's findings in Resolution 33.4:

> No more than four WHO collaborating centres should be approved as suitable to hold and handle stocks of variola virus . . . and that other laboratories should be asked to destroy any stocks . . . or to transfer them to an approved WHO collaborating centre.

In this way, and as described earlier, smallpox samples were at first transferred to only two laboratories – one at the Centre for Disease Control (CDC) in Atlanta, Georgia and another at the USSR Institute for Viral Preparations in Moscow – in 1978 and after. However, mutual suspicion between the two countries that possessed the virus were not long in coming to the surface. Each was concerned that the other was preparing stocks for use in biological warfare.

In 1996, the WHO was not a little anxious to learn that the Russian Federation had two years earlier shifted its smallpox samples to another laboratory, Vector, in Siberia, without the WHO's knowledge or permission.[3] The TWN source goes on to inform us that the WHO could only accept this as a fait accompli and inform the WHA. Although the WHO was not in a position (or so it ruled) to do anything about it, it was worried by the fact that Vector had been a focal point for research on biological weapons for the Soviet Ministry of Defence! The USA, needless to say, was highly suspicious and was convinced that Russia had secretly given over samples of the smallpox virus to another laboratory, but despite this the USA actually funded live smallpox research at Vector for two years, from 2000 to 2002. Since then it has withheld such funding.

However, the CDC – despite no longer backing Vector's programme – has itself proliferated research access to the virus. For example, it has granted access to the virus to the US Army Medical Research Institute for Infectious Diseases (USAMRIID) in Fort Detrick, Maryland. In 2002, it held viruses that are combinations of smallpox virus with rabbitpox and cowpox.[4]

As the TWN's research goes on to show, the CDC in the USA and Vector in Russia submit lists of their smallpox stocks to the WHO, but it was not until 2002 – when they started working with hybrids at CDC – that they listed the results of the hybrid experiments. On receiving that news, the WHO immediately called for their destruction, but so far the USA has consistently refused. They claim, moreover, that they actually wish to increase experimentation with these hybrid viruses.

## THE VARIOLA ADVISORY COMMITTEE (VAC)

In those euphoric days when the WHO first announced to the world that it had eliminated the curse of smallpox, and before it knew of these later complications with the USA and Russia, it set up the Committee on Orthopox Virus Infections, with the task of overseeing smallpox research. The Committee set about establishing strict guidelines for such research, but precluding any genetic engineering of the virus. In 1994 it, recommended that all remaining smallpox virus should be scheduled for destruction. In 1996, the WHA adopted this recommendation and set 30 June 1999 as the destruction date. However, before that time arrived, the USA signalled that it was not prepared to follow through on the decision because its national security demanded more research on defences against smallpox used as a biological weapon.

Pressured by the USA and Russia, in May 1999 the WHA retreated. It agreed to a time-limited 'temporary retention' of live smallpox, rescheduling destruction for the end of 2002. Because the Committee on Orthopox Virus Infections no longer had funding and had been reduced to 'ad hoc' status, the WHA also established a technical advisory committee to oversee smallpox studies in the interim period before the new destruction date. This committee, which was called the WHO Advisory Committee on Variola Virus Research, or the Variola Advisory Committee (VAC), has had a part-time staff and meetings funded by the USA since its establishment in 1999.

However, although the VAC has 18 member states, along with a variable number of observers and technical advisers, the TWN's research[1] shows that the USA and the EU nations dominate the VAC and its decisions. Moreover, actual attendance at VAC meetings has in no way reflected appropriate regional variation. In all respects, the VAC cannot help but be responsive to military and neoliberal pressures weighted in favour of the First World. These dominant influences press for VAC restrictions to be reduced, partly for psychological reasons.

The TWN convincingly argues that fewer of the scientists who were active in the field during the WHO's heroic smallpox eradication programme – people who personally beheld the horrors and human tragedy of real smallpox epidemics – are able to attend meetings in Geneva, etc., as they become older.

As the TWN report makes clear, the effect is a slow substitution of those individuals with real-world experience of smallpox outbreaks (who frequently favour destruction of virus) with a new generation of researchers whose personal ambitions include smallpox research. Consequently, these researchers frequently have a personal bias towards retaining smallpox stocks and relaxing research restrictions. Over time, the ration of smallpox 'destructionists' to 'retentionists' has changed, becoming lopsided in favour of those who, for personal or institutional reasons, would prefer to keep smallpox virus stocks and expand research with the live virus.

The dangers multiply with diffusion, as the TWN points out, and the VAC has met six times, starting in December 1999. By the third VAC meeting (in

December 2001) the roster of advisers had begun to expand from its initial ten, and a Scientific Subcommittee, which 'meets' by electronic mail, had been established to review proposed research projects.

The December 2001 meeting, held in the wake of the US anthrax letter incidents, took critical decisions leading to the situation today. First, the VAC determined that the (mainly) US smallpox research agenda could not be completed by the end of 2002, suggesting that ongoing experiments and planned research would have to be terminated in order to comply with WHA rulings. Secondly, the meeting's report records the first discussion of the US proposal to genetically engineer smallpox. The meeting concluded that a detailed risk analysis was necessary in order for the Scientific Subcommittee of the VAC to consider the proposal.

In May 2002, the WHA considered the VAC's report and again yielded on the smallpox destruction deadline. Rather than again postponing the date, this time the WHA took an even larger step backwards and agreed to an indefinite extension of the destruction order, until the USA and Russia completed an ambitious research agenda, including the development of new antiviral drugs, a new smallpox vaccine, and sequencing more strains of smallpox infection. If this is not a flagrant breaking of WHO principles, what is?

At the fourth VAC meeting in November 2002, the USA returned with proposals to genetically engineer smallpox and to insert smallpox genes in other poxviruses. The VAC responded by establishing a new subsidiary body, called the Technical Panel. This panel overlapped by at least 50% with the Scientific Subcommittee, and plainly its purpose was to weaken the restrictions on smallpox research and even access to the virus itself. These restrictive guidelines of 1994 had, of course, been promulgated precisely to prevent the USA's militarily led proposals!

The VAC was not entirely supine in the face of such pressure, and made this clear at its fifth meeting, in November 2003. Confronted with the Technical Panel's recommendations to restrict access to smallpox research, the VAC fought back by defending any decision. Instead they referred the matter to the ad-hoc Committee on Orthopox Virus Infections (Ad Hoc Pox Committee). This, of course, was the same committee that had originally called for restrictions and destruction of samples back in 1992–93. However, in September 2004 it gave up the struggle and acceded. It claimed that it was not in a position to comment on the proposed watering down of the restrictions, because the committee itself lacked the appropriate expertise.

Thus, in November 2004, the proposals to allow genetic engineering of small-pox went back to the VAC. The proposals were no longer stalled. The VAC approved the Technical Panel's recommendations, qualifying them by recommending that the genetic engineering of smallpox be restricted to the insertion of reporter genes, and prohibiting the expression of smallpox 'virulence' genes in other poxviruses. This meeting set the stage for final approval of the genetic engineering of smallpox virus.

In January 2005, the WHO Executive Board agreed to forward the VAC recommendations to the World Health Assembly. However, because of controversy when the recommendations were made public, the WHO Director General announced that he would also conduct a study of the issue. Little is known about this study, although it was (presumably) to be tabled prior to the World Health Assembly in May 2005, when a decision could be taken. It was so tabled.

## BIOTERRORISM AND THE WEAKENING OF THE WHO'S PROTECTIVE RÔLE

The reader, of course, will be very familiar with the use of fear propaganda, since the early 1990s, to render the citizen of the 'democratic' states acquiescent to restrictions on what had long been regarded as basic human rights. However, disseminating badly researched and biased reporting on the possibilities of biological warfare has been astonishingly successful in creating a more compliant and frightened citizenry. Smallpox lends itself magnificently to such attempts. Neoliberalism has been dominantly represented in this.

Acambis is a vaccines manufacturer in Cambridge in the UK, and in Cambridge, Massachusetts in the USA it quickly implemented a sophisticated marketing campaign after the events of September 11 2001. Co-opting academic researchers, the company's marketing subsidiary has sponsored international conferences and 'preparedness workshops' in Geneva, Athens, Kuala Lumpur and Mexico City. The conferences play up fears about bioterrorism. The take-home message is that stockpiling large quantities of vaccines is the answer. The company's sponsorship of the conferences is kept very low-key. Acambis secretly sponsored a website (www.smallpoxbiosecurity.org) that was aimed at convincing government officials to buy batches of smallpox vaccine. It was not until an investigation by non-profit organizations that Acambis acknowledged that it was behind the website.

Meanwhile, in Missouri in the USA, Mark Buller, a St Louis University researcher previously supported by Acambis grants, assigned himself the task of performing an experiment (with mousepox) that was deliberately designed to demonstrate how smallpox virus might be genetically engineered to make it an even more deadly pathogen. Buller chose to unveil his findings at an Acambis-sponsored conference in Geneva. He explained his actions by saying that they were a contribution to the US biodefence programme.

The University of Texas in Galveston, a medical school, promoted its ambition to construct a giant new maximum-containment laboratory to study biological warfare agents in a television news story with the disturbing title 'Warriors in Lab Coats.' Although the smallpox virus is restricted to CDC (and Vector) by WHA resolution, a university scientist terrorized viewers with dire predictions of the effects of a terrorist attack with smallpox virus. The suggestion was that residents should support the proposed facility in order to protect themselves against smallpox, a dubious assertion indeed.

In the face of this, the WHO has remained almost completely silent. As was made clear at the Alma Ata Conference in 1978, the WHO's rôle is not confined to specific health campaigns – Band-Aid reactive responses to health emergencies

– but must include the task of empowerment in mobilizing civic society in matters of public health. However, in this case and others, it has increasingly allowed its educational rôle to be taken over by commercial interests. It has offered itself up as a sacrifice on the altar of neoliberalism!

Of just as much interest to the corporate concerns of neoliberalism is almost anything to do with defence spending. It is almost irrationally lavish, as the recent experience with the 2006 BAE scandal in the UK has made plain.[5] The 'privatization' of the WHO's administration of smallpox virus samples since its global victory over the disease has, as we have seen, provided a boost to weapons research and to what former US President Dwight D Eisenhower had candidly referred to as the 'military industrial complex',[6] as the TWN's findings show in the next section.

## SINISTER PROGRESS IN MAKING SMALLPOX A WEAPON

The USA's primary argument for expanding research on live smallpox virus is the fear that it might be used as a weapon against them. However, at the same time, the proposed research projects themselves will add significantly to the risk of smallpox virus being released.

At present, tightly restricted access to smallpox virus reduces the chances of its being used as a weapon. There is no evidence that any country other than Russia and the USA has maintained stocks of the virus. All claims to the contrary have so far turned out to be untrue. For example, the fear that Iraq might have retained stocks of smallpox virus was raised in early 2003 by the US government. Two years later the CIA reported that it had 'found no evidence that [Iraq] retained any stocks of smallpox or actively conducted research into this agent for BW [Biological Warfare] intentions.'[7] The smallpox fear was misused to support the case for war, but it was not based on fact.

Independent bioweapons experts generally agree that the current risk of a deliberate release of smallpox virus is low, because the state or non-state actors with a putative interest in smallpox weapons are most unlikely to have access to the virus. Any steps that would increase access to smallpox virus, including expanding the number of individuals with access to and performing research on it, will consequently increase the likelihood of abuse. Unfortunately, the recommendations of the VAC would, if they were adopted, lead in this dangerous direction.

It is easier to mass-produce viruses for military purposes. They could do so either by creating the virus in the laboratory or by targeting mutagenesis, on an industrial scale, of some related virus. If VAC's recommendations on smallpox research were to prevail, there would be an enormous increase in the number of countries able to produce the virus industrially in this way.

This is because the VAC recommendation would allow any laboratory to possess up to 10% of the total smallpox genome, in DNA sequences of up to 500 contiguous base pairs each. Its recommended limits would only prohibit the final step, namely synthesizing the entire smallpox virus! The recommendations make it perfectly legal to synthesize smaller fragments and then to splice them together and introduce them into related viruses. Thus VAC rules would allow all that a perpetrator of biological warfare would need. Not only that, but it would be next to impossible for such activities to be detected. It would all be legal. The only way that Health For All (HFA) can prevent such retrograde steps is to insist that all existing smallpox stocks be destroyed as a matter of urgency. Only then would the WHO (and the WHA) be abiding by their mandate to 'promote and defend' global human rights.

## THE WHO IN ACTION AND BIOSAFETY

We now face the danger of smallpox all over again, largely because of the WHO's propensity for dalliance with neoliberalism. This is made clear by the fact that the VAC's own watered-down recommendations expose us to such a pandemic in two ways:
1   by the increasing possibility of accidental release of the virus
2   by the genetic engineering of less harmful viruses into extremely dangerous ones.

With regard to the first, the reader merely has to recall the above-mentioned tragic accident in Birmingham. The thing about 'accidents', of course, is that they cannot usually be predicted. The term 'accident' applies with particular force when, despite all precautions having been taken, they still occur. In this we are really talking about statistical probabilities. The only way of reducing such probabilities to zero is by removing altogether any possibility of the 'accident' concerned. The only way that highly improbable human errors can be prevented and the highest conceivable barriers to access to the danger put in place is by eliminating the source of danger itself. This has to be a policy decision, because to prevent all accidents from happening in this way, we would have to ban a host of ordinary activities which enrich our lives, and indeed which make life possible at all. Thus we would have to eschew walking, driving, sport – and even eating!

It is a matter of necessity and of the 'sum total' of social good involved. The danger we faced, once smallpox had been conquered by the WHO, was (as the WHO recognized) that if even the smallest sample of the virus existed, there also existed the mathematical probability that it might accidentally escape. Moreover, there was no conceivable value in keeping any of it alive. However, a few people and institutions stood to benefit enormously from 'just a little' proliferation of access to the virus.

These 'few people', of course, included both military researchers and pure scientists, and certain neoliberal corporations stood to make a killing for themselves and their stockholders from both of these groups. A truly empowered civil society would have said 'No way!', because any benefits that could arise would only affect a very small group of people, while exposing all of us to real danger. However, as we have seen, the WHA gradually caved in, as did the VAC. The question then arises as to why the WHO, in this way, neglected its primary mandate to put the health of all people ahead of any other considerations.

Table 5.1 gives a partial list of some of such 'leaky laboratory' accidents. And these are only a sample of those which have been 'disclosed.' There is ample evidence, as discussed below, that a not inconsiderable number of such accidents are not disclosed!

**TABLE 5.1** Some recently disclosed laboratory accidents[8]

| Organism (year) | Type | Country | Laboratory |
| --- | --- | --- | --- |
| SARS (2004) | Laboratory-acquired infection | China | Centres for Disease Control |
| Eloba (22004) | Laboratory-acquired infection | Russia | Vector |
| SARS (2003) | Laboratory-acquired infection | Singapore | Environmental Health Institute |
| Marburg (unknown) | Aerosolization incident | South Africa | National Institute for Communicable Diseases |
| SARS (2003) | Laboratory-acquired infection | Taiwan | Institute of Preventative Medicine |
| Tularaemia (2004) | Laboratory-acquired infection | USA | Boston University |
| Anthrax (2004) | | USA | Southern Research Institute |
| Tuberculosis (2004) | Laboratory-acquired infection | USA | Infectious Disease Research Institute |
| Eloba (2004) | | USA | USAMRIID, Fort Detrick |
| Q Fever (2005) | | USA | Rocky Mountain Laboratories |
| Glanders (2000) | Laboratory-acquired infection | USA | USAMRIID, Fort Detrick |
| Anthrax (2002) | Laboratory-acquired infection | USA | Undisclosed (Texas) |
| West Nile Virus (2002) | Laboratory-acquired infection | USA | Undisclosed |
| E. coli O157 (2007) | Laboratory-acquired infection | USA | Betsville Agricultural Research Centre |

To what extent has the WHO led the UN to create requirements for adequate reporting of such accidents? The answer is hardly any. In fact, only a few countries make such reporting mandatory.

Last year at Vector, where Russia holds smallpox virus stocks, a researcher stabbed herself with an Ebola virus-infected needle and later died. The CDC laboratory that holds smallpox virus has not reported any recent accidents, but public disclosure is not required by US law. At the US Army Medical Research Institute of Infectious Disease (USAMRIID), at Fort Detrick, Maryland, where

US Army researchers study smallpox, laboratory-acquired infections of glanders and Q fever bacteria as well as vaccinia, chikungunya and Venezuelan equine encephalitis viruses have occurred in recent years. In addition, the USAMRIID facility, which performed analysis of the anthrax letters (DNA sequences), did not safely manage the weaponized germs. An internal investigation revealed widespread contamination of the facility, including areas outside the high-containment laboratories, by anthrax spores.

No particularly deep insight into the mathematics of probability is needed to show that the greater the number of smallpox experiments (even if they all took place in the same laboratory), the higher will be the probability of an accident. This probability increases greatly as the number and locations of such laboratories increase. And 'containment' after such an accident occurs becomes increasingly difficult with the passage of time and the more widely dispersed the accident sites are. For instance, the above-mentioned accident in Birmingham in 1978 was contained (after secondary transmission), and this was largely attributable to the high degree of smallpox vaccination/immunity in the UK population at that time. A similar accident today could well wreak havoc in a large population, because fewer and fewer people have strong immunity to smallpox. Even if all experiments with live smallpox virus are conducted under maximum containment conditions, there is always the risk of accidental release of the virus.

The danger of inadvertently constructing highly lethal pathogens was recently demonstrated by an Australian research team experimenting with a virus that is closely related to the smallpox virus. The team genetically engineered the mouse-pox virus in an attempt to create a fertility control vaccine to control mouse populations. The result was unintended and unforeseen – all of the mice infected with the new virus strain died, even those that had been vaccinated against mousepox. It turned out that the additional gene had the unanticipated effect of turning off the immune system of the mice, making them vulnerable to lethal infection by the otherwise harmless virus. The prospect of a genetically engineered smallpox virus overcoming vaccinations and the immune system is disturbing.

Similarly, the introduction of single genes from the smallpox virus into related poxviruses may well lead to new, highly pathogenic strains. This danger is exemplified by an experiment on the influenza virus that was published in 2002. US researchers introduced two genes from a particularly virulent and pathogenic strain – the so-called 'Spanish' flu strain of 1918–19 – into another, less dangerous flu strain. In animal experiments, the artificial strain proved to be much more deadly to mice than other viruses containing genes from contemporary influenza virus.[9]

## GIVING THE WHO MORE TEETH

It can be argued that the WHO (and the VAC) have themselves been accident-prone due to having insufficient staff and/or financial support. This emerges in the TWN report[8] when it discusses the WHO's Biosafety Advisory Group (BAG).

VAC documents refer to the submission of smallpox recommendations to the WHO BAG, but do not explain what this group is and the extremely limited role and activities of the WHO laboratory biosafety programme.

The WHO has one staff member working on laboratory biosafety, with the daunting task of managing WHO activity in all laboratories, from Australia to Zambia, ranging from hospital diagnostic benches to maximum-containment research facilities, and from issues of physical infrastructure to personnel training and operating procedures.

There are no WHO advisory committees dedicated to laboratory biosafety. The WHO BAG is an informal group that provides email suggestions to WHO staff members. It is not constituted by WHA resolution, nor does it report to the WHA or any of its subsidiaries, nor is it empowered to advise the WHO. As of early 2005, the WHO BAG consisted of five individuals, two from the USA, and one each from Canada, Australia and the UK.

This emerged and was discussed at the meeting of the 60th World Health Assembly at Geneva in May 2007. At that meeting, the WHA made it clear that it wanted to agree on a sufficiently strong and detailed resolution leading to the destruction of all smallpox virus stocks. Among other things, it was agreed that a far more controlled and thorough research base had to be assumed under VAC mediation within a drive to prevent the previous tendency to allow a wide variety of geographically dispersed laboratories to have access to the smallpox various.

In particular, it was agreed that WHO member states should pay very careful attention to any resolution language concerning the scope of permissible research involving smallpox virus stocks. The kind of research that may be permitted by the WHO, including those permitted by the Advisory Committee on Variola Virus Research, includes diagnostics, antiviral drugs and sequencing. Despite this strict limitation, the USA has begun to defend its research by stating that 'scientists have yet to exhaust the research potential of live smallpox virus.' This statement misrepresents the scope of permissible research. The WHA has never authorized research until the smallpox virus has been 'exhausted' of all possible studies, nor should it ever authorize such research. No organism is ever beyond the scope of another study, so permitting research until research on the organism is 'exhausted' would be the same thing as never actually destroying the virus. This would negate the goal of all WHO members, repeated in numerous resolutions, to destroy the live virus stocks. Thus it is critical that any such misrepresentation of the scope of permissible research is rejected, and for all resolution language to clearly indicate that under no circumstances will research outside the WHO regulations be permitted. The aim of the carefully crafted resolution was to ensure that the criteria for permissible research should all relate generally and specifically to public health.

If this can be done, it will restore to the WHO a little of all the authority that it has lost, in rendering it able to address its Alma Ata mandate. Admittedly, the discussions alluded to above still represent a watered-down version of the rôles of both the VAC and the HFA, but even so they embody a strength of purpose that should contribute realistically to a general UN agreement on the destruction of all existing smallpox stocks. As usual, though, the problem is that the phraseology even of the 2007 resolution implies that the WHO consensus of 1978 could still be queried and 'modified.' Any such philosophical vacuums will quickly be filled by neoliberal and militaristic exploitation of the situation.

A discussion of the privatization of avian flu, potentially an even more dangerous global pandemic than smallpox, illustrates many of the same points about the WHO being 'bought off' by private corporations and the like as smallpox did. However, an even more sinister aspect of neoliberalism becomes evident with regard to avian flu.

## NEOLIBERALISM AND AVIAN FLU

The basic details of Indonesia's experience when it trustingly sent samples of avian flu (H5N1) virus are now well known, not only because it exposed to the world's media the link between the WHO and neoliberal interests, but also (less well known) because Indonesia's own alternative to sending samples to the WHO was for the Indonesians themselves to get on the neoliberal bandwagon and sell samples directly to the pharmaceutical corporations. This may have caused it to reverse its original decision. Images of eggs jumping from frying pans into fires spring readily to mind!

However, before going into all of the gory details, this author perceives a bright side to the still unfolding story. First of all, the WHO has not been party to making money itself out of the events. It simply passed the viral samples on to its collaborating centres for them to undertake the necessary research (including genetic engineering) and – if possible – vaccine elaboration. It was some of the scientists in the collaborating centres who went ahead and patented the results. Under WTO regulations, including use of GATS and TRIPS, this meant that the country providing the original samples could not be guaranteed access to the vaccine for its own people without incurring a financial outlay in excess of its resources.

In the account given so far, then, can the WHO only be accused of stupidity rather than cupidity? Given their original mandate, based on the UDHR and, later, on the Alma Ata Declaration, there were at least two things they could have done that would have averted the situation.

1  They could have extracted a prior agreement with potential laboratories requiring them not to patent their findings, but simply to return them to the WHO and to inform the donor country
2  They could have required such laboratories to give the donor country – at no or minimal cost – priority in rationing out supplies of any resulting vaccine.

Had the WHO taken such precautions, its own reputation would never have been called into question. It would also have been able to extricate itself more easily from the whole WTO finance-driven matrix of GATS and TRIPS. Right now there are subcommittees within the WHO devoted to solving the problem of working within TRIPS. But why should this be? The WHO should surely regard it as contrary to its own mandate (and to the UDHR) to even recognize the legitimacy of TRIPS if applied to the elaboration of global public health procedures.

Thus the WHO's contretemps with Indonesia could act as a wake-up call to both. The long-term solutions (if any can be elaborated) to the threat of a pandemic variety of the H5N1 virus contagious among humans require the relentless efforts of scientists without the intrusion of financial considerations. Hopefully that lesson has now begun to be learned. However, just as the Alma Ata Declaration recognized that solutions to global health inequities involved political redirection even more than clinical considerations, the world's governments have to appreciate that disentangling ourselves from acquiescence to neoliberalism is a precondition for achieving human rights equity generally.

## THE RÔLE OF SCIENCE

An adequate account of how scientific developments have the potential to free the WHO from WTO restrictions would require a book of its own. The TWN has published a useful series entitled the 'Intellectual Property Rights Series.'[10] However, the following brief account of the science behind much of the progress to date is intended to contextualize the issue and allow the reader to appreciate the degree to which TRIPS complicates matters unnecessarily. I shall only deal with research carried out at one of the WHO's collaborating centres – the St Jude Children's Research Hospital in Memphis, Tennessee, in the USA.

It was scientists at St Jude Children's Research Hospital who announced in February 2003 the development of a vaccine against H5N1, a new lethal influenza virus that triggered the WHO to declare a pandemic alert.

The virus appeared in birds in Hong Kong in late 2002, and subsequently killed one of two infected people with rapidly progressive pneumonia in the next month.

St Jude developed the vaccine within 4 weeks of receiving the H5N1 virus sample from colleagues in Hong Kong through the WHO.

> The announcement comes at a time when a second, as yet unidentified virus has taken several lives around the world. The unknown virus, which causes severe acute respiratory syndrome (SARS), appears to have originated at the same time and in the same place as the new 'flu.'
>
> The development of the initial ('seed') batch of H5N1 vaccine is significant because humans do not have a natural immunity to the virus, according to Robert Webster, a member of the Department of Infectious Diseases at St Jude. Rather, humans appear to become infected through contact with chickens and other birds. In the past the virus killed only the chickens it infected. But the new variant of H5N1 also killed many kinds of wild birds, which is unusual.
>
> If H5N1 were to acquire the ability to pass from human to human, there would be the potential for concern similar to that for SARS, according to Webster.

'It's likely there were two things that prevented the 1997 poultry influenza outbreak in Hong Kong from becoming more deadly – its (so far) inability to spread from human to human, and the slaughter of more than 1.5 million chickens and other birds in the open-air markets of Hong Kong, which eliminated the source of the virus', Webster said. 'In fact, the sudden appearance of SARS in the same region of the world is just another warning that the large populations of people and poultry in this region are a potential source of viruses.'[11]

It is when laboratories have to send samples and reports to one another that neoliberal considerations almost force scientists and their institutions (which themselves often depend on government and corporation grants) to protect themselves by using patent law. Robert Webster is Director of the WHO Collaborating Centre at St Jude. His is the only WHO laboratory for which the major focus is research into transmission of viral infection from other animals to people.

Webster's laboratory sent the seed H5N1 vaccine to the CDC in Atlanta and the World Influenza Center in London for further testing, in preparation for initial Phase I and Phase II trials in humans.

'It's important to move right along with these trials in case the virus begins spreading from person to person', Webster stated.

Led by Richard Webby, PhD, and Daniel Perez, PhD, the St Jude laboratory team successfully modified a technique called reverse genetics to permit them to develop the H5N1 vaccine very quickly. Using the samples of H5N1 obtained from Hong Kong, Webby mixed two genes from H5N1 with six genes from a second virus (A/PR8/34)(H1N1)). H1N1 is a rapidly growing 'master' strain of virus commonly used to make vaccines.

The genes from flu viruses produce proteins called HA and NA, which are on the surface of the virus, in full 'view' of the immune system. Webby took the modified gene for HA and the NA from H5N1 and mixed them inside a cell with six genes from H1N1. The HA gene was modified in order to abolish its ability to cause disease, and thus safer to use in the vaccine.

The genes were mixed together, and the resulting vaccine virus produced in the cell thus carried HA and NA from H5N1. However, because of the alterations to the HA, and the rest of the genes being derived from H1N1, the new virus vaccine cannot cause disease. Rather, it can only stimulate the immune system to respond to H5N1. The scientists took precautions to prevent the kind of leakage of infection that occurred with smallpox.

'The St Jude vaccine is like a gun without ammunition', said Elaine Tuomanen, MD, director of the St Jude Department of Infectious Diseases. 'The vaccine looks deadly enough for its HA and NA proteins to alert the immune system. But in reality it's carrying blanks that can't cause disease.'

However, all of this discussion about avian flu may have led some researchers to forget about a previous warning that the WHO had received about it, and that was the malady known as severe acute respiratory syndrome (SARS). In fact, SARS is likewise an avian flu, and an epidemic of it broke out in 2002, first in

Vietnam and China. Initially it only attacked fowl, but early in 2003 cases were reported of people – who had caught it from poultry – dying of the infection. The WHO was very much involved in collecting samples of the virus from Vietnam. Still, even by 2004 a vaccine for it had not yet been isolated.

Eventually Dr Malik Peiris, a physician and microbiologist researching at the University of Hong Kong, identified the SARS virus, which is the first step in being able to create vaccines against various forms of it. However, this was only achieved because Hong Kong University, through the WHO, was cooperating with various collaborating institutions and these shared findings with a variety of other laboratories. Basically the isolation of the SARS virus came about because of the availability of the research team at St Jude. Thus the reader can see that the effective prosecution of the necessary science requires a degree of openness between nations and institutions that could be seriously compromised by concerns about TRIPS.

This is highlighted even more clearly by the ongoing research on H5N1. The research itself is crucial because, if H5N1 eventually evolves a form that can be transmitted from person to person, our present global transport system will spread the pandemic much more quickly and lethally than was the case with the famous 1918 influenza pandemic.

A new variant of the bird flu virus H5N1 emerged in late 2005, and it replaced most of the previous variants across a large part of southern China, despite an ongoing programme to vaccinate poultry, according to researchers at the University of Hong Kong in collaboration with scientists at St Jude Children's Research Hospital:[12]

> The new virus, called Fujian-like (FL), appears to be responsible for the increased incidence of H5N1 poultry infections since October 2005, as well as recent human cases in China, the researchers said. FL has now also been transmitted to Hong Kong, Laos, Malaysia and Thailand, resulting in a new bird flu outbreak wave in South-East Asia that has caused human infections as well, according to the Hong Kong/St Jude team.
>
> The investigators also warned that it is possible that this new H5N1 variant will spread further through Asia and into Europe, as it evolves to form other sub-lineages that vary from place to place. This evolution into different sub-lineages also occurred during the previous two waves of H5N1 transmission that occurred during the past several years, according to the investigators. A report on these findings can be found in the November online edition of the *Proceedings of the National Academy of Sciences (PNAS)*.
>
> The findings are significant because experts believe that H5N1 is the most likely virus to trigger a human influenza pandemic (worldwide epidemic). Moreover, the increasing number of transmissions from birds to humans in the past year supports this opinion, said Robert G Webster, PhD, a co-author of the PNAS paper. Webster is a member of the Infectious Diseases Department and holder of the Rose Marie Thomas Chair at St Jude.

Based on their study of vaccinated poultry, the Hong Kong/St Jude team suggested that the vaccination itself might have facilitated the emergence of this new variant.

This emergence and rapid distribution of FL virus, despite the vaccination programme that was started in September 2005, also suggests that the current H5N1 control measures are still inadequate, Webster said.

Moreover, since November 2005, some of the 22 H5N1 human infections reported from 14 provinces in China were from infected residents of metropolitan areas such as Shangai, Wuhan and Guangzhou, which are remote from poultry farms.

'We don't know yet whether the people in those metropolitan areas were infected locally by contact with poultry or by contact with other humans', Webster said, 'but we suspect from the studies they are being infected by contact with poultry.'

The researchers found the virus in samples taken from infected chickens in 11 of the last 12 months of the present study, compared with only 4 months during 2004-05. This indicates an increase in the incidence of H5N1 infection in 2005–06 compared with previous years, which suggests that H5N1 viruses have not been effectively contained.

The investigators also conducted genetic studies of 390 H5N1 viruses isolated from poultry in the current study (30% of the total found in southern China), and found that 68% were of the FL sub-lineage.

The emergence of FL-like viruses and their success in replacing other H5N1 variants in such a short time demonstrates how difficult it is to control H5N1 in China, Webster has said.[13]

The above brief glimpse of the scientific collaboration required globally for the WHO to even begin to meet its Alma Ata mandate should make it clear to the reader how important it is for WTO restrictions, TRIPS and such multilateral arrangements as GATT and GATS not to be able to interfere with the WHO's activities. They have to be entirely separate, and patent law can have no legitimate humanitarian authority over the invention, production and exchange of medicines or of medical information.

With that in mind, we can now make some sense of the account of Indonesia's disagreement with the WHO. We shall first consider Indonesia's justification for its loss of faith in the WHO's capacity to adequately protect the Indonesian people from the threat of a potentially lethally pandemic – even though Indonesia had given the WHO the samples required for the elaboration of a vaccine. We shall then discuss what can only be described as a happy ending to the saga, as Indonesia once more agrees to cooperate with the WHO. However, it was a close run thing, and it illustrates how dangerous neoliberalism can be if we expose the UN and the WHO to its dominance.

## INDONESIA'S PLAN OF SELF-DEFENCE

A number of accounts of the issue ran in the media. The most coherent, in this author's view, was that expressed on the editorial page of an issue of the *New Scientist* early in 2007.[14] The whole incident really brought the word 'biopiracy' (and the concept) to popular attention. The *New Scientist* editorial applauded Indonesia's response to the situation, going on to say that, despite the grave medical problems that Indonesia's action might augur for world health generally, that country is '. . . doing the only thing it can do to protect its own people. It has also brought an unpalatable truth out into the open.'

This 'unpalatable truth' is that the WHO in effect acted as a middleman between pharmaceutical manufactures and the WHO's collaborative laboratories – using TRIPS regulations to achieve neoliberalism's goals. The editorial goes on to point out that if health protection, and efficiency in achieving it, were the only criteria, then it would send its virus to the best laboratories and receive a decent share in any vaccine derived from it. Indeed it sent its samples off to its high-quality collaborative laboratories, as already described, but from there on the forces of neoliberalism took over – and Indonesia found that, in the case of an avian flu pandemic, it would not necessarily be able to access supplies of the vaccine to protect its own citizens. This was because the Indonesians would only be able to acquire the vaccine on a commercial basis. Such an arrangement would exclude not only Indonesians, of course, but also the people of many other Third World countries.

The upshot was that Indonesia treated the affair as a matter of biopiracy. Along with Indonesia, many other poorer, tropical countries are 'hotspots for biodiversity.' Much of our modern pharmaceutical history has involved rich foreign countries coming into less economically favoured ones and helping themselves to herbs, and other biological materials, the curative efficiency of which had already been established over the generations by thousands of people. These highly developed countries have then set up a truly Byzantine system of laws to control exports of genetic material without agreement. Since 1995 the WTO has refined this entire process, and now the worm has finally turned!

The First World invokes TRIPS to thus control H5N1 samples under 'the rule of law.' However, money is not the only object. They also know that should an avian flu pandemic arise, the First World countries will ensure that they are protected first. Poorer countries would therefore be unlikely to receive the vaccine in time to avert the first wave of the pandemic. So, as the *New Scientist* editorial so clearly points out, by withholding the virus, Indonesia is leveraging the one resource it has to obtain flu vaccine, and possibly even to obtain its own factory. As Lily Sulistyowati of Indonesia's health ministry expressed it, 'Indonesia's state-owned drug maker Bio Farma does not have the technology and expertise to create the vaccine. We can only offer foreign pharmaceutical companies our strain of the virus.' The country says that it will do this only under material transfer agreements that ban commercial use except by prior agreement.

The editorial expresses its regret that things have come to this. Indonesia should be able to share its virus freely without feeling that it is sacrificing the one chance it has to save its people from a pandemic. Perhaps vaccine manufacture should be a global public good, not a national or private one. We need a system that works for everyone. In its absence, those material transfer agreements should be signed now. We need to see what H5N1 is up to in Indonesia.

Indonesia's announcement in February 2007 that it would not share its samples was criticized by researchers as a major departure from a 50-year-old worldwide system of free virus sharing, and one that would severely limit the ability of the WHO to monitor the ever-changing virus.

However, the country has stood firm on the need to change a system that it says keeps life-saving pharmaceuticals out of reach of poor countries.

'We must work together to change the perverse incentives that have resulted in developing countries being disadvantaged', the Indonesian health minister, Siti Fadilah Supari, said recently. She then went on to state that she also urgently wanted assistance for poor nations in developing 'domestic vaccine production.'[15]

Indonesia has had the highest number of human cases of the H5N1 strain of bird flu. Of 281 cases worldwide, 81 cases were recorded there, and 63 of those were fatal.

David Heymann, Assistant Director General for Communicable Diseases at the WHO, said that he recognized the inequalities in the current virus-sharing system. However, he also emphasized the importance of sharing viruses in order to help to protect global health.

'It is critical that all developing countries have access to pandemic vaccines', Heymann said. At the same time it is critical that the world shares its 'novel influenza viruses' for risk assessment and the development of vaccines.[16]

On 13 March 2007, Indonesia's Health Minister Siti Fadilah Supari went on record as saying that Indonesia will not share bird flu samples with the WHO without a legally binding agreement that the virus will not be used to develop an expensive commercial vaccine.

Siti Fadilah Supari, digging in her heels after a week-long stand-off with the global body, said a letter of guarantee from the WHO's Director General Margaret Chan late last month was not good enough.

'We will not share the virus before there is a Material Transfer Agreement', she told reporters, adding that she hoped one would be drafted during a bird flu meeting in Jakarta in late March 2007 between Asia Pacific health leaders and the WHO. As of today (late 2007) it is still under discussion.

Several countries are developing vaccines to protect against H5N1, the bird flu virus strain blamed for 167 human deaths worldwide – more than a third of them in Indonesia.

The virus remains mainly an animal disease, but experts fear that it may mutate into a form that spreads easily among humans, potentially killing millions.

Dr Margaret Chan, only a few months into her new position as Director General of the WHO, said in a letter to Dr Supari, dated 28 February 2007, that the WHO would use Indonesia's strain of the virus 'only for public health risk assessment.'

Fortunately for the entire human population, Indonesia has since reversed its position.[17]


## INDONESIA NOW COOPERATING WITH THE WHO

On 15 May 2007, Indonesia relented and once again started to send avian flu virus samples to the WHO, which submitted them to one of its collaborating laboratories. However, the shipment was small, containing only three samples from two patients. Indonesia has confirmed 15 or so human cases since the start of the impasse, which is over affordable access to pandemic vaccines.

It was not clear whether more clinical specimens would be sent later, or whether this was a one-off gesture.

> 'I am pleased to announce to all of you that Indonesia has resumed sending its H5N1 specimens to the WHO collaborating centre in Tokyo', Indonesian Health Minister Siti Fadilah Supari told the WHO's annual general meeting, the World Health Assembly, in Geneva in May 2007.
>
> The director of the WHO collaborating centre, Dr Masato Tashiro, said his laboratory began work last week to try to grow viruses from the specimens.
>
> 'Probably this week we will get – I hope – viruses', Tashiro, Director of the Department of Viral Diseases and Vaccine Control for Japan's National Institute of Infectious Diseases, said from Tokyo.

Supari, who is demanding equitable access to affordable H5N1 vaccine for developing countries, placed a motion calling for a new system of virus sharing, one which affords more rights to countries that provide virus samples to the WHO system. The resolution was brought forward by 17 countries, including Algeria, Laos, Malaysia, Peru, Iraq and North Korea.

It should be noted that the WHO had been running its influenza surveillance programme, which has been in existence for more than 50 years, by operating on a principle of free sharing. Flu viruses from around the world are submitted free of charge to WHO reference laboratories. Viruses that are deemed to be important new strains are turned into vaccine strains and provided free of charge to vaccine manufacturers.

There was no objection to this system when it was used to make seasonal influenza vaccine. Annual flu shots are a public health tool used by wealthy countries. They have not been a priority for developing countries that have many pressing needs and stretched health budgets. However, the picture has shifted with the development of H5N1 vaccines, which are being stockpiled by several countries, including the USA. Other wealthy countries, such as Canada, have signed long-term contracts with manufacturers to procure first access to vaccine when a pandemic occurs.

At the heart of the proposed WHO compromise is an effort to put together a virtual vaccine stockpile from which developing countries could draw if necessary. WHO Director General Dr Margaret Chan said that she was heartened at the response she was receiving from potential donors to the notion of a vaccine stockpile: 'I am in dialogue with development partners and with executives from all the leading influenza vaccine companies. I am greatly encouraged by their commitment.'

The agency's senior official for pandemic influenza, Dr David Heymann, has said that a stockpile of between 40 million and 60 million doses is on the drawing board. The idea would be to provide developing countries with limited amounts of vaccine for essential workers, such as police, military and healthcare staff.

Thailand, which has been sympathetic to Indonesia's efforts but was not a signatory to the resolution, has said that it would need enough vaccine to protect 600 000 people or about 1% of its population. However, Supari said that Indonesia would need 22 million doses of vaccine, enough to protect roughly 10% of that country's population. Meeting this demand would drain about one-third to one-half of the WHO's proposed stockpile.

Of course, if it were not for TRIPS and other patent law considerations, the WHO could use more collaborating laboratories to ensure adequate supplies for all without having to comply with financial limitations. At present this is the problem that the WHO faces. With current production methods and capacity, global demand for vaccine will far outstrip global supply in a pandemic, experts insist. And most if not all manufacturers have already signed contracts promising their output to developed countries which are paying to ensure access to that capacity.

To date, no company or country has publicly announced a contribution of vaccine to the virtual stockpile project.

In this account of Indonesia's anger at the WHO's procedures, the WHO could not claim to have acted entirely honourably, even if one throws in a huge proportion of innocent naivety about business practice. The next section considers some of these wider implications.

## THE RIPPLE EFFECT ON WORLD HEALTH GENERALLY

In a 'blog' by Chan Chee Khoon[18] published by Singaling, the wider implications of the Indonesian contretemps are considered. When Indonesia's Health Minister initially decided against sharing Indonesian samples of the bird flu virus, she argued that a better arrangement had to be made to protect the citizens of donating countries.

In breaking with the existing practice of freely sending flu virus samples to these laboratories, she expressed dissatisfaction with a system which obliged WHO member states to share virus samples with collaborating centres, but which lacked mechanisms for an equitable sharing of benefits – most importantly affordable vaccines developed from these viral source materials by patent-seeking commercial entities.

To consolidate regional support for this initiative, a meeting of Asia-Pacific developing countries was convened in late March to explore mechanisms for more equitable access to vaccines produced from virus-sharing arrangements. The Indonesian decision elicited unease, but also sympathy from a cross-section of the global community, including the above-mentioned editorial in the *New Scientist*.

On 29 March 2007, immediately after an interim agreement for Indonesia to resume sending flu virus samples to the WHO, health ministers of 18 Asia-Pacific countries issued the Jakarta Declaration, which called upon the WHO 'to convene the necessary meetings, initiate the critical processes and obtain the essential commitment of all stakeholders to establish the mechanisms for more open virus- and information-sharing and accessibility to avian influenza and other potential pandemic influenza vaccines for developing countries.'

These proposals were tabled at the 60th World Health Assembly in Geneva (May 2007) as part of a resolution calling for new mechanisms for virus sharing and for more equitable access to vaccines developed from these viral source materials.

It was here that the WHO's culpability emerged. In the course of the deliberations, it emerged that the WHO had violated the terms of the 2005 WHO guidelines on sharing of viruses, which required the consent of donor countries before its collaborating centres could pass on the viruses to third parties such as vaccine manufacturers. Indeed the WHO's collaborating centres themselves, as well as third parties, had sought patents covering parts of the source viruses used in the development of vaccines and diagnostics.

The Indonesian stand-off with the WHO comes on the heels of Director General Margaret Chan's admonishment to the Thai public health ministry, in February 2007, over the issuing of compulsory licences for HIV/AIDS and heart medications. In the course of a visit to the National Health Security Office in Bangkok, she had publicly urged the Thai health authorities to seek instead a negotiated compromise with pharmaceutical companies over high drug prices. This perceived tilt in favour of neoliberalism drew strong criticism from health advocates in Thailand and elsewhere.

They pointed out that the Thai ministry 'has been in regular contact with the industry over the high prices of its drugs in Thailand', but these negotiations have led nowhere. The best price for originators of Efavirenz, for example, is still twice the price available from Indian generic sources (US$500 per patient a year vs. US$224). The best offer for the originators of lopinavir/ritonavir is US$2000 per patient a year, five times more than the WHO's estimate of manufacturing costs. The Thai Health Ministry estimates that the price of clopidogrel would fall by over 90% if it was made generically. These are substantial price differences in a country where the average annual wage is US$1400 a year.'

The implications for equity of access to primary healthcare are abundantly clear. It is uncertain whether these episodes amount to tactical shifts, let alone a more fundamental realignment between the WHO, member states, corporate actors and health activists on the issue of access to essential medicines. However, the ramifications are clear for the interlinked concerns of global health equity and international health security.

The Indonesian government's stance in particular was notable on three counts:

❒ It was explicitly a critique of the WHO's balance of pragmatism, which it felt was overly accommodating of corporate priorities, to the detriment of the health and well-being of a key constituency that the WHO was mandated to defend, namely the under-developed communities among its member states.

❒ It was an exercise of leverage by a source country of biological materials, seeking to redress the inequities of access to what may be vitally important health inputs (avian flu vaccines) developed from these source materials.

❒ It was seeking equitable benefits from commercial developers not just for its nationals, but for other communities as well who were likely to be sidelined by commercially driven product development and distribution systems.

The way forward for the WHO, and for the UN as a whole, is plain to see but full of complexities. What it boils down to, as will become evident in subsequent chapters, is that we somehow have to separate the WTO and – except for provision of finance as requested by the WHO and similar human-rights-related agencies – the IMF and the World Bank, with the WHO deciding what the World Bank's health investment priorities should be. Such a radical shift would have to be reflected in the legal structures (e.g. relating to patents) of individual UN member states, and argued through as Security Council resolutions. The issues cannot be resolved within the WHO itself.

## REFERENCES

1 Third World Network. *The Genetic Engineering of Smallpox*; www.smallpoxbiosafety.org (accessed 20 July 2007).

2 ProMED-mail. *Laboratory Safety and Disease Dissemination*, 29 May 2004; www. promedmail.org (accessed 21 July 2007).

3 Third World Network, op. cit., p. 4.

4 Third World Network, op. cit., p. 5.

5 MacDonald T. *Health, Human Rights and the United Nations*. Oxford: Radcliffe Publishing; 2007. pp. 178–85.

6 Eisenhower DC. The military industrial complex. In: *Speeches of the Presidents*; http:// coursesa.matrix.msu.edu/~hst306/documents/indust.html (accessed 21 July 2007).

7 Central Intelligence Agency (CIA). *Report of the CIA's Iraq Survey Group*; http://cia. gov/cia/reports/iraq_wind_2004 (accessed 21 July 2007).

8 Third World Network. *Destruction of Smallpox Virus Stocks* (an update for the 60th World Health Assembly Conference in May 2007); www.smallpoxbiosafety.org/ news220107.html (accessed 21 July 2007).

9 Tumpy T, Garcia-Sastre A, Mikulasova A *et al.* Existing antivirals are effective against

influenza viruses with genes from the 1918 pandemic virus. *Proc Natl Acad Sci USA.* 2001; **99**: 13849–54.

10 Third World Network (TWN): Khor M. *Rethinking IPRs and the TRIPS Agreement* (2001). Oh C. *Trips, Drugs and Public Health: issues and proposals* (2001). Ha-Joon C. *IPR and Economic Development* (2005). Khor M. *Intellectual Property, Competition and Development* (2005). Chee Yoke L. *Malaysia's Experience in Increasing Access to ARVs: exercising the government's use option* (2006).

11 Webster R. *Special Reverse Genetics Used for Vaccine Against H5N1*; www.stjude.org/media/0,2561,453_5484_4638,00.html (accessed 21 July 2007).

12 Webster R. *Control Measures Fail to Stop Spread of the New H5N1 Virus*; www.stjude.org/infectious-diseases/0,2535,427_2054_22024.html (accessed 23 July 2007).

13 Ibid., p. 2.

14 Self-defence over bird flu is no crime (editorial). *New Scientist.* 2007; **17 February:** 3.

15 Bird Flu Guard. *Indonesia Defiant on Refusal to Share Bird Flu Samples*; http://birdfluguard.blogspot.com/2007_03_01_archive.html (accessed 23 July 2007).

16 Ibid.

17 World Watch News. *Indonesia Sharing Bird Flu Virus.* Broadcast on BBC News 24, 16 February 2007.

18 Khoon C. *Singaland: furthering the common good*; http://singaland.bloodspot.com (accessed 23 July 2007).

# Chapter 6

# The UN's dalliance with nuclear power

## RÔLE OF THE INTERNATIONAL ATOMIC ENERGY AGENCY (IAEA)

Moving away from 'natural disasters' and pandemics, we now ask whether the UN, and even the WHO, have sold out to another less well-known UN agency, namely the International Atomic Energy Agency (IAEA), and the latter to the rich and powerful nuclear lobby. Such a scenario may be difficult to imagine. After all, the UN and its WHO are there to promote and defend human rights, including health. Their respective mandates make this quite clear, as does the UN's Universal Declaration of Human Rights (UDHR).

The IAEA is one of the least understood and spoken about of the UN's panoply of agencies, and (from its point of view) maybe this is how it wants things to be, because nuclear power compromises the ideals of the UN at three general levels:
- financial
- political
- psychological.

As the reader will appreciate, the economics and politics of nuclear energy – even if devoted to such peaceful purposes as household energy supply – have enormous financial implications. Whenever a nation adopts the 'nuclear path' by deciding to generate a substantial portion of its domestic energy needs by means of nuclear power plants (NPPs), wealthy nuclear power corporations are on the doorstep, hats in hand. However, they face a deep-seated psychological problem. Ordinary people are, by and large, fearful of the nuclear option. Some of their fear is irrational, but some of it is based on a growing realization that the major threat to health and safety lies not in the building of the necessary infrastructure, nor in the actual use of nuclear power, but in how to safely discontinue the use of such a facility when necessary. It is now widely known that we have not yet elaborated a completely safe way of disposing of the used rods once they are no longer required as a power source. This issue is constantly being debated by nuclear physicists and related scientific and technical pundits.

Some indeed argue that so far we have not really developed a completely safe and foolproof method of disposal, and that until we do so, the nuclear pathway cannot really be regarded as feasible. Others have adopted a more sanguine approach. They have discussed a variety of solutions – from coating the rods in a thick sleeve of silicon and burying them deep in ground that has no significant water run-off, to blasting the material into outer space! However, they are sufficiently certain that a safe method will be found that we should not let that consideration be a barrier to using nuclear power. After all, it has many advantages in that it does not add carbon dioxide to the atmosphere. However, there is still the problem of safe disposal of the rods, which can remain highly radioactive for as long as 250 000 years.

Those who stand to make huge profits from nuclear power are extremely concerned that large numbers of the population should not be fearful of nuclear power. And this is where the IAEA comes in. Most of us only hear about it as an agency that monitors the danger of nuclear proliferation for military use. One of its positive rôles is to referee global access to nuclear power. Thus the IAEA played a part in ascertaining whether or not Iraq was really developing nuclear facilities under Saddam Hussein, concluding finally that it was not doing so. More recently, it has been active in trying to prevent Iran from developing an independent nuclear capacity.

The fact that nuclear accidents have occurred – one has only to think of the Chernobyl disaster in the former Soviet Union – keeps alive the popular worry about nuclear power. Obviously such accidents raise serious implications for world health, and should attract the attention of the WHO. However, as will be described in this book, the IAEA has been accused of preventing the WHO from public comment or policy making based on Chernobyl, and similar accidents. If this is true, whose interests is the IAEA really defending in imposing this gag on the WHO? It is certainly not protection of the world's health that lies at the bottom of it. It is much more likely that both the IAEA and the WHO are acting in the interests of the neoliberal corporate powers, which stand to profit so handsomely from nuclear development for industry and commerce.

However, the entire picture is much more complex than this and – linked to high-level corporate financial interests – has from the beginning been consideration of statecraft and politics. Until the atomic bombs fell on Hiroshima and Nagasaki, scientists had very little real idea about the severity of harm that the bombs would cause. It was certainly appreciated that they would be more destructive than anything yet devised in the red routines of war, but the long-term genetic effects were rather sketchily understood.

Between 1945 and 1986, both the military and the scientific establishment learned a great deal about man-made radiation and its potential for genetic destruction. Also, however, the potential for the peaceful application of nuclear fission as an energy source became clearer. Not every country can produce uranium of sufficient quality for the manufacture of nuclear weapons, with the result that countries that could do so quickly found themselves in a most favourable economic position. For instance, Australia happens to hold about 40% of easily accessible uranium, and it is significant that, while selling the material widely to many other countries, Australia itself has been one of the most conservative countries in terms of adopting nuclear power as an energy source for domestic use, as we shall see later.

The popular view of nuclear energy, informed as it was by news reports of long-term genetic damage caused by the nuclear bomb that was dropped on Japan, gave rise to an instinctive – and possibly irrational – fear of its use among lay people worldwide. Even as ordinary citizens gradually came to appreciate the many economic and even environmental advantages of nuclear power as a source of domestic energy, this was accompanied by a lurking fear of accident or sabotage endangering the world. Films, books and the media certainly capitalized on this. However, by 1986 most people had become used to the idea that nuclear energy might be a 'good thing' and that its application should be pursued. The so-called 'nuclear lobby' consisted, on the whole, of highly educated people – many of them with advanced degrees in physics. The latter gave them an almost cultic standing in the intellectual community of the day and, by and large, they were trusted.

However, on the morning of 26 April 1986 – and over the ensuing few weeks – this trust was shattered by the accident at Chernobyl in the former Soviet Union. That event – as we shall see – gave rise to two very different reactions, which only added to lay doubts about nuclear energy for domestic use.

First, the government of the (then) Soviet Union was anxious to play down the event and to minimize the impact of the event on the health of the people in the vicinity of the disaster. The leader of the day, Mikhail Gorbachev – despite the programme of glasnost – did everything he could not only to minimize the reporting of death rates in the region of Chernobyl itself, but also to minimize estimates of the area affected. He was particularly anxious to deny significant health impacts on other countries, concerned by reactions of the worldwide anti-nuclear lobby – the 'I-told-you-so' brigade. They were angered by estimates that greatly magnified the number killed outright, the number whose health was adversely affected, and the geographical extent of these effects.

In this, as we shall see, the UN and several of its agencies quickly became involved. In the weeks and months following the disaster, the UN and the WHO released estimates of the damage done that virtually reflected the former Soviet Union's figure. These gave the impression that actual death rates were much lower than had at first appeared, and that the adverse effects on the health of survivors were surprisingly slight. The claims from countries as far away as Canada that they had suffered significant health damage were largely dismissed as being the result of fear-mongering.

Why did the UN react in this way? Initially one suspects that the reasons were political. The former Soviet Union was undergoing rapid reforms in the areas of democratic governance and accountability under Gorbachev, and it was considered important not to torpedo these tendencies so early in the piece. However, other reasons soon became apparent. In the USA, in Europe and in many other parts of the First World, considerable advances in the application of nuclear power for domestic use had already been made. Nuclear power stations had been built, and the corporate interests involved had begun to profit enormously from the enterprise. Research by various groups from 1986 until the present day suggested that UN agencies have been highly complicit in being guided in their pronouncements by the needs of the nuclear lobby. This suggests a second reason for the UN to be less than forthcoming about the matter. However, before dealing with this, let us first gain an insight into what might be called the 'incontestable facts.'

## THE CHERNOBYL ACCIDENT

There is no shortage of accounts of the disaster itself – and very little disagreement as to the details. For this account, the author consulted a number of these sources and found that the BBC News Report for 13 July 2006[1] summarized the situation particularly clearly. The event occurred on 25 April 1986, when reactor number 4 at the Chernobyl Nuclear Power Plant blew up. Forty-eight hours later, the entire area was evacuated. Over the following months there were hosts of alarming stories of mass graves, and frightening warnings of myriad deaths from radiation sickness.

The BBC report then went on to give what the author has called the 'official' account. The programme, *Horizon*, stated that a number of scientists argue that 20 years after the accident there is no credible scientific evidence that any of these predictions are coming true.

The 20th anniversary of the world's worst nuclear accident, in April 2006, saw the publication of a number of reports that examined the potential death toll resulting from exposure to radiation from the Chernobyl accident. Immediately after the event, the environmental group Greenpeace had said that the figure would be close to 100 000. Another environmental group, Torch (The Other Report on Chernobyl), had predicted an extra 30 000–60 000 cancer deaths across Europe.

However, 20 years on, according to figures from the Chernobyl Forum, an international organization of scientific bodies that includes a number of UN agencies, deaths directly attributed to radiation from the Chernobyl accident currently stand at 56 – less than the weekly death toll on the UK's roads.

The Chernobyl Forum is generally positive in its commentary on the after-effects of the accident at Chernobyl, and states that reports which suggest these after-effects should cause concern are alarmist, inspired by a mixture of Green activism and a generally uninformed fear of anything nuclear. Their report goes on to say:

> When people hear of radiation they think of the atomic bomb and they think of thousands of deaths, and they think the Chernobyl reactor accident was

equivalent to the atomic bombing in Japan, which is absolutely untrue', says Dr Mike Repacholi, a radiation scientist working at the World Health Organization (WHO).[2]

The BBC report, whose coverage of the after-effects is largely derived from the Chernobyl Forum, goes on to point out that scientists involved in the Forum expect the death toll to rise, but not far.

'We're not going to get an epidemic of leukaemia', Dr Repacholi told *Horizon*, 'and we don't expect an epidemic of solid cancers either.'

So why have the predictions varied so wildly?

Both scientific and public attitudes to radiation are still dominated by the devastating effects of the atomic bombs that were dropped on the Japanese cities of Hiroshima and Nagasaki by the USA more than half a century ago.

However, the Forum is at great pains to suggest that no fair comparison can be made between the Chernobyl accident (they never refer to it as a 'disaster') and what happened when nuclear bombs were actually dropped on cities. They say that when the latter occurred, at least 200 000 people died almost immediately from the blast, and thousands more were exposed to higher levels of radiation than anyone had ever been exposed to before. The survivors of Hiroshima and Nagasaki became the most intensely studied people in the world.

According to Professor Antone L Brooks of Washington State University, USA:

> The detonation of the A-bomb was the first time that scientists had an opportunity really to look and to see the health effects of radiation; how much radiation was required to produce how much cancer.[3]

In 1958, using data largely drawn from these bomb studies, scientists came up with an answer. It was called the *linear no-threshold (LNT) model*, and it suggested that all radiation, no matter how small, was dangerous. It became the internationally recognized basis for assessing radiation risk.

Exposure to nuclear radiation is usually measured in 'millisieverts' (mSv) or 'sieverts' (Sv), with the former being one-thousandth of the latter. The exposure, in sieverts, is dependent on the mass of the person, as it is a measure of exposure per kilogram.

The millisievert (mSv) is commonly used to measure the effective dose in diagnostic medical procedures (e.g. X-rays, nuclear medicine, positron emission tomography and computed tomography). The natural background effective dose varies considerably from place to place, but is typically around 2.4 mSv per year.

For acute full-body equivalent dose, 1 Sv causes slight blood changes, and 2.5 Sv causes nausea, hair loss and haemorrhage, and will cause death in many cases. More than 3 Sv will lead to death in 50% of cases within 30 days, and with a dose of 6 Sv survival is unlikely.

These measures are used constantly in discussions of nuclear exposure, and give the reader a ready idea of 'safe' or 'unsafe' dosages. Thus, returning to the problem of comparing exposure levels after the atomic bombs fell on Japan and after what happened at Chernobyl, we must appreciate that the data from Hiroshima and Nagasaki were for very high levels of exposure – often several thousand millisieverts, whereas the Chernobyl Forum points out that no significant data existed for lower exposures, especially below 200 millisieverts. However, as the reader probably knows, exposure to nuclear radiation is dangerous at almost any level. The Chernobyl Forum takes the view that scientists who were opposed to the use of nuclear radiation simply 'guessed' that if high levels of radiation were dangerous, lower levels would also be hazardous. The Forum argues that this assumption is unwarranted. However, as the author will show, this greatly oversimplifies the issue.

The Forum argues that with regard to Chernobyl, most people received radiation doses below 200 mSv. In their view, this makes Chernobyl the first opportunity to observe the effects of large-scale exposure to low doses of radiation. They consistently argue that the evidence from Chernobyl shows that low dosages are not particularly hazardous. They even state that low doses of radiation are a very poor carcinogen, and that people have therefore been worrying needlessly.

Some of the contributors to the Forum's findings even claim that the overall impact of the Chernobyl accident may well have been beneficial to the health of those affected. The above-mentioned BBC *Horizon* programme quoted Professor Ron Chesser, of Texas Tech University, USA, who has spent 10 years studying animals living within the 30-kilometre exclusion zone surrounding Chernobyl. He has found that, far from low-level radiation having carcinogenic effects, it appears to boost those genes that protect us against cancer: 'One of the thoughts that comes out of this is that prior exposure to low levels of radiation actually may have a beneficial effect.'

Today, although most radiation scientists are reluctant to sign up to this phenomenon, known as *radiation hormesis*, there is a growing body of opinion that it is time to rethink the LNT model and with it our attitude to radiation exposure below about 200 millisieverts.

However, a number of radiological protection scientists still advocate the use of the LNT model. In April, the WHO's International Agency for Research on Cancer (IARC) published a report that used the latest LNT-based radiation risk projection models to update the estimated cancer deaths from Chernobyl. It concluded that about 16 000 people across Europe could die as a result of the accident.

Dr Peter Boyle, director of the IARC, put the row over the figures into perspective when he pointed out that 'Tobacco smoking will cause several thousand times more cancers in the same population.'

The Chernobyl disaster was about as bad as a power-station accident gets – a complete meltdown of the reactor core – yet the lessons of the accident suggest that among the myriad issues surrounding nuclear power, the threat to human health posed by radiation has been overstated. That is, if we believe the Chernobyl Forum!

All of this is most reassuring, but there is a huge body of scientific opinion that comes to the opposite conclusion. This raises the question of the credentials of the Chernobyl Forum. How was it established? Does it represent any obvious interest groups? To what extent is the UN involved?

## THE CHERNOBYL FORUM

Eighteen years after the Chernobyl nuclear power plant accident, people in the region still live with widely varying reports about what impact the accident will have on their families' future health and on the environment. The IAEA-initiated 'Chernobyl Forum' is working to give people in the affected villages greater certainty, by issuing factual, authoritative statements on the health effects caused by radiation exposure from the reactor explosion, and also its environmental consequences.

The Forum – consisting of eight UN organizations, and Belarus, Russia and the Ukraine – met in Vienna on 10 and 11 March 2004 at IAEA headquarters. The IAEA Director of Radiation and Waste Safety, Mr Abel González, said that conflicting information had caused tremendous confusion and suffering:[4]

> People living in the affected villages are very distressed because the information they receive – from one expert after another turning up there – is inconsistent. People living there are afraid for their children. The aim of the Forum is not to repeat the thousands of studies already done, but to give them authoritative, transparent statements that show the factual situation in the aftermath of Chernobyl.

The Forum was set up in 2003 following discussions between IAEA Director General Mohamed El Baradi and the Prime Minister of Belarus. It is part of broader efforts to help to implement the UN strategy on 'The Human Consequences of the Chernobyl Nuclear Accident – A Strategy for Recovery.'

At its meeting in Vienna in March 2004, initial reports were presented by the Forum's expert groups for 'health' (led by the WHO) and the 'environment' (led by the IAEA). It was expected that the Forum would issue its findings at a conference to be held in 2005 or 2006, but such a conference had not been convened as of December 2007.

Another key aspect of the Forum's work is to advise on, and help to implement, programmes that mitigate the accident's impact. For example, this could include:

❏ remediation of contaminated land
❏ special healthcare of the affected population
❏ monitoring long-term human exposure to radiation
❏ environmental aspects of decommissioning of the Chernobyl nuclear reactor and the shelters erected for the clean-up crews after the accident
❏ addressing environmental issues related to radioactive waste from the accident.

The UN organizations involved in the Forum include the IAEA, the Food and Agriculture Organization, the UN Office for the Coordination of Humanitarian Affairs, the UN Development Programme, the UN Environment Programme, the UN Scientific Committee on the Effects of Atomic Radiation, the WHO and the World Bank.

The Forum is part of ongoing IAEA efforts to mitigate the effects of Chernobyl. Since the 1986 accident it has assisted with technical activities, environmental and agricultural monitoring and rehabilitation.[5]

Except for the occasional blog or other extraneous comment, the scientific community – or that part of it which is not beholden to the nuclear industry – takes a very different view. This began within days of the accident, with local scientific reporters naturally among the first to express their well-informed fears. The former Soviet Union was able to silence most of these, and thus their voices were not heard by the UN or its agencies. The IAEA, of course, had to be admitted by the former Soviet Union, and it was there within two days of the event.

However, as indicated at the beginning of this chapter, the remit of the IAEA is much wider than is suggested by its rôle as an assessor and moderator of nuclear proliferation. And, as shown in the foregoing section, the Chernobyl Forum includes other UN agencies along with the IAEA. Bearing this in mind, then, let us examine the contrary points of view.

One of the first to sound an alternative note was the Soviet scientific reporter Alla Yaroshinskaya. At first her reports were based specifically on what she witnessed, and she lived only 24 km from the site. Naturally she was alarmed, and said so. The negative reaction of the Soviet authorities was not entirely unexpected, but within weeks her written reports were being dismissed as 'rubbish' and 'uninformed' hysteria by powerful political voices in the west. This encouraged her to dig deeper. In 1990 she came across secret documents about the event which revealed a cover-up of massive proportions along with an officially sanctioned policy of calculated misinformation – 'official lies', so to speak.

The state and party leadership had knowingly played down the extent of the contamination and offered a sanitized version to the outside world. In 1991, five years after the accident, a series of laws was adopted to protect the victims of radiation. Scientists have now begun to find serious flaws in these, too. As recent studies show, the human and environmental damage shows no sign of abating.[6]

One of the facts that she uncovered was that, despite its rapidly developing nuclear energy programmes, particularly those associated with nuclear weapons, the former Soviet Union was the only nuclear power in the world that lacked any nuclear safety laws! Both the USA and the UK adopted such laws in 1946, and a year earlier France did, for instance. Only in 1984 did the former Soviet Union get round to it, but it was never implemented, due to bureaucratic inertia, even after the Chernobyl accident! There was never any legal entitlement to compensation, even if the law had been enforced. Yet in the former Soviet Union dozens of nuclear accidents occurred annually at both military and civilian nuclear establishments. None of these were ever reported.

Thus it was quite natural in the former Soviet Union that neither the government of the Soviet Union nor the local authorities were prepared to take legal responsibility for the ecological, social and other problems caused by the Chernobyl accident – even though Gorbachev's policies of glasnost and perestroika were already in place. However, the scale of the accident and the changes that had taken place in society by that time made it impossible to conceal the fact of the accident altogether. People in the affected territories repeatedly demanded the introduction of legislation to cover their health problems, ecological damage, and compensation for material losses arising from the accident.

In April 1990, the Supreme Soviet reviewed the situation concerning the consequences of the liquidation of the Chernobyl accident, and noted the discrepancies. Yaroshinskaya points out that the accident at the Chernobyl nuclear power plant is, in terms of its consequences, the gravest disaster of the present time, affecting the destinies of millions of people residing in a vast territory. The ecological effect of the Chernobyl accident has made the country face the necessity of solving new, exceptionally complex, large-scale problems that affect virtually all spheres of social life, many aspects of science and manufacturing, culture, ethics and morality.

It appears that the government of the former Soviet Union was more anxious to protect its people from information than from nuclear health risks! Legislation was slow in being enacted, was very limited, and Soviet citizens were not widely aware of it. In fact, the author was surprised, on a brief visit to Russia in 1991, to find that educated civilians to whom he spoke informally about Chernobyl were not aware of how they stood legally with regard to a possible nuclear accident.

One law actually authorized a programme for 1991–92 of immediate measures to deal with the Chernobyl aftermath. It assigned the Council of Ministers the duty of drafting a 'Law on the Chernobyl Catastrophe' and submitting it to the Supreme Soviet in the fourth quarter of 1990. This law was to define the legal status of the catastrophe victims, the participants in containment and clean-up operations, individuals who lived and worked in the affected areas, and those compulsorily resettled. It would also cover the 'legal regime of the disaster area, discipline of population residence and activities, military service, formation and functioning of state administrative bodies, and public organizations in the affected area.'

However, as the next relevant decree of the Supreme Soviet on 9 April 1991 noted, 'There has been no possibility at present to adopt the Law on the Chernobyl Catastrophe and the Law on Nuclear Energy Use and Nuclear Safety due to the delay in submitting the drafts of these laws.' Only in 1991, five years after the accident, were fully adequate legislative acts adopted, defining the responsibility of the government for the damage inflicted on citizens by a nuclear enterprise adopted in the former Soviet Union.

However, these laws applied primarily to the affected population, and only dealt indirectly with environmental problems. Yet compared with the legal vacuum of the previous five years, they represented a significant step forward. This is all the more important as no one had ever faced such social and environmental problems before. Nuclear accidents in other countries, such as Three Mile Island in the USA and Windscale in the UK, could not be compared to the far-reaching consequences of Chernobyl. However, almost 20 years after the Chernobyl accident, scientists, specialists and ecologists have begun to question the 'Chernobyl' laws of Russia, Belarus and Ukraine. A great many studies have exposed the current system of social-economic and medical measures to harsh criticism, particularly with regard to the calculations of the dose of radiation delivered to the population, which still constitute the basis for compensation and assistance.

## OFFICIAL ATTEMPTS TO DISCREDIT ALLA YAROSHINSKAYA

From 1992, when she first wrote a book about the cover-up,[7] Yaroshinskaya found herself not only *persona non grata* in her own country, but also widely and vociferously discredited in the west. To her very great credit, she vigorously rebutted many of these criticisms.

She was not allowed to publish what she found during the Gorbachev era, despite calls for Glaznost. When Yeltsin took over, Yaroshinskaya was elected a member of the Russian Parliament, the Duma, and during those years she became the Chairperson of the Chernobyl Investigation Commission, which obtained access to even formerly top secret Politburo reports on what happened in Chernobyl. Those were truly massive and terrible events.

As a 20-year anniversary memorial to Chernobyl's appalling effects, Yaroshinskaya has published a follow-up version of her earlier book, called *The Big Lie*, in which she once again documents these 'forbidden truths', largely showing that the vast number of deaths and morbidity which were caused in the former states of the Soviet Union are far higher and more extensive than the Western press and even the UN reports will admit.

One of dozens of attacks on her credibility follows. It can be found in a Department of Public Information of New York report (a UN report), and is datelined as from Washington and under the authority of the IAEA, the WHO and the UN Development Programme.[8] One could hardly ask for stronger UN support than that for the following résumé of the report's 'findings', roundly rebutting Yaroshinskaya's views. The report claims that, after nearly two decades, only 4000 people (at the very most) would eventually die of the effects of the accident, and that this figure was reached by an international team of 100 scientists. Very few non-UN scientists agree with these findings. After stating that up to 4000 people *could* die, only 50 had done so as of mid-2005! This is so unbelievable that this author wonders why they picked such an unlikely figure, for even with careful monitoring by former Soviet Union security personnel, dozens of foreign reporters had – by interviewing bereaved Ukrainians – determined much higher figures. Moreover, the WHO report goes on to state that of these 50 deaths, almost all of the cases had been highly exposed rescue workers.

The new figures are presented in a landmark digest report, *Chernobyl's Legacy: Health, Environmental and Socio-Economic Impacts*, just released by the Chernobyl

Forum. The digest, based on a three-volume, 600-page report and incorporating the work of hundreds of scientists, economists and health experts, assesses the 20-year impact of the largest nuclear accident in history. The Forum is made up of eight UN specialized agencies, including the IAEA, the WHO, the UN Development Programme (UNDP), the Food and Agriculture Organization (FAO), the UN Environment Programme (UNEP), the UN Office for the Coordination of Humanitarian Affairs (UN-OCHA), the UN Scientific Committee on the Effects of Atomic Radiation (UNSCEAR), and the World Bank, as well as the governments of Belarus, the Russian Federation and Ukraine.

> This compilation of the latest research can help to settle the outstanding questions about how much death, disease and economic fallout really resulted from the Chernobyl accident', explains Dr Burton Bennett, chairman of the Chernobyl Forum and an authority on radiation effects. 'The Governments of the three most affected countries have realized that they need to find a clear way forward, and that progress must be based on a sound consensus about environmental, health and economic consequences and some good advice and support from the international community.'
>
> Dr Bennett continued: 'This was a very serious accident with major health consequences, especially for thousands of workers exposed in the early days who received very high radiation doses, and for the thousands more stricken with thyroid cancer. By and large, however, we have not found profound negative health impacts to the rest of the population in surrounding areas, nor have we found widespread contamination that would continue to pose a substantial threat to human health, within a few exceptional, restricted areas.'
>
> The Forum's report aims to help the affected countries understand the true scale of the accident's consequences and also suggests ways the governments of Belarus, the Russian Federation and Ukraine might address major economic and social problems stemming from the accident. Members of the Forum, including representatives of the three governments, will meet on 6 and 7 September 2005 in Vienna at an unprecedented gathering of the world's experts on Chernobyl, radiation effects and protection, to consider these findings and recommendations.
>
> But, says Dr Michael Repacholi, Manager of the WHO's Radiation Programme, 'the sum total of the Chernobyl Forum is a reassuring message.'
>
> He explains that there have been 4000 cases of thyroid cancer, mainly in children, but that except for nine deaths, all of them have recovered. 'Otherwise, the team of international experts found no evidence for any increases in the incidence of leukaemia and cancer among affected residents.'
>
> The international experts have estimated that radiation could cause up to about 4000 eventual deaths among the higher-exposed Chernobyl populations, i.e. emergency workers from 1986–87, evacuees and residents of the most contaminated areas. This number contains both the known radiation-induced cancer and leukaemia deaths and a statistical prediction, based on estimates

of the radiation doses received by these populations. As about a quarter of people will die from spontaneous cancer not caused by Chernobyl radiation, the radiation-induced increase of only about 3% will be difficult to observe. However, in the most exposed cohorts of emergency and recovery operation workers, some increase of particular cancer forms (e.g. leukaemia) in particular time periods has already been observed. The predictions use six decades of scientific experience with the effects of such doses, explained Dr Repacholi.

Dr Repacholi concludes that 'the health effects of the accident were potentially horrific, but when you add them up using validated conclusions from good science, the public health effects were not nearly as substantial as had at first been feared.'

The report's estimate of the eventual number of deaths is far lower than earlier, well-publicized speculations that radiation exposure would claim tens of thousands of lives. However, the 4000 figure is not too different from estimates made in 1986 by Soviet scientists, according to Dr Mikhail Balonov, a radiation expert with the International Atomic Energy Agency in Vienna, who was a scientist in the former Soviet Union at the time of the accident.

Before considering the majority scientific assessments, which support Yaroshinskaya's estimates, let us conclude this section with a few more UN/WHO/IAEA assurances in the form of questions and answers as printed in their report:[9]

**How much radiation were people exposed to as a result of the accident?**

With the exception of on-site reactor staff and emergency workers exposed on 26 April, most recovery operation workers and those living in contaminated territories received relatively low whole body radiation doses, comparable to background radiation levels, and lower than the average doses received by residents in some parts of the world having high natural background radiation levels.

For the majority of the five million people living in the contaminated areas, exposures are within the recommended dose limit for the general public, although about 100 000 residents still receive more. Remediation of those areas and application of some agricultural countermeasures continues. Further reduction of exposure levels will be slow, but most exposure from the accident has already occurred.

**How many people died and how many more are likely to die in the future?**

The total number of deaths already attributable to Chernobyl or expected in the future over the lifetime of emergency workers and local residents in the most contaminated areas is estimated to be about 4000. This includes some 50 emergency workers who died of acute radiation syndrome and nine children who died of thyroid cancer, and an estimated total of 3940 deaths from radiation-induced cancer and leukaemia among the 200 000 emergency workers from 1986–1987, 116 000 evacuees and 270 000 residents of the most contaminated areas (total about 600 000). These three major cohorts were subjected to higher doses of radiation amongst all the people exposed to Chernobyl radiation.

The estimated 4000 casualties may occur during the lifetime of about 600 000 people under consideration. As about a quarter of them will eventually die from spontaneous cancer not caused by Chernobyl radiation, the radiation-induced increase of about 3% will be difficult to observe. However, in the most highly exposed cohorts of emergency and recovery operation workers, some increase in particular cancers (e.g. leukaemia) has already been observed.

Confusion about the impact has arisen owing to the fact that thousands of people in the affected areas have died of natural causes. Also, widespread expectations of ill health and a tendency to attribute all health problems to radiation exposure have led local residents to assume that Chernobyl-related fatalities were much higher than they actually were.

### What diseases have already occurred or might occur in the future?

Residents who ate food contaminated with radioactive iodine in the days immediately after the accident received relatively high doses to the thyroid gland. This was especially true of children who drank milk from cows that had eaten contaminated grass. Since iodine concentrates in the thyroid gland, this was a major cause of the high incidence of thyroid cancer in children.

Several recent studies suggest a slight increase in the incidence of leukaemia among emergency workers, but not in children or adult residents of contaminated areas. A slight increase in solid cancers and possibly circulatory system diseases was noted, but needs to be evaluated further because of the possible indirect influence of such factors as smoking, alcohol, stress and unhealthy lifestyle.

### Have there been or will there be any inherited or reproductive effects?

Because of the relatively low doses to residents of contaminated territories, no evidence or likelihood of decreased fertility has been seen among males or females. Also, because the doses were so low, there was no evidence of any effect on the number of stillbirths, adverse pregnancy outcomes, delivery complications or overall health of children. A modest but steady increase in reported congenital malformations in both contaminated and uncontaminated areas of Belarus appears to be related to better reporting, not radiation.

### Did the trauma of rapid relocation cause persistent psychological or mental health problems?

Stress symptoms, depression, anxiety and medically unexplained physical symptoms have been reported, including self-perceived poor health. The designation of the affected population as 'victims' rather than 'survivors' has led them to perceive themselves as helpless, weak and lacking control over their future.

This, in turn, has led either to over-cautious behaviour and exaggerated health concerns, or to reckless conduct, such as consumption of mushrooms, berries and game from areas still designated as highly contaminated, overuse of alcohol and tobacco, and unprotected promiscuous sexual activity.

### What was the environmental impact?

Ecosystems affected by Chernobyl have been studied and monitored extensively for the past two decades. Major releases of radionuclides continued for ten days and contaminated more than 200 000 square kilometres of Europe. The extent of deposition varied depending on whether it was raining when contaminated air masses passed.

Most of the strontium and plutonium isotopes were deposited within 100 kilometres of the damaged reactor. Radioactive iodine, of great concern after the accident, has a short half-life, and has now decayed away. Strontium and caesium, with a longer half-life of 30 years, persist and will remain a concern for decades to come. Although plutonium isotopes and Americium 241 will persist perhaps for thousands of years, their contribution to human exposure is low.

A great deal more of this material is available and easily consulted on the Internet, but what has been cited above provides enough for the thoughtful reader to conclude that, at least since the late 1980s, the UN, the WHO and other agencies have been acting less and less in the interests of those they were intended by the UDHR to protect, and more and more in the interests of political convenience and of the corporations representing the nuclear interests. At this point, then, let us consider just one example of contrary opinion.

Many people, not only in the Ukraine, would profoundly disagree with the barely credible and somewhat patronizing comments of the Chernobyl Forum and its UN supporters.

Both the UN report and the Russian authorities themselves have been energetic in issuing denials of negative reports about the environmental effects of the Chernobyl event. Yaroshinskaya roundly condemns the entire report as a lie.[10]

She reports that the official Ukrainian government figures show that 142 000 people died within the first decade after the Chernobyl accident. This figure did not include the deaths in Belarus, Russian and other affected areas. Current estimates for Chernobyl-related deaths in the Ukraine are around 620 000 deaths and millions suffering long-term radiation exposure and acute re-exposure events, also from Chernobyl. The death estimates for Belarus' 1986 population of 10 million will be about 2 million, as 25% of the land area of Belarus was widely (and much still remains) too contaminated for safe habitation, and represents far worse contamination of Belarus than any other state. Thus if the situation is bad in the Ukraine, it is far worse in Belarus, which lies just over the border from Chernobyl – a mere 10 km in fact. The initial radioactive clouds of smoke from the burning reactor blew north for days – carrying the worst radioactivity – directly over Belarus. Kiev is about 70 km south of Chernobyl.

The deaths in Belarus were not even reported by their hard-line Soviet-style officials in Minsk, thus preventing the data from easily being made public. There the situation is clearly much worse than in the Ukraine. One sees no play given to that fact in the press, either. If the number of deaths caused by the Chernobyl accident were about 620 000 in the Ukraine, then in Belarus the corresponding figure was about 1 million by 2006. This is also consistent with ongoing population declines in the region. Yaroshinskaya also reported the deaths of 100 000 of the 650 000 clean-up workers associated with the building of the 'sarcophagus' and the initial attempts to stop the graphite fires at Chernobyl. She also documents, from official records at the clinics and hospitals, how the number of deaths was 'officially' reduced by not allowing autopsies and by artificially changing the 'radiation-level' exposures. Those people who did not die in hospitals were 'sent home', where they died and thus did not officially meet the criteria for treatment for radiation. Their illnesses were attributed to 'other causes', which also acted to cover up the true mortality and morbidity associated with the Chernobyl accident. The review of Yaroshinskaya's book, *The Big Lie*, shows this repeatedly and convincingly:

> The records of tens of thousands (at least) of those who were exposed at Chernobyl have simply disappeared, as well. Without the records, then how can one tie, 'officially', such a death to Chernobyl? 'It's nothing less than a bookkeeping trick used by crooks to cover up the actual numbers', she claims. These persistent and existing attempts to cover up the events at Chernobyl cast real doubt on the 'official' versions. As does any cursory review of the total amounts of radiation released there, of about 1–2 billion curies at least, and possibly as much as 5–6 billion curies.
>
> One curie from the core reactor radiation can kill, if delivered effectively to their bodies, 1 million adults, and a greater number of children. Thus these vast amounts of radiation, even if reduced by 1000-fold, are still capable of killing trillions of people, if effectively delivered to human beings. That is more than enough to create the human and environmental disaster which is being seen there. She reports that hundreds of tons of radioactive reactor core were released in the fires, and those massive smoke clouds pouring out of the reactor core radiated at 10 000 REMS/hour, for 10 days! Reactor core blocks found in the control room by Medvedev were measured at 15 000 REMS per hour, as the reactor was in the last stages of operation, due to massive build-up of radioactive isotopes in the core rods. The meltdown significantly added to that vast amount of radioactivity, as well. A 'REM' is a unit of radiation dose that would produce the same effect in a person as one roentgen of X-rays or of gamma rays.
>
> Because the reactor was at its end of cycle-point, where it was being readied to be shut down, and the reactor core rods replaced, it was full of Pu (Plutonium). All plant life within miles of the reactors died. Studies at Oak Ridge, Tennessee,

show that even 50 years later, areas of land exposed to high-level radiation from Co-60 (Cobalt 60) have not yet recovered, and remain sterile, devoid of life. The amount of radiation of Pu alone from Chernobyl will likely result in uninhabitable regions there for about 200 000 years, and perhaps longer. That is not a trivial amount of radiation release (the half-life of Pu is 24 000 years). The magnitude of the disaster has never been nationally reported in the USA, let alone Russia. It's widely known, though, in Ukraine, Belarus and Russia, however.

One can read these official documents and the supporting extracts of these data which Yaroshinskaya not only showed repeatedly in her first book, but which have also been massively confirmed even to this day in the Ukraine and Russia. The official UN figures are very suspect, because they depend upon an inaccurate and tainted source, namely the official Soviet and Russian Government figures, not the actual events, as Yaroshinskaya details:

> You can believe UN officials, or you can believe the actual, on-ground, on-site events. The author prefers primary sources, as most do and for the reason that they are more closely tied to real and direct data than such official 'lies' are.
>
> The UN, the WHO, and Soviet, Russian and US media reports are simply wrong. They even ignored the massive NorthAm radioactive fallout over Idaho and in New England, which caused a significant rise in thyroid problems in children there just after Chernobyl. Sadly, ignoring the evidence of these Soviet and current denials of events is just more of what has been going on. Yaroshinskaya's books seek to 'redress this grievance' by showing more of the whole truth, which happened at the time and is still going on, as the Sonsnovy Bor reactor accident, never reported in the US, shows. One need only read the voluminous relevant documents and citations. And if one ignores this vast sea of evidence? One is reminded of the thief who stated that two of his 120 convictions for theft were not necessarily true or proved. He was still a thief, regardless . . .

One can forgive Yaroshinskaya for her combination of cynicism and anger, especially if the reader consults some of the more eminent scientific authorities who categorically refute the UN 'official' view. Back in 1996, Walter Huda published a bibliography of commentaries on Chernobyl, which this author recommends that the reader in search of more detail should consult.[11] Dr Hude is a medical physicist who obtained a doctorate in physics at Oxford University and then another doctorate in medical physics at Hammersmith Hospital London. After spending some time as a medical physicist, in particular in oncology in Canada, he is now Director of Radiological Physics there. He has also lectured in the Ukraine (his native country) and, one might say, he knows rather a lot about the issues.

## THE LONG-TERM VIEW

The health effects of Chernobyl continue to kill and to maim. These effects were not only limited to the immediate location of the radiation release, nor even to the 1 million young men (called Liquidators – rather ironically as they liquidated many of themselves) who were dragooned into cleaning up the nuclear rubble, and into risking their lives still further when they had to build mammoth sarcophagi in which to dispose of the corpses. The total environmental destruction, the damage to the ecosystem, the effects of low-level radiation and the social and psychological impact of Chernobyl should not be underestimated. Even today, low-level radiation ingested by the general population in the form of food and milk is causing malformation, mutilations and cancer deaths, as well as countless non-cancer diseases in the affected populations. Due to genomic instabilities caused by radiation, the full effects of the accident will only develop within the next six generations, which shows that Chernobyl is more than just a temporary accident. It continues to kill – every year.[12]

Worse than all this, even at the time of writing (2007) we cannot claim that the Chernobyl accident is only a ghost of the past. It still threatens global health – and will continue to do so for hundreds of thousands of years. We cannot know for sure what the future holds, especially if the region suffers a major earthquake or other disaster. The failure of our UN agencies to properly inform us would pass as little more than a very sick joke were it not for the fact that it has probably already had such deadly political effects. By this I mean that most thinking people – due to lack of specific information, through the controlled media's almost total silence on the matter for two decades – have been left with a rather relaxed view of the use of nuclear energy.

Thus, in the UK, the people are walking dream-like into an insane situation in which they regard the 'scrapping' of their nuclear submarines (Tridents), and the replacement of the latter, with equanimity. However, if nothing else, Chernobyl should have taught us that nuclear power – whether it be for domestic or military use – is not really safe. For one thing, how is a nuclear submarine 'scrapped'? The expense is exorbitant enough, but how can the old submarines be 'scrapped' in a way that is not fraught with environmental implications?

As this chapter has already made clear, the 'official' figures of the IAEA do not reflect the real situation. The IAEA, which is responsible for 'the worldwide promotion of peaceful use of nuclear technology' (according to the IAEA Charter) and composed mainly of scientists from nuclear-energy states, has no inherent interest in addressing the true casualties and health effects of the Chernobyl disaster. Instead, it propagates the myth of a benign and manageable nuclear accident. According to IAEA figures, as we have seen, only 50 people died as a result of the Chernobyl accident, while the total number of deaths may rise to 4000. Plausible and scientific evidence from all affected regions, compiled by national cancer registries and supported by western scientists, show numbers that greatly exceed these obviously downplayed statistics – more than 500 000 invalids, more than 50 000 deaths among the liquidators, thousands of childhood deaths and malformations all over Europe, countless cases of thyroid cancers, all not counting the psychological and social impact of the catastrophe and the subsequent resettlement and stigmatization. And the risk of another accident like Chernobyl is still out there.

Indeed, the Chernobyl disaster has shown the whole world the ugly face of nuclear power – the one that the nuclear industry is trying to hide and the one that opponents had been warning about for many years before the meltdown. Chernobyl should have been the turning point of the world's nuclear policy, yet it appears that it was not even the first major nuclear accident. And since then, several others have occurred in the UK, Germany, the USA and Japan. None were of the magnitude of Chernobyl, yet according to scientists the next accident is inevitable – it is only a matter of time.

## EVIDENCE FROM OUTSIDE THE FORUM

Many references have been made thus far to the vast body of evidence – over 250 refereed scientific papers and books that this author has accessed – with regard to the real effects of Chernobyl. There follow specific references to eight of these studies, from which the reader can gain some insight into what can only politely be classified as 'biased reporting' by the agencies represented in the Chernobyl Forum.

1  Epidemiological analysis of demographic consequences of radioactive irradiation of inhabitants of 12 radioactive contaminated regions of Ukraine. Omelyanets NI *et al.* Scientific Centre of Radiation Medicine, AMS of Ukraine, Kiev.

Review of all data for 20 million people in contaminated zones up to 1998 shows that for both acute (i.e. immediate post accident) and chronic irradiation there are 'extremely adverse combinations of high infant and general mortality with low birth rate.' If the Low Level Radiation Campaign's (LLRC) understanding of non-standard English syntax is correct, the increased mortality arises from 'radiation' being recorded as the cause of death, and current figures for non-cancer illnesses, combined with unfavourable demographic factors, should be taken as the harbinger of a soon-to-be-realized increase in cancer similar to that already seen for thyroid cancer.

2  Sexual structure of the inhabitants of the country and its influence on reproduction health of a nation. Omelyanets SN. Supreme Rada of Ukraine Committee on Chernobyl Disaster Problems, Kiev.

A disproportion of sex ratios, beginning at birth and increasing throughout life, threatens to deepen the demographic catastrophe already seen in a rapidly declining population. An uncharacteristically high but statistically significant proportion of boys is born, but mortality in boys is uncharacteristically high and the excess continues to grow. It continues into manhood with 'supermortality' of able-bodied men. 'In connection with the early extinction of men in the senior age groups, the [proportion] of women . . . sharply grows.' A 3.9-year reduction in life expectancy was seen in the eight years to 1998 – by which time expectancy was 61.2 years for men, 72.7 years for women.

3 Oncologic brain damage epidemiology in children. Orlov Yu A *et al.* AP Romodaniv's Institute of Neurosurgery, AMS of Ukraine, Kiev.
'Rather substantial' increases in brain tumour frequency have been recorded in children between two 5-year periods before and after Chernobyl.

4 Unstandard approaches to Chernobyl disaster epidemiology: the territorial-time-span analysis of leukaemia diseases. Osechinsky IV *et al.* Haematology Research Centre, AMS of Russia, Moscow.
Earlier work by the same authors had shown that leukaemia and lymphoma SMRs in 8 years after Chernobyl in the 'most contaminated' territories relative to an unspecified control were not substantially different from 1.0. No trend with dose was observable in the less contaminated territories. Present work involves aggregating data for blood diseases in cows and people relative to radiation and chemical industry plant. Again, no consistent dose/response trend has been found.

5 The cytogenetic consequences in children of continuous residence in towns contaminated by the Chernobyl accident (1986–1991): a methodological and epidemiological report. Pilinskaya M. Scientific Centre for Radiation Medicine, AMS of Ukraine, Kiev, with Graduate School of Public Health, University of Pittsburgh.
Preliminary report on work to score possible chromosome aberrations in children with significant ophthalmic problems controlled against children without. No results have been obtained yet.

6 Results and aims of epidemiological analysis of health of population residing [in] the contaminated territories. Pirigova EA *et al.* Scientific Centre for Radiation Medicine, AMS of Ukraine, Kiev.
Overview of declining health (citing WHO findings that 18.9% of men and 14.8% of women are healthy). Shows increasing morbidity and high rates of registered disability.

7 Epidemiological study of malignant neoplasm among the population affected after the Chernobyl accident: results, problems and perspectives. Prysyazhnyuk A *et al.* Scientific Centre for Radiation Medicine, AMS of Ukraine, Kiev, Ukrainian Research Institute of Oncology and Radiology, Ministry of Public Health of Ukraine, Kiev.
'The 10-year period after the Chernobyl accident is well known as a latent period.' This stresses the importance of further monitoring.

8 A new study of radionuclide contamination of maternal milk in Italy. Risica S. Italian National Institute of Health, Rome.
Two studies had been carried out in Rome and near Lake Como to investigate caesium transfer from food to mothers' milk. No results reported here. In 1997 samples were collected from four areas. Caesium contamination of some tens of mBq per kg was found. No results are available for strontium yet.

Brief summaries of other studies have been provided by Walter Hude, of the Department of Radiology, University of Florida, and can be found online at www. brama.com/Ukraine/chornbib.html.

## GREENPEACE'S ANALYSIS OF THE EVENTS

Although Greenpeace has a long record of opposition to the nuclear industry, its integrity is generally respected internationally, and its analysis is regarded as being sober, well judged and not sensationalist. Also, in many of its publications it has reflected support for the UN as our most important guarantee of world peace. Therefore its judgement on the way that the Chernobyl accident has been treated deserves consideration.[13] Greenpeace has been quoted as saying that the health effects of the Chernobyl disaster 20 years earlier have been grossly underestimated.

Official UN figures predicted a maximum of 9000 cancer deaths due to Chernobyl. However, Greenpeace claims that 'unbiased' studies not released by the Forum show that the average number of predicted deaths will be around 93 000! Furthermore, emphasizing that there are often problems with the diagnosis, it reveals that other Chernobyl-related illnesses could take that toll up to 200 000. Greenpeace campaigner Jun Van de Puffe told a Reuters journalist that one problem was that there is no accepted statistical methodology for calculating the number who might have died from these other diseases.[14]

There is no question about the fact that the explosion and subsequent fire at the Chernobyl nuclear power plant had been the world's worst nuclear accident. It was responsible for emitting a cloud of radioactive particles across a whole swathe of European countries, and this affected even more distant regions. Despite the evacuation of the immediate area by USSR authorities, several million people still live in contaminated areas.

In view of all of this, the question may (indeed, must!) arise as to how the UN arrived at its much smaller figure of 4000–9000 extra cancer deaths. Their figure came – as we have seen – from the UN-led Chernobyl Forum. The full UN figures are as follows:

| | |
|---|---|
| Acute radiation sickness (ARS) deaths in 1986 | 28 |
| ARS patients who died later | 19 |
| | |
| (However, the UN report even suggested that the number 19 was too high, as some of them died of cancers unconnected to Chernobyl!) | |
| Others who died in the actual explosion | 2 |
| Child thyroid cancer deaths from 1992–2002 | 15 |
| Predicated extra cancer deaths | 4000 |

These figures not only grossly underestimate the categories listed, but they also ignore such categories as deaths of previously non-radiated personnel in getting rid of the corpses (of which there were only two, according to the UN report!). However, in its report, Greenpeace's consulted range of medical sources estimates that 270 000 cases of cancer will be caused by the fallout, of which 93 000 are expected to be fatal. The Chernobyl Forum's response is to accuse Greenpeace, and a whole army of medical researchers and statisticians from some of the world's leading universities, of being 'alarmist'. They state that 'A tendency to attribute all health problems to exposure to radiation has led local residents to assume that Chernobyl-related fatalities were much higher.'

Much more generous was the counter-response of Mr Lee Harwood, medical physics adviser to Greenpeace. He said that 'There may be technical reasons for the huge discrepancy.' However, he also alleged that the nuclear industry had a 'vested interest in playing down Chernobyl because it's an embarrassment to them.'

Dr Oxana Lozova, who works at a children's hospital in the Rivne district, 300 km (190 miles) west of Chernobyl, said that many generations appeared to be affected.

'I think the fallout from Chernobyl has affected the immunity of those who were young children at the time of the disaster', she told the BBC's Moscow correspondent, Damian Grammaticas. 'We now have to deal with people who are a lot weaker than their fathers and grandfathers were. They're falling ill at an age when they really should still be quite fit.'

Speaking on the BBC News website, the WHO said that comparing the Chernobyl Forum and Greenpeace reports was like 'comparing apples and oranges.'

'The Greenpeace report is looking at all of Europe, whereas our report looks at only the most affected areas of the three most affected countries', said WHO spokesman Gregory Hartl.

'The WHO felt it had recourse to the best national and international scientific evidence and studies when it came up with its estimates of (up to) 9000 excess deaths for the most affected areas. We feel they're very sound.'

Mr Hartl rejected accusations of bias toward the nuclear industry in the report.

'We are acting as (neither) an apologist nor an attacker of the nuclear industry,' he said.[15]

The original report found that more than 600 000 people received high levels of exposure, including reactor staff, emergency and recovery personnel, and residents of the nearby areas.

The reader is, of course, free to make up their own mind. To aid this endeavour, let us touch briefly on the cancer issue, mentioned several times earlier in this chapter. In November 2004 the *Swiss Medical Weekly* – internationally regarded as thoroughly reliable – printed a paper submitted by scientists at the Clinical Institute of Radiation Medicine and Endocrinology Research in Minsk, Belarus. It unequivocally showed that between 1990 and 2000, cancer rates rose 40% above the pre-Chernobyl figures. Considerations of space limit a very full account of the paper, but the following short summary brings out the salient findings, as well as illustrating the ease with which the data are analysed.[16]

To set the context, the reader should be aware that Belarus has had a National Cancer Registry for as long as the UK has had one. The increases in cancer rates after 1986 in Belarus were all statistically significant.

The scientists' findings completely contradict the predictions of the International Council for Radiological Pollution (ICRP) and the pronouncements of the IAEA and the WHO. In 2001, Chris Busby reported to the Belarus government that cancer rates would increase by 125% over the lifetimes of the exposed population.

Now, 18 years after the accident, 40% of that increase is apparent. The relative risks all have high statistical significance.

Increases in the various oblasts (regions) were as follows:

❐  Brest – 33%
❐  Vitebsk – 38%
❐  Gomel – 52%
❐  Grodno – 44%
❐  Minsk – 49%
❐  Mogilev – 32%
❐  Minsk City – 18%
❐  all Belarus – 40%.

However, the view of conventional radiation protection 'experts' is that very little if any cancer has resulted or will result from the fallout. This view was expressed, for example, in 2000 by the UN Scientific Committee on Effects of Atomic Radiation (UNSCEAR):[17]

> Apart from the substantial increase in thyroid cancer after childhood exposure observed in Belarus, the Russian Federation and Ukraine, there is no evidence of a major public health impact related to ionizing radiation 14 years after the Chernobyl accident. No increases in overall cancer incidence or mortality that could be associated with radiation exposure have been observed. The risk of leukaemia, one of the most sensitive indicators of radiation exposure, has not been found to be elevated even in the accident recovery operation workers or in children. There is no scientific proof of an increase in non-malignant disorders related to ionizing radiation . . . For the most part [the public] were exposed to radiation levels comparable to or a few times higher than the natural background levels. Lives have been disrupted by the Chernobyl accident, but from the radiological point of view, based on the assessment of this Annex, generally positive prospects for the future health of most individuals should prevail.

As the next section shows, it is not only in the interests of the Chernobyl Forum, and related UN agencies, to keep the truth from emerging. Many national governments in the First World are anxious to avoid antagonizing the wealthy and powerful figures in the nuclear industry. These people stand to make an enormous profit from both domestic and military expenditure on nuclear installations. The last thing they want to do is to disrupt the smooth routines of the lives of masses of citizens with information about nuclear dangers.

Many examples of such national cover-ups could be described, but we shall just consider the situation in Scotland, as described in an article published in the *Glasgow Morning Herald*:[18]

> The Scottish Cancer Registry, desperate to keep leukaemia data secret, is going to the House of Lords to try overturning orders by the Information Commissioner and the Court of Session to release it. In an earlier move they published a fudged analysis of the data. It seems obvious that they fear the data will eventually be dragged into the light and that people will see higher risks near the coast of the Solway Firth, which is contaminated by Sellafield and by the testing of depleted uranium weapons at the Dundrennan firing range.

The article goes on to address the nuclear industry's claims that low levels of radiation exposure are nothing to worry about:

> For 50 years the nuclear establishment has claimed its discharges are pretty harmless. They admit that there's no safe dose, so that even the smallest amounts of radiation can cause genetic damage leading to cancer, leukaemia or birth defects, but according to the official view not even the Chernobyl disaster has caused any visible effects. Officially, it caused the deaths of a few highly irradiated firemen, and up to 2000 additional thyroid cancers, which are mostly treatable. And that's it, they say.
>
> We have a different story to tell. The nuclear age is also the cancer age. The first visible population effect was the increase in childhood leukaemia which began during World War One and rose in line with radium production for decades. The Cold War orgy of nuclear bomb tests, which spread man-made radioactivity all round the globe, was accompanied by a change in infant mortality rates which accounted for the deaths of tens of thousands of children. Variations in the amounts of radioactive fallout were reflected in subsequent cancer rates, and we are now living through a cancer epidemic.

Cancer and leukaemia clusters have been found in association with nuclear sites and with places where radioactive discharges are deposited – for example, mud banks and estuaries. The effects of Chernobyl, especially those reported from Belarus, the Ukraine and Russia, are a holocaust.

Officials deny that any of this can be attributed to radioactivity but, as has been explained earlier, the denials have no scientific basis. This is because:

❐   the underlying scientific model is based on external irradiation
❐   risk is quantified in terms of dose
❐   dose is now acknowledged to be meaningless for many types of radioactivity when they are inside the body.

This is the largest and longest running health scandal of all time. The Low Level Radiation Campaign has been working to uncover it since 1992, taking the lid off cover-ups, lies, data withheld, data revised, gross errors by cancer authorities, bad science, bowdlerized reports, bullying in committees, legal threats, and dissenting scientists being libelled and barred from conferences. As what is believed to be a direct result of this, the authorities can no longer deny the truth, and we are now witnessing a slow-motion paradigm shift.

## THE WHO'S ABDICATION TO RULE BY THE IAEA

As the author implied earlier in this chapter, our WHO has not been a completely 'innocent victim' in the gradual selling off of its ideals to the highest bidder. We have already seen that by the late 1980s the WHO had started to sell its soul to the WTO, but its ambivalence with regard to its original mandate goes back much further – at least to 1959. This comes across in an email sent to delegates at the WHO conference in Geneva in May 2007, and to delegates at the People's Health Movement conference the week before.[19] In it the author, Claudio Schuftan, reminds us of the WHO's supine acquiescence to the IAEA and the nuclear power lobby. The email is reproduced below:

> Public Health Catastrophe in Chernobyl.
> WHO guilty of non-assistance to populations in danger.
>
> Demand to amend the agreement of 28 May 1959 between the World Health Organization (WHO) and the International Atomic Energy Agency (IAEA).
>
> FOR FREE AND INDEPENDENT INFORMATION ON THE RISKS OF NUCLEAR POWER AND ITS EFFECTS ON THE HEALTH OF POPULATIONS.
>
> We request that revision of the agreement of 28 May 1959 be put on the agenda of the next World Health Assembly in order for WHO to recover its independence and its authority vis-à-vis the IAEA and present the facts on the long- and short-term health consequences of the Chernobyl catastrophe.
>
> Through this agreement, WHO has abdicated its authority in the area of population health in favour of the IAEA, the sole objective of which is to promote the nuclear industry. As a result, the tragic health consequences of this nuclear accident have been deliberately covered up.
>
> The IAEA, which has no medical function, must abandon the prerogatives it has exercised for 47 years in the area of radioprotection of populations. WHO must recover complete independence from the IAEA in research and publication of information in order to assure the protection of populations subjected to nuclear contamination.
>
> We demand full information on the consequences – past, present and future – of the Chernobyl accident, which concerns millions of inhabitants of the planet,

and effective, long-term assistance to all victims of low-dose, ionizing radiation, the major cause of the public health catastrophe at Chernobyl.

For further information and petition for signature, see website:
www.independentwho.info
Emails: yann@forget-me.net and omsindependante@gmail.com

Initiated by: Les Enfants de Tchernobyl-Belarus, la CRIIRAD, le Réseau Sortir de Nucléaire, ContrAtom Genève, SDN Loire et Vilaine, Brut de Beton Production.

This has been a lengthy chapter, and it barely scratches the surface of the entire nuclear power issue. Any kind of adequate examination of that – and it is far from an 'academic' issue – would require much more than a chapter in a book. Yet it is a crucial issue of immediate practical consequence, because the debate about nuclear power for both domestic and military applications is now current. In the UK, we are faced with a government that is committed to renewing the nuclear submarine force (Trident). This of course violates the Nuclear Non-Proliferation Treaty and belies the argument for having it in the first place, which was to make the former Soviet Union reluctant to send nuclear weapons against Britain. However, that risk no longer exists. We now live in a world in which there is a real danger of terrorist groups using nuclear weapons against the UK. But we have no way of knowing from where such an attack will come, and the potential perpetrators are not psychologically disposed to worry about retaliation! In the former Soviet Union, after all, we had a rational 'enemy', so policy could be modified out of fear of reprisal.

In fact, by rendering the UK more nuclear, we are actually increasing the risk of a fanatical attack, whatever the risks to the attackers. However, we also increasingly endanger both the environment and ourselves the more frequently we construct nuclear installations of any kind. The same now applies in an ever increasing number of countries. In this the world is, in a sense, playing with probability theory or – perhaps more to the point – Russian roulette!

With regard to domestic issues of nuclear power for electricity supply, it is significant that we have not seriously either applied or experimented with more sustainable sources of energy. These are issues that we must reflect on, and we must persuade our governments to actually meet the needs of ordinary citizens – you and I – rather than continuing to bankroll powerful corporations. The UN (under its own UDHR) and the WHO mandate to protect our health have in many ways sold out to the highest bidders. It is up to an informed population to change things.

In Chapter 9 of this book, the author will briefly consider a few other areas of UN and WHO action that conflict with their foundational documents. There are many other such individual areas, to each of which a chapter could be devoted. However, the primary purpose of Chapter 9 is to identify the global health risks of neoliberalism – a philosophy guaranteed to prevent equity in global human rights, as the author will argue. Only when we are clear about the philosophical issues involved can we take practical steps to make of the UN (and its agencies) the international mediator that its founders intended.

## REFERENCES

1 British Broadcasting Corporation (BBC). *Chernobyl's Nuclear Nightmares*. BBC *Horizon* Programme, broadcast 13 July 2006.

2 Ibid.

3 Ibid.

4 IAEA News Center. *Chernobyl: clarifying consequences*; www.iaea.org/NewsCenter/News/2004/consequences.html (accessed 23 July 2007).

5 Ibid., p. 2.

6 Yaroshinskaya A. *The Big Lie: the secret Chernobyl documents*; www.eurozine.com/article/2006-04-21-Yaroshinskaya-n.html.40k (accessed 23 July 2007).

7 Yaroshinskaya A. *Chernobyl: the forbidden truth*. Omaha, NE: University of Nebraska Press; 1999. pp. 17–31.

8 UN Department of Public Information. *Chernobyl: the true scale of the accident*. www.un.org/News/Press/docs/2005/dev2539.doc.html (accessed 24 July 2007).

9 Ibid., pp. 4–9.

10 UpLink. *Environmental Effects of Chernobyl on Humans*; http://uplink.space.com/showflat.php?Cat=&Board-Phenomenon (accessed 24 July 2007).

11 BRAMA. *Annotated Chernobyl Bibliography*; www.brama.com/Ukraine/chernbib.html (accessed 24 July 2007).

12 Committee of Concerned Medical Staff and Students. *Truth about Chernobyl Fatalities*. Dusseldorf, Germany: Medical School, Heinrich Heine University; 2006.

13 BBC News. *Greenpeace Rejects Chernobyl Toll*. Broadcast 18 April 2006.

14 Ibid.

15 Ibid.

16 Okeanov A, Sosnovskaya E, Priatkina O. National Cancer Registry to assess trends after Chernobyl accident. *Swiss Medical Weekly*. 2006; **18 July**. www.chernobyl.info/index-php?userhash=24884087&nav/D=221&11D=2 (accessed 13 December 2007).

17 UN Scientific Committee on Effects of Atomic Radiation (UNSCEAR). *Sources and Effects of Ionizing Radiation*. New York: UN General Assembly; 2000. pp. 51–94.

18 MacDiarmid H. Leukaemia risk covered up by Scottish Cancer Registry. *Glasgow Morning Herald*, 10 July 2007. p. 4.

19 Schuftan C. Email sent to all members of the Public Health Movement, 23 May 2007.

# Chapter 7

# Neoliberalism and the human right to health

## NEOLIBERALISM ENDANGERS HEALTH

Of all the technical, economic and political arguments that can be marshalled against neoliberalism, and the UN's determined dalliance with it, one is unquestionable, namely that neoliberalism is very bad for one's health. Again, there are many reasons for this, but one supremely logical one undergirds them all. Neoliberalism, as we know, results in winners big time. There are First World corporation bosses who profit handsomely from it, of course, but there are also entrepreneurs in the Third World, through whom the corporations concerned have to mediate their activities, and those people also do very well out of the transaction, ending up with enough US dollars to live as millionaires in their own country. However, simple mathematics tells us that – given that the amount of money is finite – the existence of such big 'winners' implies that crowds of 'losers' are also produced, most of whom live in the Third World.

In other words, neoliberalism is highly competitive, and with winners at one end and losers at the other, there is no way that it can result in equity of income distribution. However, the UN's UDHR, and the WHO's commitment to the Alma Ata ideals, both tacitly imply that the realization of these goals is achieved by struggling for equity. A competitive system, by its very nature, cannot be expected to result in equity!

Enough of the logical theory – now let us briefly consider some of the health consequences of neoliberalism. A number of research studies have been conducted on this, and the work of Vicente Navarro[1] and of Di McIntyre and Gavin Mooney[2] springs to mind. Many others have also independently done sterling work in this field, including Susan George, whose research has already been cited. One example of neoliberalism's malign impact on health has been the privatization of water (*see* Chapter 3). This issue will only be examined cursorily in the present context. The author draws on a blog by Steve Hayes addressed from his home in Tshwane in Gauteng, South Africa.[3] Hayes is a church deacon and may therefore see things from a theological point of view, but this in no way detracts from the cogency of his work.

Haynes addresses the issue from a Third World perspective, living as he does in South Africa. However, before considering his observations, it is important that the reader appreciates that the First World has also felt the adverse impact of neoliberalism on health, even in the most wealthy countries. This issue will be dealt with later on. However, it must be realized that privatization is not the only way in which neoliberalism is experienced. It also creates commercialization. What is the difference? According to Hayes in his above-mentioned account from South Africa, one of the factors that contributed to a serious decline in healthcare in South Africa was the nationalization of all church hospitals in the 'homelands' in 1973. This has been documented by Dr Darryl Hackland, who had been Medical Superintendent of Bethesda Hospital (Methodist) in Zululand, and after it was nationalized became a senior official in the KwaZulu Department of Health. The church hospitals were run by 'private enterprise', but the difference was that they were not run for profit. That is, some privatization enhances community life because it is not commercial.

In the 1980s there was a re-privatization of health services. However, this did not take place in the poorer areas of the country, but in the rich ones. The government at the time (under PW Botha) followed the Reagan/Thatcher ideology, and encouraged the formation of commercial clinics, in which doctors owned shares. It was privatization for profit.

Medical Aid schemes have been infected as well. They were formerly socialist bodies, owned and run by their members as a form of mutual aid. Now many of them are owned by outside shareholders. They no longer speak of members, but 'customers.' They no longer provide healthcare, but 'products.' They advertise, and refer to themselves as 'financial services providers.' Beware of any 'financial services provider' that tries to sell you a 'product'! Whenever anyone uses the term 'product' for a service – financial or otherwise – it is a pretty sure indication that they are simply out to rip you off.

Thus if a government that was determined to mediate on the side of equity of access to primary healthcare simply got rid of private medical facilities, it might thereby unwittingly subvert the emergence of 'communities of concern.' Cuba provided a good example of a more useful and enlightened approach to this kind of thing. The revolution took place at the beginning of 1959, but until 1964 private Catholic hospitals were allowed to continue so long as they did not deny treatment to people simply because they could not pay.

Arguments about how a country's healthcare system should be run very often entrap the system in some kind of neoliberal net because priority is accorded to issues such as 'patient choice', 'financial efficiency', etc., when the focus should only be based on one criterion, namely what will ensure sufficient social and cultural empowerment of the community with regard to access to healthcare.

Many people are aware of the drastically perilous state of health to be found in a number of African countries, and perhaps even realize that neoliberalism – the same competitive neoliberalism that is making some people in those same countries obscenely rich – is condemning thousands of their own countrymen and women to illness and unnecessary death. Thus, because it depends for its operation on competition, it effectively divides communities. The more effectively neoliberalism is grafted on to a culture, the wider becomes the gap between the rich and the poor in the same community. We notice this more spectacularly in countries in which a high proportion of the population already live on the edge of economic ruin.

However, neoliberalism – with its logically inbuilt necessity for competition – also splits communities in First World countries. A recent report[4] from the Rowntree Trust in the UK makes this quite clear. As society becomes more consumerist, neoliberalism flourishes. Community ethos tends to become lost in a welter of competition in conspicuous consumption. People become judged and valued less and less on their community impact and more and more on what consumer power they command. The ethos of the society based on consumerism enhances neoliberalism, and vice versa, and the community becomes more and more a two-track society. At both levels, the negative impacts on health at the broadest level become obvious. The people at the top level have to develop a highly individualistic approach that allows them not to feel the loss of social contact with many of their compatriots – to ascribe the gap to laziness on the part of the poor and some kind of moral superiority on their own part. Their physical health – considered very narrowly – is bound to be better, but their social and psychological health is steadily undermined until they become little more than ciphers – 'walking billboards' advertising the consumerist values that are basic to effective neoliberalism.

The people at the bottom suffer much more physical deprivation, and also the psychological effects of sporadic and insecure employment. However, they too are motivated by consumerism, placing their hope in spectacular lottery wins, while they contribute abundantly to the consumerist culture by smoking more than the people at the top. With their gaze set on dreams of sudden wealth, they relentlessly pay for their dreams and their loss of community by shorter lives.

## THE JOSEPH RESEARCH REPORT

The findings cited above show starkly how poverty and wealth are distributed in the UK in 2007, and how they have changed over almost four decades. There is now an increasingly well understood link between wealth and postcode, which itself is an incentive to individualism, competition and an erosion of community spirit. The Rowntree study has built on a volume of well-documented research in previous studies. In addition, census and survey data were used to construct consistent 'small area' measures of poverty and wealth changes over the 37-year time span of the study. The researchers developed the following four consistent measures of the households studied:

1   'core poor' (people who are income poor, materially deprived and subjectively poor)
2   'breadline poor' (people living below a relative poverty line and, as such, excluded from participating in the norms of society)
3   'asset wealthy' (estimated using the relationship between housing wealth and the contemporary inheritance tax threshold)
4   'exclusive wealthy' (people with so much wealth that they can exclude themselves from the norms of society).

By estimating the numbers of poor and wealthy households, the authors have counted the number of households that fall into a fifth group, between the second and third listed above – those that are neither poor nor wealthy (i.e. 'normal' or 'average' households). Figure 7.1 illustrates the distribution of these households in 2000.

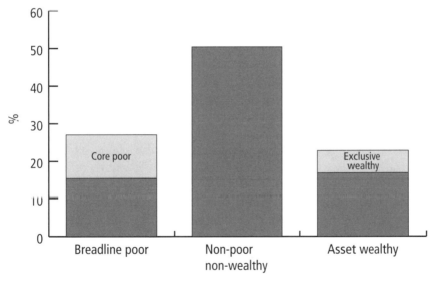

**FIGURE** 7.1 Distribution of households in 2000. The left-hand column indicates the 'poor' (both 'core' and 'breadline', as described above), while the right-hand column indicates the 'wealthy' (both 'asset wealthy' and 'exclusively wealthy', as described above).

Analysis of the fifth category in terms of internal detail would contribute little to the analysis, but the reader will probably be surprised to note that there has been a real deficit of research on the actual geography of wealth in the UK, despite frequent informal references by real estate agents, etc., to 'north' and 'south' (and even 'east' and 'west'). This study has formalized the analysis by developing new measures of wealth, and has mapped poverty and wealth over recent decades. It assesses whether the UK's population has become more or less polarized with regard to area poverty and wealth.

Figure 7.2 charts the national proportions of poverty and wealth for each time period. The proportions of households that were core poor and breadline poor declined during the 1970s, but then increased again during the 1980s. The 1990s saw the two poverty measures diverge, with the breadline poor continuing to rise, and the core poor falling to around 11% of households. In 2000, more than a quarter of households were breadline poor.

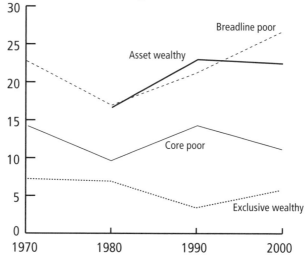

**FIGURE** 7.2 Poverty and wealth measures for the UK for the period 1970–2000.

The asset wealthy increased substantially during the 1980s, and then changed little in total number between 1990 and 2000. Over a fifth of households fall into this category. The exclusive wealthy declined slightly during the 1970s, and more sharply during the 1980s, but then increased in number from 1990 to 2000. Throughout this period, the personal wealth held by the wealthiest 1% of the population grew as a proportion of the national share (from 17% in 1991 to 24% in 2002). The 'fifth' category, between groups 2 and 3, fell from about 66% of all households in 1980 to just over half (50%) by 2000. This exacerbates the sense of a two-tier society, rendering the golden grail of 'equity' less achievable.

The key focus of the Rowntree study was to assess the changing spatial distribution of poor and wealthy households over the last few decades. The poverty and wealth measures were specifically designed to be calculated for small areas of the UK. Since standard small areas, such as census wards, change substantially over time, the analyses use a consistent set of 'tracts', allowing the comparison of spatial statistics over time.

## INCREASING POLARIZATION, SEGREGATION AND SPATIAL CONCENTRATION

Poor, rich and average households became less and less likely to live next door to one another between 1970 and 2000. As both the poor and the wealthy have become more and more clustered in different areas, so the spatial concentration of 'average' households (non-poor, non-wealthy) has also increased. The only group for whom geographical polarization has not increased is the core poor, among whom spatial inequality declined slightly between 1990 and 2000. Exclusive wealthy households appear to be increasingly concentrated in a small number of areas.

**TABLE 7.1** Index of dissimilarity

|  | 1970 | 1980 | 1990 | 2000 |
|---|---|---|---|---|
| Core poor | 12.3% | 15.6% | 15.3% | 14.1% |
| Breadline poor | 14.7% | 16.7% | 17.1% | 18.3% |
| Non-poor, non-wealthy | – | 15.4% | 16.7% | 19.8% |
| Asset wealthy | – | 34.9% | 34.5% | 40.1% |
| Exclusive wealthy | – | 43.6% | 60.6% | 59.7% |

Table 7.1 shows the inexorably increasing separation of breadline poor from asset wealthy subgroups in the community as a whole. Taking an overview of all five groups, we see that both poor and wealthy have separated further over the 40 years. The only group for whom geographical polarization has not increased is the core poor, among whom spatial inequality declined slightly between 1990 and 2000. It is noteworthy that the exclusive wealthy households have the highest index of dissimilarity for all years (with a very high increase observed between 1980 and 1990), which suggests that they tend increasingly to be concentrated in a small number of areas.

Much of the above has been suspected by public health workers in the UK since 'privatization reforms' have become a major preoccupation of governments.

## CAN THESE PROBLEMS BE SOLVED 'INTERNALLY'?

Whether discussing a less developed country (LDC) or a highly developed country like the UK, the following question must be raised. How can we increase social cohesion, and prevent the fracturing of communities, without actually moving away from neoliberalism? If it is true that, as we are often told, neoliberalism represents the way of the future, and its global spread is only a matter of time, then we must answer this question. The alternative is to conclude that these problems arise from neoliberalism, and that in fact neoliberalism *is* the problem. There have been heroic attempts to solve the problems within neoliberalism and, again referring to the First World context, we shall now consider some of them.

All such 'solutions' involve somehow 'mixing' different classes artificially. For instance, in the USA a very marked index of social segregation is based on race. The same is true in the UK and in various other countries, but the USA has the longest experience of trying to solve the problem by government intervention. For instance, the reader has probably heard of 'bussing' – preventing students from being compelled to attend their neighbourhood schools, which would all tend to be monoracial (either black or white) – by assigning masses of pupils from schools in one area to schools in another area. This would prevent the long-held ideal that every child should be within walking distance of his or her local school. The simple argument is that the system would serve to 'blur' social and class distinctions. However, at the end of the school day – and during vacations – the pupils would return to their racially, socially, culturally and economically segregated ghettos. In all, whether in the USA or in the UK, Lois Weiner[5] has concluded that such forced moving for fixed periods of time is ineffective. The Joseph Rowntree study agreed with this view.

## THE ROWNTREE TRUST'S CONCLUSIONS

It seems from the Rowntree Trust's review of the evidence that creating mixed neighbourhoods treats a symptom of inequality, not its cause. The problem is poverty – what makes people poor and what keeps them poor – not the type of neighbourhood in which people live. However, neoliberalism depends upon disparity between neighbourhoods and ghettoism.

Trying to create mixed neighbourhoods requires substantial resources that could be used directly to relieve poverty. The onus of proof should be on the advocates of mixed neighbourhoods to demonstrate that they are an effective way of relieving poverty and reducing social exclusion. A careful examination of the evidence does not provide much support for this conclusion.

There is a danger that trying to create mixed neighbourhoods diverts efforts away from tackling the underlying causes of poverty and social exclusion, lulling us into a comforting but false belief that we are doing something positive.

Effective policies for tackling poverty would include income redistribution. It seems fair that richer people should pay to tackle poverty effectively. However, that does not mean that we should completely ignore the welfare of the more affluent. The evidence from a number of studies strongly suggests not only that mixing neighbourhoods does not effectively help the poor, but also that it detracts from the welfare of the better off because it makes it more difficult for them to find neighbourhoods populated by other compatible households with similar tastes and lifestyles. Mixing neighbourhoods is not so much a redistribution of social welfare as its confiscation.

There has been an increasing polarization in the job market, and the pay-off to high-level skills has risen, leaving the low skilled and less educated behind. As the rich have got richer relative to the poor, so residential segregation has intensified. Indeed what evidence there is shows an associated polarization in house prices.

Redistribution of resources and opportunities from the richer to the poor seems to have had less emphasis in recent years. However, this is likely to be a more effective – certainly a more cost-effective – way of helping the poor than trying to ensure that they live in more affluent neighbourhoods. Before returning to Third World phenomena linked to neoliberalism, let us look briefly at US findings.

## THIRD WORLD PERSPECTIVES ON NEOLIBERALISM

Not only does neoliberalism, by promoting competition between nations, produce winners and losers, but – unsurprisingly – the bulk of winners are First World corporations and individuals, while the losers tend to live in the Third World. In fact, and as the author pointed out as late as May 2007,[6] the Millennium Development Goals (MDGs) will not be met in most of the Third World – primarily as a result of IMF Structural Adjustment Policies backed up by WTO neoliberal policies. Larry Elliott,[7] writing in the *Guardian*, also drew attention to this, but in addition made clear the UN's anxiety to interpret the dismal figures in a way that was more favourable to its policies.

He reports that the whole of sub-Saharan Africa – the poorest region of the world – will fail to meet the goals set 7 years ago for eradicating global poverty by 2015. The UN made the same prediction in late July. In a progress report at the halfway point to the target date for hitting the MDGs, the UN said that the world was failing in the battle to combat hunger, reduce infant mortality and put every child in school.

'The results presented in this report suggest that there have been some gains and that success is still possible in most parts of the world', UN Secretary-General Ban Ki-moon said. 'But they also point to how much remains to be done.'

Boosted by the economic progress in China and India, the UN said that the proportion of people living on less than a dollar a day had fallen from 23.4% in 1999 to 19.2%, and the world was on track to hit the 15.8% target for 2105. However, the 23.4% benchmark for Africa would not be met. And, as the author has pointed out previously, a decline in the numbers of people living on less than US$1.00 per day – achieved by increasing the number living on less than US$2.00 a day – is hardly cause for joy!

Slower progress had been made on halving the number of children under five who are underweight from the figure of 33% in 1990. The percentage has come down to 27%, with 46% of under-fives in Africa registered as underweight. Infant mortality is down by only one-sixth, compared with the UN's target of a two-thirds cut.

Although the UN has a target of universal primary education, it said that 30% of children in sub-Saharan Africa and 12% globally were out of school.

The UN has a target of halving the number of people without access to clean water and sanitation by 2015, the need for progress being greatest in sub-Saharan Africa and South Asia.

WaterAid said that instead of being overlooked by donors, investment in water and sanitation was vital as part of an integrated approach to tackling poverty. In Bangladesh, a country that has made water and sanitation a priority, there had been a dramatic reduction in waterborne diseases, according to this charity.

By contrast, Malawi had cut the proportion of spending on water and sanitation at the same time as it had increased investment in health and education.

Mali spends just 6% of a US$1.6 billion (£800 million) annual budget on water and sanitation.

The *Business Report* published on 29 March 2007 by Share the World's Resources[8] addresses the issue in the following terms. It explains that the context of the widening health gap is due in part to neoliberal competition between countries but, using South Africa as an example, competition between sub-sections of the South African community is also promoted by neoliberalism. In fact, statistics in the USA and South Africa show that the rich are increasingly accounting for a disproportionately large share of borrowings from banks. However, unlike the middle-income earners who borrow to finance their living costs, the rich often use debt as a financial tool. This is one way in which the gap between the rich and the poor is widened.

Too much inequality is not good for any society – much more so in a country where much inequality is a result of racial discrimination. Most of the debt owed by the rich is for mortgage bonds on primary or secondary residences. 'After buying up second [and third and fourth] homes and funding ever more lavish lifestyles, today's risk-friendly rich are embracing debt as a way to expand their fortunes and fund increasingly acquisitive lives', the *Wall Street Journal* observed in an editorial published on 26 January 2007.[9]

As already cited, Share the World's Resources point out that figures from the Federal Reserve Board's surveys of consumer finances showed that the richest 1% of Americans held 7% of the nation's debt in 2004, with a total of US$650 billion (R5 trillion) of borrowings, up from 5% in 1998, the journal said. The survey is conducted every three years, and reported in the *Wall Street Journal*, to provide detailed information on the finances of US families.

From the same source, we learn that the richest 1% are households with net worths, including primary residences, of at least US$6 million. Debt for this group grew faster than for any other group in the Federal Reserve Board's survey. It grew by 150% between 1998 and 2004.

In a report published in July 2007, WaterAid said that education – particularly that of girls – suffered in those countries that lacked clean water and sanitation:

> Although rarely recognized by education policy makers, a large part of the explanation for this high dropout rate is inadequate water and sanitation. Girls miss school because they spend hours fetching water for their families. With the onset of puberty, they face the embarrassment of menstruation in schools where toilets are unclean, have no doors and are shared with the boys in their class.

The report added that in countries with high child mortality rates, diarrhoea accounted for more deaths than did any other cause – more than pneumonia and more than malaria and HIV/AIDS combined:

> Over 90% of diarrhoeal deaths are attributed to poor hygiene, sanitation and unsafe drinking water.[10]

Naturally people – particularly in the Third World – are receiving a rapid education in neoliberal social economics! In Asia, long known for its apparent success in making neoliberalism work well for it, it only took 10 years or perhaps less for people to realize that instruments like IMF Structural Adjustment Policies had little of lasting value to offer.

## ASIA WAKES UP TO NEOLIBERALISM

The above has been well explained by Marwaan Macan-Markar.[11] In fact, his findings suggest that Asian government and humanitarian agencies are, in effect, telling the IMF and the World Bank to get out of South Asia. It was in 1997 that the now famous 'Asian Economic Crisis' struck, turning many Tiger economies back in their tracks, and exposing their citizens to levels of financial insecurity and poor health that they had long thought were gone for good. The crisis first made itself felt in Thailand, but spread rapidly to eight other south Asian Tiger economics. Desperately they called on the UN for help. And the UN responded!

In rode the IMF with the customary swagger of a powerful moneylender. For the next two years it supplied over US$38 billion in loans to the affected countries, according to available reports. This financial bailout and other economic prescriptions to the affected countries, such as Indonesia, South Korea and Thailand, were given on conditions that the Washington DC-based international financial institution (IFI) thought were best, including strict austerity measures.

However, times have changed. A meeting on Monday in Manila, hosted by the Asian Development Bank (AsDB), conveyed the tone of contempt with which finance and economic officials from the affected countries now view the IMF. It is a view built around the region's rapid economic recovery over the past decade and its abundant foreign reserves to stave off a repetition of a similar crisis. The officials from Thailand, Malaysia, South Korea and the Philippines who spoke at the meeting are also warming to the idea of an Asian Monetary Fund created through regional financial cooperation as an alternative to the IMF.

'Looking ahead, we need to take responsibility. Asia now needs to be the one to manage the global financial system', said Thai Finance Minister Chalongphob Sussangkarn.

However, as this author has pointed out in a previous publication,[12] the solution is unlikely to lie in that direction. Neoliberalism is a system independent of the culture of its hegemony, and owes loyalty to no nation. Ostensibly China is a communist society, yet it could assume hegemony of global neoliberalism tomorrow, while lessening its negative impacts on health and human rights.

In terms of community health, the welfare of women is pivotal. Their influence is broad in terms of the care of the next generation, and of making vital decisions about domestic spending on food, education, healthcare, etc. Yet it was women (and hence an entire generation of children) who were the first victims of the crisis. Working women in countries like South Korea, Thailand and Indonesia were among the worst hit as companies went bankrupt, according to the International

Labour Organization (ILO). These women were among the first to be retrenched, to lose social welfare from the state and, if hired later, were only taken back as part-time, contractual labour.

The cold stares that the IMF received at its Washington meeting in July 2007, add to a growing trend pointing to its irrelevance in the developing world, says Bello, of Focus on the Global South: 'Countries are looking for other sources of finance than the IMF. China has emerged as a major player.'

This shift away from an IFI set up 60 years ago to give loans to countries struggling with financial problems was brought to a head by the end of 2006. Rather than borrowing from it, more developing countries are paying back past loans. From lending over US$100 billion annually up to four year ago, the IMF was reported to have given US$20 billion in loans annually in the years since.

## FOCUSING ON THE BOTTOM

Much of the frothy rhetoric about neoliberalism being the 'end of history' and 'the only rational way forward' was evident during the Reagan (in the USA) and Thatcher (in the UK) years. In a previous book,[13] the author describes a statistical measure, known as the Gini coefficient, which allows a systematic comparison of population incomes globally or between sub-populations of one country. The Gini coefficient has thus rendered a systematic way of comparing incomes accurately. In 2006, Kanshil Basu[14] used the Gini coefficient when writing a paper that investigated three stages to answering the questions in this chapter's title.

1   He provided a brief historical overview of the background and function of the World Bank, the IMF and the WTO.
2   From this, he showed how financial globalization under neoliberal auspices has increased inequities.
3   Then, based on these two points, he proposes a solution based on focusing on the bottom 20% of incomes.

Points 1 and 2 have already been thoroughly discussed in the preceding pages, but his third point warrants scrutiny.

In the first stage, he considers the phenomenon of increasing global inequality. Secondly, he describes the channels to which income inequality increases due to globalization. Finally, he proposes the bottom quintile income of a poor country as a focus for policy makers, and calls for a new international organization that helps to coordinate inter-country anti-inequality policies

On the one hand, the world has become more globalized and much more prosperous in the last five centuries. On the other hand, inter-regional inequality has grown. If one tracks per capita GDP of the large regions of the world, the growing disparity is obvious. The richest region was 1.8 times richer than the poorest half a millennium ago, whereas currently the richest region has a per capita income that is 20 times the income of the poorest region.[15]

Basu uses the Gini coefficient to explore income inequality. He finds different results depending on the way in which the Gini coefficient is computed. If we compare per capita income, the Gini coefficient increased over the last decades. However, if we compare the income of countries as whole, the Gini coefficient has been declining almost monotonically since the late 1960s. The latter is driven in large measure by the strong economic growth in China since the late 1970s, and in India since the early 1990s.

Basu states that one of the biggest problems of rapid globalization is that the wages of unskilled labour in poor countries will lag behind the wages of skilled labour. Therefore income inequality within poor nations increases as a consequence of global finance.

**TABLE 7.2** Quintile incomes of nations, 2002

| Country | Per capita income (US$, PPP)* | Percentage of income accruing to poorest 20% | Quintile income (US$, PPP)* |
|---|---|---|---|
| Norway | 36 690 | 9.6 | 17 611 |
| USA | 36 110 | 5.4 | 9750 |
| Switzerland | 31840 | 6.9 | 10 985 |
| Japan | 27 380 | 10.6 | 14 511 |
| Finland | 26 160 | 9.6 | 12 557 |
| Sweden | 25 820 | 9.1 | 11.748 |
| South Korea | 16 960 | 7.9 | 6699 |
| South Africa | 9810 | 2.0 | 981 |
| Trinidad and Tobago | 9000 | 5.5 | 2475 |
| Malaysia | 8500 | 4.4 | 1870 |
| Russian Federation | 8080 | 4.9 | 1980 |
| Romania | 6490 | 8.2 | 2661 |
| Peru | 4880 | 2.9 | 708 |
| China | 4520 | 4.7 | 1062 |
| Guatemala | 4030 | 2.6 | 524 |
| India | 2650 | 8.9 | 1179 |
| Bangladesh | 1770 | 9.0 | 797 |
| Sierra Leone | 500 | 1.1 | 28 |

* PPP = Purchasing Power Parity

He criticizes the traditional objective of policy makers to maximize each country's per capita income. He proposes another normative criterion which he calls the 'quintile axiom' – that is, policy makers should be concerned about the income of the poorest 20% of the population. Evaluating an economy using the bottom quintile income makes a large difference in absolute numbers, and changes the rankings of countries sharply, as shown in Table 7.2. The first column shows the annual per capita income. The third column shows the annual per capita income of the poorest 20% of the country. For example, using per capita income yields a similar picture for Norway and the USA. However, the bottom quintile income of the USA is almost half that of Norway, indicating that the poor in Norway are better off than the poor in the USA. In other words, social policies that emphasize individualism, competitiveness and less government social intervention tend to produce less cohesive societies, whereas societies characterized by a narrow disparity between rich and poor, and in which government mediation plays a large social rôle, tend to be more cohesive and psychologically secure.

Basu's defence against critics that this measure, unlike the UN Development Programme's Human Development Index, does not consider the non-income aspects of development is that, in general, quintile incomes will have a closer relationship to other well-being indicators, such as infant mortality, life expectancy, and so on, than per capita incomes. Basu is interested in suggesting a measure that is simple and easy to understand.

Basu urges the need for a new international organization, or a division of an existing international organization, that helps to coordinate inter-country anti-inequality policies. Achieving greater global equity may require the use of policy interventions that are coordinated across countries: 'Unilateral effort by a country is likely to cause flight of capital and skilled labour from the country and impoverish those who stay behind.' Economics game theory calls this a 'Prisoner's Dilemma.' That is, for each country it is individually rational not to engage in actions that reduce global inequity, although the world as a whole would benefit from them. The WTO, the ILO and the UN Development Programme are agencies designed to reduce such coordination problems. However, there is no such agency for anti-poverty and anti-inequality issues.

Previously in this book we have referred to the European Network on Debt and Development (Eurodad). Its analysis of the negative impacts of neoliberalism on health – and other human rights – warrants a critical overview, as Eurodad has been gathering data and analysing them specifically with a view to closing the health equity gap – a good embodiment of the policies of the People's Health Movement (PHM), discussed in Chapter 1 – for years.

## CAN EURODAD PROVIDE A USEFUL CRITIQUE?

Eurodad[16] is a network of 53 non-government organizations (NGOs) from 16 European countries working on issues related to debt, development finance and poverty reduction. The Eurodad network offers a great platform for exploring issues, collecting intelligence and ideas, and undertaking collective advocacy.

The network has recently focused on multilateral debt cancellation, debt sustainability, aid quality, conditionality and harmonization, and export credit debts. Work is continuing on these issues, and increased attention is being given to illegitimate debt and to tracking aid spending by the different European countries. The main institutions targeted by the Eurodad network are European governments, the World Bank, the IMF and the Organization for Economic Co-operation and Development.

Eurodad's aims are as follows:

❑ to push for development policies that support pro-poor and democratically defined sustainable development strategies
❑ to support the empowerment of the people of LDCs to chart their own path towards development and ending poverty
❑ to seek a lasting and sustainable solution to the debt crisis, appropriate development financing, and a stable international financial system conducive to development, without prior acquiescence to neoliberal interests.

Eurodad coordinates the work of NGOs working on these issues, and collaborates actively with civil society worldwide to attain these goals. Eurodad has existed since 1990, and is registered as a non-profit organization in both the Netherlands and Belgium.

Staff at Eurodad's office in Brussels monitor and analyse policy debates at the international level, and link with members and LDC-oriented groups to gather and disseminate experiences from the national level. They also analyse policy trends and options to feed into advocacy, campaign and awareness-raising work by Eurodad's members and other contacts around the world. An external evaluation of Eurodad's work from 2004 to 2007 was very positive about the way that Eurodad balances and carries out these varied rôles, and made a number of recommendations for further improvements. These improvements, like Eurodad's work in general, will be overseen by the Eurodad Board and also by the General Assembly.

Whether by design or fortuitous circumstance, the work of Eurodad has been of huge importance in tracing the channels through which neoliberal influences have been tightening their grip on UN and WHO policies through the use of Independent Finance Institutions (IFIs). They explain the initial connection between the World Bank, the IMF and IFIs as follows.

The World Bank and the IMF were created in the aftermath of World War Two to direct investments to the neediest countries of the world (the World Bank) and to ensure international monetary cooperation (the IMF). These IFIs have changed their rôles over the last few decades, becoming international advocates of controversial economic policies in developing countries.

The IFIs sit at the heart of the global aid architecture. The World Bank is a major source of finance for developing countries, and the IMF has a crucial function in 'signalling' which countries receive more funding from both official and private sources. These rôles yield incredible power for the two institutions, which have spread their wings well beyond their original mandates. The governance of the World Bank and the IMF is severely skewed towards rich countries which dominate decision making in these institutions.

After receiving severe criticism, the IFIs claim to be undergoing semi-permanent reform. Ownership and consultation have become their mantras – but is this only old wine in new bottles? Eurodad monitors closely key policy processes within these institutions to help to bring about this much needed reform. In the light of this, Eurodad – more than many other NGO and government umbrella groups associated with practical aid in the field – has developed an insight into the vexed issue of 'sustainable debt' and world trade and human rights.

Eurodad believes that current practices in the way that a country is deemed to have 'sustainable' or 'unsustainable' debts by the international financial community are wrong both on a theoretical level and on a practical, results-oriented level. The approach adopted by the IFIs and the international creditor community simply assesses whether, given certain analyses of economic growth, external trade dynamics and the availability of financial resources, a debtor country is able to service its obligations. It says very little about the consequences for human development that such payments entail. Sadly, this very limited concept of debt sustainability has been adopted by the international community.

Its work in this area involves advocating a concept of debt sustainability which takes into account the resources that developing countries need in order to tackle the eradication of poverty and get on track towards reaching the internationally agreed MDGs. Eurodad, its network members and colleagues in the Third World work to expose the limitations of the IFIs' approach, both in general and in its application to particular countries. They believe that in order to move forward, debt sustainability needs to be redefined as the level of debt that allows a country to achieve the MDGs and reach 2015 without an increase in debt ratios. This was highlighted only recently by the UN Secretary General in his major report submitted for decision to Heads of State and government at the September 2005 High Level Meeting on Finance for Development.

Sooner or later we can be optimistic that the IFIs and their shareholder governments will be forced to recognize that their approach to debt sustainability is too restrictive and indeed damaging for Third World countries, and will therefore accept the practical and ethical necessity of a needs-based methodology.

To make the point, let us consider a few examples. For instance, the issue of debt generally – whether sustainable or otherwise – is put into meaningful perspective and can be recognized as nothing but a method by which wealthy nations, through neoliberalism, gain dominance over LDCs, not only in terms of disposal of their natural assets, but also over their social policies.

Debt is both a symptom of a skewed global financial system and a cause of imbalances and poverty. Debt has long been used within and between countries as a way to maintain power over individuals and governments. Eurodad considers debt to be a political and ethical issue, not merely one of financing, and they are keen to push for cancellation of debts while exposing the responsibilities of creditors and supporting lasting changes to the international financial architecture.

Many countries have been caught in a debt-poverty trap over the last three decades. Although civil society campaigning has made an impact and has ensured that some debts have been cancelled, the overall problem has barely been addressed by existing initiatives and mechanisms. Rich country governments and creditor institutions such as the Paris Club, the World Bank and the IMF still wield disproportionate power.

Eurodad's work on debt is focused on the following areas:

1   promoting multilateral debt cancellation for all LDCs. Eurodad monitors official initiatives, analyses key debates and informs and stimulates advocacy
2   tracking and scrutinizing bilateral debt, private debt and export credit agencies. Eurodad exposes dubious deals and calls for new, fair and transparent loan contraction and arbitration processes
3   working to reveal that many debts are illegitimate and that co-responsibility should be assumed by creditors
4   advocating a needs-based approach to debt sustainability to replace the orthodoxy based on repayability.

The hand of neoliberalism is most conspicuous in the realm of Structural Adjustment Policies (SAPs) being imposed as a condition for loans, as we have seen throughout this book.

Aid to developing countries nearly always comes with conditions attached, to which Third World governments must adhere in order to receive the funding. Even if some measures are necessary to ensure that money will not be misappropriated, a large number of SAPs impose specific economic policies on developing countries, determining fiscal and monetary choices and pushing for privatization of essential services and for other controversial policies, such as trade liberalization.

Civil society organizations have campaigned to stop development agencies imposing economic policy conditions as part of aid. Donors' economic policy conditions are politically intrusive, undermine democratic oversight, and fail to take account of the national context. Many of the policies have had negative impacts on poorer people. After much debate, some development agencies have claimed that they will reduce conditions and only apply them in areas which will aid poverty reduction. However, recent official and civil society reports show a lack of progress.

One could select as examples a number of LDCs, but in this context the author will only consider two, namely Ecuador and Haiti.

## ECUADOR IN THE HANDS OF THE MONEYLENDERS

In November 2005, the election of Rafael Correa as Ecuador's President sent a shiver of anticipatory dread down the spines of corporate CEOs worldwide, but especially in the USA. Until then it was thought that Ecuador was so thoroughly economically compromised (especially after it was forced to 'dollarize' early in 2005 as an IMF conditionality) that it could never disentangle itself from neoliberalism. However, Ecuador was not standing alone in its opposition to the neoliberal impact on its domestic programme in health and education. In a somewhat similar manner, a shift 'to the left' brought like-minded governments to power in a number of Latin American countries. Venezuela is an outstanding example.

Ecuador's unexpected emergence on to the same stage has been analysed by Gail Hurly.[17] She puts Ecuador in the context of a tiny, defenceless country that produced a leader and policies that could radically change its story. This small and often overlooked Latin American country has been in the media spotlight in recent months. It has many rich country governments, multilateral institutions and the international capital markets in a state of anxiety about what steps the government will take to honour (or not) regular payments on its external debt burden. This follows the election of Rafael Correa to power, as mentioned above. Correa's leftist government was elected after it made promises not to sign a controversial free-trade agreement with the USA, and a commitment to reduce the country's external debt burden of US$10.97 billion.

In some of the world's major mainstream newspapers, such as the *Financial Times* of 16 February 2007 ('Ecuador threatens to become the first debtor with the ability to pay'), journalists and commentators have suggested that Ecuador in fact 'has the ability to repay' its external debt. They argue that the country's debt ratios are 'low by emerging market standards', with an external debt-to-GDP ratio of approximately 38%. Should the Correa Government choose to default, it could 'set a dangerous precedent.' What these articles have in common – and neglect to mention – is that external debt service as a percentage of government revenues is extremely high in the country. This, coupled with high and worsening social indicators and serious questions with regard to the legitimacy of many of the creditors' claims, casts serious doubt on the robustness of these newspapers' conclusions.

In 2006, payments on Ecuador's external debt reached a massive 38% of government revenues (the UN recommends that developing nations should spend not more than 10–13% of revenues on external debt repayments). Ecuador owes US$4.38 billion to multilateral institutions such as the Inter-American Development Bank and the World Bank, US$2 billion to bilateral lenders and US$4.15 billion in government bonds. Spain is Ecuador's largest bilateral creditor, with a total of US$396.8 billion in claims on the country (*see* Table 7.3). Ecuador, despite high (and worsening) poverty indicators, has to date been excluded from all bilateral and multilateral debt cancellation initiatives, and has been eligible instead for (repeated) debt restructuring deals. Ecuador has visited the Paris Club a total of eight times between 1983 and 2003. According to the Debt Management Department in the Ministry of Finance, only one visit was made to refinance the capital on the country's loans with Paris Club creditors. The rest rescheduled interest and interest-on-interest only.

Various non-transparent decisions to bail out the private sector by buying back its debt via the issuing of government bonds (essentially transforming private debt into public sovereign debt), followed by the restructuring of these same bonds – several times over – at higher interest rates, has also been mired in controversy, as is explained in a new report by Ecuador's Special Investigation Commission on External Debt (CEIDEX).

A glance at Tables 7.3 and 7.4 clarifies Ecuador's overall financial situation.

It is little wonder then that the government wants (and has committed) to end this absurd cycle of continuously high debt service payments coupled with repeated debt refinancing deals of various kinds.

**TABLE 7.3** Ecuador's creditors in Europe as at 31 March 2007

| Creditor | Original contracts | Restructured Paris Club debt | Total |
|---|---|---|---|
| Belgium | 16.3 | - | |
| Denmark | 158.0 | - | |
| France | 83.7 | 95.5 | 179.2 |
| Germany | 16.5 | 40.6 | 57.1 |
| Italy | 69.4 | 271.0 | 340.4 |
| Spain | 378.2 | 18.6 | 396.8 |
| UK | | 99.8 | 99.8 |

*Source:* Eurodad. Ecuador in the spotlight as government seeks to renegotiate debt on its terms. 5 August 2007. Ministry of the Economy and Finance.

**TABLE 7.4** Selected social indicators, 2003

| | |
|---|---|
| Population living in poverty (rural areas) | 81% |
| Child malnutrition | 50% |
| Primary healthcare coverage | 30% |
| Levels of academic achievement | Average of 6 years of schooling completed nationally. This declines to 3.9 years in rural areas |

*Source:* Jubilee 2000 Red Guayaquíl (a local NGO).

## Correa's commitments

In April 2007, at an international seminar on the illegitimacy of the country's external debt, organized by Jubilee 2000 Red Guayaquíl and supported by a range of local and international organizations, Ricardo Patiño, Ecuador's Minister for the Economy and Finance, announced ambitious new budget plans for the period 2006–10. These include bold measures to reduce the percentage of national revenues dedicated to external debt repayments. Between 2007 and 2010, Correa's government intends to reduce external debt service from 38% of the central government budget to 11.8% (*see* Tables 7.3 and 7.4).

In parallel, amounts invested in the social sectors and the development of basic infrastructure will be dramatically increased. How the government intends to secure these ambitious reductions in external debt service has been the subject of intense political speculation by the international community. Some creditors fear that the government will choose to default, leaving them in a quandary as to how to react. Others have pointed to the fact that to date Ecuador has honoured its external debt service obligations.

Meanwhile Minister Patiño moved to secure fresh debt swap agreements with Spain and Italy in May 2007. What is clear, however, is that the government has ruled no option in or out at this stage. Indeed, the government announced that it would be fleshing out its external debt policy over the next few months, and it has established an advisory group composed of academic and civil society experts to advise and recommend various options as they relate to bilateral, multilateral and commercial debt stocks. Eurodad has been invited to contribute to this group. Ricardo Patiño also announced that it had already made an agreement to link its financial development to Venezuela's newly nationalized oil sales.

This author spent some time in Ecuador in the summer of 2005, and witnessed at first hand the level of desperation that the latest acquiescence to US financial power (through dollarizing the country's currency in line with IMF and WTO pressure) had inflicted on the poor, and especially on ethnic minorities. However, by comparison with Haiti – where the author had worked for a year – Ecuador was 'rich.' Haiti absolutely plumbed the depths of hopelessness – and still does – after the USA had intervened and forced its elected leader to flee. Let us therefore turn our attention to Haiti. As the reader is probably aware, that country is in such dire economic straits that it is classified by the UN as a Heavily Indebted Poor Country (HIPC).

## WILL HAITI'S CLASSIFICATION AS AN HIPC REALLY HELP?

Haiti has reached decision point under the HIPC Initiative of the World Bank and the IMF. According to the country's decision-point document, debt relief under the HIPC Initiative will total approximately US$140.3 million in net present value terms, with an additional US$243 million under the Multilateral Debt Relief Initiative (MDRI) when Haiti eventually reaches completion point. Provided that the final details on Inter-American Development Bank (IDB) participation in the MDRI are agreed in January 2007, Haiti could obtain a further US$333 million in debt cancellation. The country's authorities say that they hope to reach completion point in September 2008. However, if this is delayed by just one year (which has been commonplace for many other countries, usually due to the complex and heavy burden of numerous conditionalities), Haiti will forego US$18.6 million in debt relief.

Haiti's debt is large and unsustainable for such a fragile economy. Moreover, some of the debt could easily be classified as illegitimate. Haiti's total public and publicly guaranteed debt stood at US$1.3 billion in nominal terms at the end of September 2005. Multilateral creditors accounted for 82.2% of the total (International Development Agency (IDA) accounting for 37.9% and IDB accounting for 40%). The Paris Club accounts for 14.4%, with Italy, France and Spain being the largest bilateral creditors (with 5.2%, 4.8% and 2.9% of claims, respectively). In March 2002, the World Bank in an independent evaluation of Bank assistance to Haiti from 1986 to 2001 concluded that 'the development impact of IDA lending had been negligible.' Yet under the current system the country is forced to bear the responsibility for these joint failures alone, and this debt has sat on Haiti's books ever since. Worse still, in 2005 Haiti used US$40 million of its scarce international reserves to clear arrears to the IDA on precisely these same debts. The case for debt cancellation is therefore extremely strong. Haiti must have debt relief as of now!

There is no question that Haiti urgently needs comprehensive bilateral and multilateral debt cancellation. Some could argue therefore that Haiti's progression to decision-point status under the HIPC Initiative should be welcomed. Haiti is the poorest country in Latin America and the Caribbean, and amongst the poorest in the world. Income per capita stood at just US$450 in 2005, according to the World Bank. Around 78% of Haiti's population live on less than US$2 per day, and 54% live on less than US$1. Just 53% of adults are literate, and only 55% of 6- to 12-year-olds attend school. Both health and education services are provided by predominantly non-public entities. This means that most of them charge fees which citizens just cannot afford. Yet Haiti was only recently 're-categorized' as an HIPC by the World Bank, and had until now, and for no apparent reason, been left out of all international debt reduction initiatives despite such dire (and deteriorating) socio-economic indicators and development challenges. So should this new development for Haiti be embraced?

Debt relief under the HIPC Initiative will undoubtedly contribute to creating a certain degree of fiscal space for much needed poverty-related expenditures. Indeed, in the country's decision-point document the Haitian Government has stated its intention to use debt-relief savings in the education, health, water supply and sanitation sectors, environmental protection and natural disaster avoidance. Individual expenditure priorities include the training of new teachers, provision of new teaching materials, a school feeding programme, improving the availability of drugs, extending immunization, purchase of supplies for maternity clinics, and improved potable water supply in rural areas. These are ambitious aims which are (understandably) likely to fuel domestic expectations, yet the World Bank and the IMF admit that there will be 'relatively limited resources from HIPC assistance', and in 2006–07, even after the provision of HIPC Initiative assistance, debt service as a percentage of government revenue will reach as much as 14.6%.

But in a rich world how could such a thing happen? Why are there such 'limited resources' from HIPC assistance, despite such clear need?

The World Bank and the IMF have assessed the amount of debt reduction to be granted to Haiti in order to reduce the country's debt to export ratio to the debt sustainability threshold of 150%. However, a more detailed examination of Haiti's decision-point document reveals that the IMF and the World Bank have assumed average economic growth rates of 4.2% between 2006 and 2025 in order to arrive at a cancellation figure of US$140.3 million. Worryingly, however, Haiti's growth has averaged just 1% over the last 10 years. This logically begs the question of why such optimistic economic growth rates have been forecast.

The World Bank and the IMF argue that, despite overall low growth rates over the last half century, these have largely reflected periods of political instability. If one excludes these periods of political turbulence from the economic simulations, growth has averaged around 4.5% annually, in particular in the 1970s fuelled by investment in light manufacturing and the development of tourism. However, given the IFIs' track record in accurately projecting the growth performance of countries within the HIPC Initiative programme, many civil society campaigners may question whether these assumptions are at all valid.

It is true that Haiti will benefit from a more comprehensive write-down of its IDA debt under the MDRI, but this will only be granted at the very earliest two years down the line, upon satisfactory completion of the HIPC Initiative. Interim debt service relief in the mean time is based on the above assumptions. Moreover, there are no IMF loans eligible for inclusion in the MDRI, because they were disbursed after the cut-off date of the end of 2004. In November 2006, the IMF approved US$109.5 million in new loans for Haiti under the Poverty Reduction and Growth Facility (PRGF). These new disbursements will be covered by neither the HIPC Initiative nor the MDRI, and will go straight back on to Haiti's balance sheet.

This is ironic, because in the same decision-point paper, the World Bank and the IMF make an undisputed case for urgent and deeper debt cancellation. The IMF and World Bank have conducted a detailed debt sustainability analysis of Haiti, and flag the potential for future debt distress in the event of lower export or economic growth rates. These 'stress tests' reveal the real extent of Haiti's sustained socio-economic vulnerability. The document projects that if economic growth does not increase by the projected 4.2%, and is instead a full 2 percentage points lower, Haiti will once again be unsustainable by 2025. Worse still, if export performance is lower than projected, Haiti could once again be unsustainable as soon as 2011, according to the paper. Thus, argue the IMF and the World Bank, Haiti's export performance is vital to economic reinvigoration and to avoid future unsustainable debt. However, the emphasis on exports, while food security remains a key concern, may sound alarm bells for many local groups. In addition to these vulnerabilities, Haiti will remain extremely dependent on often volatile external donor assistance for over 50% of the government budget.

Finally, on the issue of sustainability, some might say that it comes as no great surprise that the IMF and the World Bank are quick to point the finger at Venezuela and highlight its potential rôle in aggravating Haiti's debt sustainability profile over the medium term. Haiti has recently concluded an agreement to obtain new concessional finance from Venezuela under the PetroCaribe Agreement. Under the deal, Haiti will pay 60% of the price of its oil imports up front, and will pay the remaining 40% over 25 years with a 2-year grace period at 1% interest. The grant element is highly concessional at an estimated 49%. Despite the highly concessional nature of the deal, the World Bank and the IMF say that they are concerned that repayments to PetroCaribe could reach as much as 1% of GDP in 2013. If Haiti does not use the resources from PetroCaribe in investment projects which generate a high return, this deal could worsen the country's medium-term outlook. Clearly such deals must be closely scrutinized, but it is also obvious that these concerns actually highlight the need for more, not less, and immediate, not 'somewhere down the line', debt cancellation from all of Haiti's multilateral and bilateral creditors.

Haiti faces a bewildering array of conditionalities over the next 2 years if it is to reach completion point on schedule. These span macroeconomic conditionalities, public financial management and governance, tax policy and administration, social sectors and external debt management. The IMF and the World Bank describe these conditionalities as 'essential to the success of the HIPC Initiative.' However, Haiti's weak institutional capacities, continued security concerns and lack of trained personnel probably mean that many of these detailed reforms – which span the entire range of government activities and interventions – will be a challenge to implement. So what are some of the economic, governance and social conditions with which the Haitian Government will have to comply in order to progress through the HIPC Initiative?

There are plans 'to improve the management of public enterprises and road maintenance. The Government will modernize public enterprises to increase their efficiency and maximize their profitability. Particular emphasis will be given to improving governance and transparency.' Whether this means privatization is not clear. The central bank will be reformed and part of it will be sold in a recapitalization operation. Investment and tax laws are to be revised in order to spur private sector development, which the World Bank and the IMF describe as 'key' to economic growth in the country. In many other HIPCs, this has generally translated into corporate tax breaks which have not spurred the increases in private investment and job creation that were hoped for, nor have they generated significant revenues for the host government.

And like other HIPCs before it, Haiti will also undertake significant public sector reforms, including the 'rationalization of employment and salary policy.' In other countries, such as the Honduras, this meant large lay-offs and wage ceilings for public sector employees, which in turn have generated significant social unrest. Further reforms span strengthening customs controls and public expenditure management, increasing agricultural productivity and diversification, protection of private property rights, strengthening procurement procedures and key audit reforms. Although some of these measures will arguably improve transparency and accountability, enabling local citizens to hold their government to account, the Haitian authorities have openly voiced their concern that these reforms will be difficult to implement and will delay much needed debt cancellation.

## What next?

Several groups in Haiti and elsewhere have protested that the HIPC Initiative is not what Haiti needs. Haiti needs immediate debt cancellation. The only condition some groups feel should apply is that the funds freed up via cancellation be open to public scrutiny and invested in priority-area poverty reduction expenditure. No more than that. Given the above considerations, the case for this position is extremely strong. Regrettably, it seems as if the international community has opted for the 'business as usual' approach. Paris Club creditors – which hold 14.4% of claims on Haiti – met and confirmed their commitment to reduce Haiti's debt stock, but only 'as soon as Haiti reaches the completion point.'

Neoliberalism strikes again! In July 2007, Belgium, Canada, Denmark, France, Germany, Italy, the Netherlands, Spain, the UK and the USA met and agreed on a restructuring package for Haiti rather than an immediate and comprehensive cancellation. Under the terms of the package, interest payments have been deferred until 2010, and just US$7.2 million have been written off. More claims will only be written off if Haiti satisfactorily completes all the requirements of the HIPC Initiative. We may also assume that this 'exceptional' assistance will count towards donors' ODA. Given Haiti's critical state, it is all very sad, and it represents yet another wasted opportunity to do the right thing now in support of Haiti's people and the MDGs. In this context, civil society organizations locally and around the globe will continue to campaign vigorously for the cancellation of Haiti's debts today – and not tomorrow.

It is said of Wolfgang Amadeus Mozart that during the last year of his tragically – and unnecessarily – brief life, he was suffering severe and debilitating attacks of colic. The medical treatment of the day (1791) consisted of doses of a mercury compound! Poor Wolfgang, who one assumes had even less medical insight than did the physicians of his day, reacted when the colic attacks persisted by taking more of the lethal medicine, until it eventually killed him. Haiti's experiences with neoliberally inspired IMF and WTO practices, along with those of other HIPCs, are analogous to those of the great composer. Can their salvation really lie in 'more of the same', or must an alternative way forward be found? For when we speak of 'sustainable debt', much rests on what we mean by 'sustainable.' If disadvantaged countries continue along the neoliberal road, as people like Gavan Mooney and Vicente Navarro have shown, their debt becomes even less 'sustainable' and, closely correlated with this, the health and well-being of their citizens become increasingly mortgaged to banks and corporations in the First World. Truly, the WHO has been auctioned off!

However, before we discuss the signal contributions of Navarro and Mooney in more detail, let us look at how Eurodad regards debt sustainability.[18] When is an emerging or developing country's debt 'sustainable'? Considering the debt crisis that has characterized much of the last three decades, this may sound an odd question to ask. The humanitarian catastrophes that the world witnesses every single day, and the overwhelming lack of resources that these countries can devote to basic human needs such as health, education, shelter and security – not to mention minimal state infrastructure – simply seem to point to the fact that no debt at all is sustainable when considering the developing world.

Indeed, during the 1980s and early 1990s it had already become so obvious that much Third World indebtedness was unsustainable, and in many cases just plain unpayable, that First World creditors – and their supranational arms such as the World Bank and the IMF– implicitly acknowledged this with limited debt cancellations being granted through the Paris Club process. This was then followed, trying a slightly more systemic approach, by the two (1996–99) HIPC Initiatives and, finally, by the recent MDRI (in 2005), which – falsely – claims '100%' relief for the poorest of the poor.

Unfortunately, reality does bite. Even this latter round of relief – which encompasses a mere 27 out of more than 50 indebted poor countries and covers only three multilateral institutions (the IMF and the World Bank, as well as the

African Development Bank) out of 19 – does not do enough to free debtors from the slavery of debt and enable them to stand financially on their own feet. Once again the notion of sustainability that is applied merely considers the financial capacity to repay their creditors, and withholds any inclusion of, for instance, the availability of resources needed to cater to at least the basic needs of their people, and thereby achieve the MDGs. It is an approach that does not put forward the type of generalized, open and dynamic solution to a problem that will resurface again within a few years. Moreover, it is a logic which by limiting its angle to the financial side of things does not guard against renewed unsustainability and the resulting recurrence of the debt crises.

Hence one fundamentally sound path forward is the elaboration and subsequent implementation of a type of debt sustainability – within a fair and transparent process – which at any point in time would make available resources against those needed to satisfy a developing country's basic necessities. Those needs can be established by whichever MDGs have been agreed to by both debtor and creditor governments. Only then should the financial resources in excess, and what can be considered for debt repayment, be calculated. This method, to be applied to every country struggling to reach these objectives, is the only way to guarantee that basic yet unyielding principles of equity and justice are achieved. The understanding of the importance of the antagonistic kinds of 'sustainability' is key to the conception of an alternative to the creditors' approach. To do so, it is crucial to realize that it is not a neutrally technical question to be left to specialists, but rather an intensely political one that basically asks on what grounds the rich can be repaid when the poor are starving.

One final but profoundly important point is that the actual legitimacy of the debt, and its ultimate sustainability, has necessarily been addressed in the foregoing analysis. This is somehow set aside. On the contrary, these threads actually complement and reinforce each other. Indeed, it is this author's conviction that the evaluation of whether a debt is sustainable begins only after all illegitimate debts have been taken off the books, because these simply should not enjoy any status, and should therefore be declared void. After having excluded all illegitimate debts, it could nonetheless be the case that a country's debt is still unsustainable when considering it from the human needs perspective, and this justifies the constructive and positive integration of these two notions.

The notions of debt sustainability and illegitimate debt appeal to two very distinct concepts of justice. Illegitimate debt tries to take into account the historical dimension of debt. It aims at an analysis of how debt was accumulated and whether this process of incurring debt took place in accordance with certain ethical standards. As the object in question is a process over time, we shall call the according concept of justice 'historical justice.' The concept of sustainability appeals to the moral question of what is needed to secure human development in the future. To do so it appeals to the concept of 'justice as fairness' – that is, what would be an appropriate level of debt considering the various restrictions placed on debt service by ethical questions concerning human development.

As debt sustainability and illegitimate debt are based on two different moral concepts, there are no reasons why one notion of justice should be comparable to (or even more important than) the other. Both are essential, and both have to be pursued with great vigour and confidence.

## A SUMMARY OF RECENT NEOLIBERALISM VS. HEALTH ARGUMENTS

As was stated at the beginning of this chapter, two books are of critical value in coherently and exhaustively putting forward the virtually unassailable argument that not only is neoliberalism not the only way left for rationalizing the world's economic problems, but also it can be shown statistically that it is bad for the health of people to whom it is applied. These books are:

1 McIntyre D, Mooney G, editors. *The Economics of Health Equity.* Cambridge: Cambridge University Press; 2007.
2 Navarro V, editor. *Neoliberalism, Globalization and Inequalities: consequences for health and quality of life.* Amityville, NY: Baywood Publishing Co.; 2007.

The author was fortunate enough to have attended the first day of a conference in Copenhagen in July 2007, at which all three of these authors spoke about their work. Navarro's presentation emphasized the fact that First World advocates of neoliberalism are the way forward for LDCs, and conveniently forgot that none of the OECD (Organisation for Economic Cooperation and Development) countries got where they are today by reducing government expenditure on public sector services! Navarro cited a comment made by John Williamson, known as the 'father of the neoliberal Washington Consensus', who reportedly said that 'We have to recognize that what the US government promotes abroad, it does not follow at home.'[19] In fact in most of those countries there has been a growth of public expenditure – not a decline, and certainly not starting off with next to none. Expressed as percentages of GNP and also per person, the figures for the USA are as follows. In 1980, 34% of the GNP (or US$4148 per person) was so spent, while in 2003 the corresponding figures were 37% of the GNP (or US$13 758 per person).

In addition, and again using the USA as an example, there has been an increase in taxes as a percentage of the GNP. The taxation figures (minus payroll tax) were 32% for 1980 and 36% for 2003. Altogether federal input into public expenditures increased from 21.6% of GNP to 23% of GNP. In fact, during Ronald Reagan's presidency, taxes increased twice. He increased the tax burden (in peace time) of a greater number of people than did any other US president. His 'conservative' credentials, it is true, resulted in a tax reduction for the richest 20%, but they resulted in tax increases for everyone else.

And, as this author has pointed out in a previous book,[20] US citizens do not have a universal, free-at-point-of-access healthcare system as people in the UK do. Yet US citizens pay just over 14% of the GNP on their tax for healthcare, while in the UK the figure is about 7%. In other words, as far as healthcare is concerned, the more closely a society is run on neoliberal principles, the less effective it is in providing healthcare. In the USA, about 30% of the people have no access to private health insurance (because they cannot afford the premiums), while only 43% of the remainder benefit from government-provided healthcare (under Medicaid and Medicare), and these systems – even at that – are not comprehensive. In fact, the degree of access differs from state to state – for example, a particular medical condition may be covered in Oregon but not in California. Obviously the introduction of private finance for such social services as health and education renders them less economically efficient!

As Navarro also points out, neoliberalism – both within a country and in its foreign dealings – distorts not so much the actual amount of reduction in 'social expenditure' as the way in which it is allocated. Thus in 1980 in the USA, public expenditure was as follows: 38% to persons; 41% to the military; and 23% to private enterprise. In 2000, the corresponding figures were 32% to persons (a decrease), 45% to the military (an increase), and 23% to private enterprise (an increase). Navarro also pointed out many of the international impacts of neoliberalism on health that we have already discussed earlier in this book, such as higher mortality rates, etc., but in particular illustrating how the 'dominant class' (in, say, the USA) interrelates with the 'dominant class' in, say, Saudi Arabia. That is, as observed before, neoliberalism is not constrained by loyalty to national country or culture, but by profits to be made. This should surprise no one, but does not recommend it as a good basis for equitable global economics.

One telling example used by Navarro to illustrate the point was the situation in Bangladesh. In that country (as in many others) the root of persistent malnutrition in the midst of 'relative' plenty is the unequal distribution of land. That word 'relative' is important in this context. In Bangladesh, few people are 'rich' by First World standards, but severe inequalities do prevail and they are reflected in highly skewed land ownership. For instance, the wealthiest 16% of the people control two-thirds of the land, while about 10% of Bangladeshis survive on less than an acre of land. To follow the argument, though, the reader must be reminded of the fact that the 'dominant classes' of various countries and cultures, have a greater affinity with First World 'dominant classes' than they do with their own countrymen.

New agricultural techniques, and the associated machinery, are sold by the First World 'dominant classes' (who thereby become even richer) to the 'dominant classes' in Bangladesh, thus enhancing the latter's scope for domination. This favours the larger farmers, for instance, putting them in a better position to buy out those who have so little already. In addition, the government in Bangladesh is dominated by land owners (about 75% of Members of Parliament are big land owners). In the UK, the USA and many other First World countries the basic situation is not that different, except that the 'medium of domination' in those countries tends to be industrial ownership rather than land ownership.

Moreover, food aid officials in Bangladesh admit that only a fraction of the huge tonnage of food given as aid actually reaches the poor. The food is given to the government, which in turn sells it at subsidised prices to the military, the police and others in the 'dominant class.' Despite the heart-breaking poverty that one sees in Bangladesh, in reality there is more than enough for everyone in the country. In fact the land is so good for agriculture that even if the population increases greatly over the next two decades (which has been predicted on the basis of current trends) there would still be enough food for all – if it was equitably distributed. Again, however, this raises the question that has already been considered several times in earlier chapters of this book. How can market forces and competition under neoliberalism result in such equity?

These considerations bring us right back to the Alma Ata Declaration and its insistence that healthcare must be a political activity (based on social and cultural data) rather than a purely clinical one. Neoliberalism and privatization have nothing to offer in this and, if introduced, only produce health inequities. In other words, healthy people cannot really remain healthy unless their health is a universal social good. As Navarro said in his Copenhagen presentation, 'To improve your health, you have to improve other people's health.' This does not only apply to communities. We are called upon to render it global by participating in worldwide groups, and to realize ourselves through others.

He ended his presentation in the following words, in which the political, economic and social context is realized in the Alma Ata (Health for All) concept:

### Political, Economic and Social Context as a Basis For Health

1. **Participation and democracy** – to encourage a sense of participation and collective life. Alienation is not good for health.
2. **Economic and social security** – to feel sure, and not be worried and anxious about your job, standard of living or retirement.
3. **Good, safe and healthy working environment** – to have a satisfactory job.
4. **Good, safe and healthy residential environment** – to like and enjoy your house and your community.
5. **Good, secure and favourable conditions during childhood and adolescence** – choose well your parents. If you can't, then make sure that children and adolescents are healthy and have equal opportunities.
6. **Good public health services and good, accessible and comfortable medical care services.**
7. **Effective protection against communicable diseases** – maintain basic hygiene practices.
8. **Good eating practices and safe food** – enjoy eating, do it moderately, and avoid food poisoning. Denounce unhealthy conditions in eating places.
9. **Safe sexuality and good reproductive health** – enjoy sex, in moderation, and don't get pregnant or make someone else pregnant unless the two of you want it. And if you get pregnant, make sure you stay healthy in case you want to have the child.

10. **Avoid tobacco and drugs like the pest** – you can take wine (preferably from Catalonia), however, with moderation. Red wine is healthier than white wine. [At this point the author would comment that, according to recent medical studies, much more than a glass of red wine a day can have negative consequences, strongly supporting the caveat 'with moderation.' *Medical News Today*[21] reported, about two weeks after Navarro's comments, on a large-scale study which suggested that drinking more than a unit of red wine a day (an average wine glassful) could increase one's risk of bowel cancer by 40%.]

11. **Physical exercise** – it is very good to allocate at least half an hour a day to it. Even better if you walk for one hour. Don't leave all the physical exercise for the weekend. It is not good!

12. **Be solidarious and believe strongly in some good causes** – to be self-centred, narcissist or neurotic – a regular Woody Allen type – is not good for your health. You should commit yourself with others who also want to change society. Political and social commitment (particularly to parties who believe in redistributing resources) is very good for your health and for the health of the community and of your society. Solidarity is cool and healthy.

## REFERENCES

1 Navaroo V, editor. *Neoliberalism, Globalization and Inequalities: consequences for health and quality of life.* Amityville, NY: Baywood Publishing Co.; 2007.

2 McIntyre D, Mooney G, editors. *The Economics of Health Equity.* Cambridge: Cambridge University Press; 2007.

3 Hayes S. *Health and Healing: private profit from public misery*; http://methodius.blogspot.com/search/label/neoliberalism (accessed 10 August 2007).

4 Joseph Rowntree Trust. *Poverty and Wealth Across Britain From 1968–2005*; www.jrf.org.uk/KNOWLEDGE/findings/housing/2077.asp (accessed 28 June 2007).

5 Weiner L. www.wpunj.edu/newpol/issue38/weiner38.htm (accessed 28 June 2007).

6 MacDonald T. *The Basic Human Right to Health: dream or possibility?* Oxford: Radcliffe Publishing; 2007. pp. 197–8.

7 Elliott L. Anti-poverty targets in Africa will not be met, UN warns. *Guardian*, 3 July 2007, p. 3.

8 Share the World's Resources. *The Wealth Gap Widens as the Rich Use Debt as a Financial Tool. Business Report, 29 March 2007*; www.stwr.net/content/view/1743/37 (accessed 10 August 2007).

9 Roberts G. The rich get richer – everywhere (editorial comment). *Wall Street Journal*, 7 July 2007, p. 6.

10 The rich man's debt trap (editorial). *Wall Street Journal*, 26 January 2007, p. 9.

11 Macan-Markar M. *Decades After Meltdown IMF Less Relevant in Asia*; www.stwr.net/content/view/2010/36 (accessed 10 August 2007).

12 MacDonald T. *Health, Human Rights and the United Nations: inconsistent aims and inherent contradictions.* Oxford: Radcliffe Publishing; 2007. p. 175.

13 MacDonald T. *Basic Concepts in Statistics and Epidemiology.* Oxford: Radcliffe Publishing; 2007. pp. 141–7.

14 Basu K. *Globalization, Poverty and Inequality. What is the relationship? What can be done?*; http://ucatalas.ucsc.edu/blog/?p=52 (accessed 12 August 2007).

15 World Bank. *World Development Indicators.* Washington, DC: World Bank; 2004.

16 Eurodad. *Aims and Objectives of Eurodad*; www.eurodad.org/whatsnew/articles.aspx?id=844-21k (accessed 8 August 2007).

17 Hurley G. *Tiny Ecuador in the Spotlight as Government Seeks to Renegotiate Debt on its Terms*; www.canim.org/article.php3?id_article-2669 (accessed 13 August 2007).

18 Eurodad. *To Pay or To Develop: debt sustainability handbook*; www.eurodad.org/debt/report.aspx?id118&item=0482 (accessed 13 August 2007).

19 Williamson J. *What Washington Means by the Policy Reform.* Washington, DC: Institute for International Economics; 1996.

20 MacDonald T, op. cit., pp. 30–34.

21 Lifetime and Baseline Alcohol Intake and Risk of Colon and Rectal Cancers in the European Prospective Investigation into Cancer and Nutrition (EPIC). Main article in the *International Journal of Cancer*, 31 July 2007. Printed on-line: www.medicalnewstoday.com/article/78391.php-48k (accessed 13 December 2007).

# Chapter 8

# Is the WHO mandate workable?

## THE 'REALISTIC' VIEW

The WHO mandate, as we know, was crystallized in the Alma Ata Declaration of 1978, which recognized that 'health' was as much (if not more than) a political as a clinical issue. This realization allowed the WHO to elaborate an ambitious scheme for dramatically reducing the global health equity gap by the end of the millennium. It was called the 'Health for All' (HFA) 2000 Campaign and – as the WHO was a UN agency – part and parcel of the UN's commitment to human rights as proclaimed in the latter's UDHR. At the time, many critics regarded this as ideological 'pie in the sky' sloganeering and totally 'unrealistic.'

As we have seen in the preceding chapters, this has consistently been the view of the rapidly burgeoning forces of neoliberalism. In fact, in a recent issue of the *Lancet*,[1] one of that journal's book reviewers describes how she had been so angered by an editorial in *The Economist*, which dismissed much chatter about social and economic rights as nonsense, that she wrote in to them, opposing their view and asking if they had ever heard of the Universal Declaration of Human Rights. She goes on to comment:

> The response I got from one of the editors left me stunned. 'I am of course aware that economic and social rights feature in the UDHR and elsewhere. The 'right' to a job, education, health, etc. sounds superficially attractive, but in practice it is either pernicious or meaningless. It would be more honest if the defenders of these economic, social and cultural rights would come straight out and say that they believe that socialism is the answer, and campaign for it, rather than dressing up their demands for more state intervention in the legalistic language of rights.'

Of course many of those who make such demands do indeed believe that socialism is the answer – and they may well be right. It is certainly difficult to think of any other way of achieving it, unless we are prepared to believe in such urban myths as the trickle-down effect! However, leaving that aside for the moment, that *Economist* writer's stance is just one other example of the dangerous assumption that somehow the human race has reached the end of social history and that neoliberalism is the acme of untold generations of wrestling with the problem. It is the very best humanity can do. It can best be summed up in the oft-repeated comment that 'It is unrealistic!'

We are constrained to ask the following question. Are there any existing and tangible alternatives to neoliberalism? Without implying any necessity for brutal totalitarianism, the present author would say that an outstanding alternative to the inevitability or ultimate 'realism' of neoliberalism does exist already, and that is Cuba. Of course, neoliberalism is not only the antithesis of Cuban social policy, but can also only survive in a world without the Cuban counter-example around to disturb it. However, Cuba is an awkward customer. It not only runs, eminently successfully, an HFA policy in its own country, but it has also had the temerity to share it with others worldwide. That is, Cuba has shown us not only that there is nothing intrinsically unrealistic about HFA, but that HFA cannot be established without something very similar to an 'Alma Ata insight' behind it.

## CUBA: THE ROAD TO ALMA ATA

Much has been written both about Cuba's remarkable educational system and how it was achieved and, likewise, about its impressive healthcare system. The latter has put Cuba – an economically insignificant little country – on as high a health index as the UK, and with better health indices than the USA. Without the 'benefit' of neoliberalism, it has the highest health index of any Third World country.[2] No other country in the world has one fully qualified family health specialist physician – along with a small team of health promotion advisers and social workers – available for every 200 or so people anywhere in the country. However, even more alarmingly (for the neoliberal realists) this came about *because* Cuba found by direct experience that 'health' is inseparable from civic society, community economics, politics and education. That is, they had found the 'Alma Ata Road' even earlier than 1978!

Even worse (again, from the neoliberal perspective), their 'social policy', 'community policy' or whatever you wish to call it insists that they share their community health breakthrough freely with other countries (which shows a complete disregard for neoliberalism!). And these 'other countries' are by no means all Third World countries, as US citizens and others from the First World have benefited from Cuba's medical generosity. It is here that their application of the link between health and politics (which in 1978 became the basis of the Alma Ata Declaration) became manifest in the Cuban experience.

In the two years immediately following the 'triumph of the revolution' (as Cuban propaganda delights in phrasing it!), from 1959 to 1961, Cuba mounted a most extraordinary literacy campaign. It is described in detail in a previous book by the author,[3] and was so remarkably successful – and continues to be – that it attracted worldwide attention, regular UNESCO analysis,[4] and was also exported to other Third World countries. Cuba realized, even back then, that literacy was basic to effective community involvement and the promotion of public health.

However, even Cuba could never have anticipated just how fertile this connection would turn out to be in developing a community consciousness and the awareness of the essential 'indivisibility' of health rights worldwide called for by the Millennium Development Goals (MDGs). For, unlike literacy campaigns attempted in other countries, the Cuban campaign did not lapse back into widespread illiteracy again once the campaign itself had run its energetic course. The reason for this is that, in the context of the Cuban Revolution, the transition from illiteracy to literacy had an immediate impact on the social, cultural and political rights of the beneficiaries. A peasant had barely become literate him- or herself, when he or she was then expected to teach someone else! The slogan was 'Each one, teach one!.' Masses of those literacy students, perceiving the significance of literacy for health and community involvement, demanded more and more, as the author describes, and the whole country became engaged in a learning revolution.[5]

In 1959, there were only two universities and one medical school in Cuba. By 1974, there were 18 of each! And Cuban doctors and other health workers were already fanning out to all parts of the Third World. These achievements were firmly based on the social character of the Cuban education system which, from pre-school level (*circulos infantiles*) upward, emphasized 'respect and responsibility for one another' and 'internationalism.' Almost every school system in the world has some kind of ritual to start the day. In the USA, for instance, all students swear allegiance to the flag. In Cuba, the students say in unison '*Seremos como Che. Somos internacionalistas!*' ['We shall be like Che. We are internationalists.'] This kind of indoctrination has an impact over the years, especially as these values are also promoted outside school, in the wider community.

From such roots, Cuba has developed a system of social/ public health that encompasses much more than individuals being treated for specific medical conditions. Indeed, when this author lived and worked in Cuba, it seemed to exemplify the broad principles of health promotion, with its emphasis on empowerment. With so few people on any one doctor's list, and with doctors living in the same neighbourhood, there is an easy social ambience based on mutual recognition and respect. The doctor's children would be attending the same school as those of his or her patients, and they would all recognize one another. The doctor routinely visits the homes of all of the people on his list – remember that he only has around 200 – and dispenses advice not only about health, but also about childcare, behaviour problems, etc. As an editorial in *Public Affairs Magazine* commented as far back as 2000, the story of Cuba's healthcare development between 1959 and 1999 surpassed even the most optimistic expectations.[6]

The turn-around in Cuba's healthcare delivery system these past four decades is the marvel of the world. Every world authority, including many of our own, has taken note. In 1959, as the embryonic revolutionary government started its rebuilding processes, there were three medical schools in Cuba, six blood banks, and an expected death of all other vital medical services. They obviously served the wealthy. Of the 9000 physicians, nearly 6000 fled for points north, and Fidel had to stop the medical haemorrhage. He applied a 'Band-Aid' by making a 'deal' with the archdiocese that ran a medical school in Santa Clara, and then started major initiations in healing and rehabilitation.

The original polyclinic system that opened up satellite health stations on all parts of the island, some of which had never seen a single medical officer, was discontinued in the 1980s in favour of the now established family health care system. The island today has 39 medical training centres, 75 blood banks and full services that reach the most remote parts of the country. Mountain-top villages, accessible only by horse and wagon or chain-driven vehicles, have doctors and nurses in attendance at all times.

The most remote areas have full service hospitals and clinics, with transportation available to the tertiary medical centres in Havana and other urban centres.

## THE GLOBAL IMPACT OF CUBAN HEALTHCARE

Cuba's achievements with regard to healthcare in its own country give us some idea of what the WHO could do if it were not impeded in the ways we have already documented by the UN's involvement with neoliberalism. However, even more remarkable has been Cuba's influence on healthcare in other areas of the world. This influence has expressed itself broadly in two ways – first, by Cuba acting as a global medical facility to which other nations can send 'difficult' cases, and secondly, by Cuba acting as a doctor on call, sending medical teams to countries that require basic health services to be set up.

With regard to Cuba acting as a global clinic, one can cite many examples. For instance, as far back as 2003, the *World Press Review* printed an article[7] by a Russian medical specialist writing from Havana. He marvelled that, even though Cuba was a poor Third World country itself, with not a lot to offer in its shops, it was so ready to reflect its social policy of internationalism. The following observations are drawn from his report.

> In the Havana airport, pale people in wheelchairs and groups of children with a feverish glint in their eyes are barely noticeable among noisy crowds of tourists. There are not too many of them, but there are some on almost every foreign plane landing at the airport of the Cuban capital. These are the people who have come to Cuba seeking medical treatment.

Numerous Cuban clinics and sanatoria are successfully treating thousands of cancer patients every year. Over a period of 10 years, 18 000 citizens of Russia and the Ukraine have undergone treatment in Cuba without having to pay a single kopeck. So how did a small tropical republic manage to create the best healthcare system in Latin America?

'You are asking where the billions of dollars we receive from foreign tourists go? You think the money is spent on new uniforms and false beards for Fidel?' laughs a government official in Havana. 'Take a tour of our hospitals, clinics, and rehabilitation facilities – you will find the answer to your question there. Exactly half of all the currency earned in our country goes toward the healthcare system, and it is our policy to spare no expense for that purpose. Maybe there is no gasoline in Cuba to fill the car up before heading off to work in the morning, and they don't have meat for lunch everywhere, but at least the people are healthy.'

This brings out another aspect of a health policy that is free from restraints imposed by neoliberalism – and that is Cuba's remarkable advances in medical diagnoses and treatment. These were dealt with in part by the author in 2002[8] and, with regard to more recent advances, in an important analysis by Fawthrop.[9] Generally speaking, though, we can say that without doubt the successes of Cuba in the area of healthcare are amazing, especially if one takes into account the fact that the country was on the verge of economic collapse after the former Soviet Union ended its generous financial aid programme. Physicians from leading clinics in the USA come to Cuba in secret (officially it is forbidden for US citizens to visit Cuba) to acquaint themselves with Cuban experience and practices, according to officials at the Russian Embassy in Havana. They illegally purchase medications, such as the famous Cuban vaccine for meningitis, which is produced nowhere else in the world. Then there are the Cuban physicians who have developed a drug to treat hepatitis B. With regard to treatment for cancerous tumours, the Cubans are well ahead of many of the world's developed countries.

Che Guevara, the renowned revolutionary, who once owned a popular, inexpensive clinic in Argentina, is taken to be the founding father of the Cuban healthcare system. It was he, a physician by profession, who launched the reforms that eventually transformed the country into the leader in healthcare throughout Latin America. The formula was incredibly simple – no matter what happened in the country, reducing expenditure on the health of the people was categorically forbidden. Even immediately after 1991, the year in which aid from the former Soviet Union was ended – when plants stopped operating, public buses didn't run, and shops were empty – no one in the government even suggested reducing healthcare expenditure.

The powerful combination of an educational system strongly oriented toward mutualism and internationalism and a medical system guided by what are easily recognized as 'Alma Ata-type' principles has made a huge impact globally in drawing people to Cuba itself, as described above. However, even greater has been the impact of Cuban health teams travelling around the globe performing medical services that very often a WHO crippled by Structural Adjustment Policies (SAPs) and other neoliberal intrusions cannot. As we know, from 1948 to 1988 the WHO itself was making great strides with its health teams doing similar work. Indeed, this is what the WHO was intended to be all about.

Cuba's international efforts have taken two distinct forms – first, sending in health teams to establish primary healthcare, to build clinics, train local people, etc., and secondly, sending in emergency teams to respond to health emergencies created by major natural disasters, such as earthquakes, tsunamis, hurricanes, etc. These activities will be discussed in greater detail below, but first let us examine a few practical impacts of Cuba's health philosophy in Cuba itself.

## LOCAL EFFECTS OF CUBAN HEALTHCARE

Since 1959, Cuba has made extraordinary advances in the development of 'hi-tech' approaches to both diagnosis and treatment. It has also made significant contributions in the field of genetic engineering. At the level of treatment, Cuba has gained an international reputation in surgery. This is a very pronounced aspect of Cuban medicine and, as this author[2] has frequently pointed out, it has distinguished Cuban health input even since pre-revolutionary days. The difference now, though, is that before 1959 much of the required training was carried out abroad, especially in the USA. If one glances through a directory of surgeons in the American Medical Association (AMA), one cannot help but notice the high frequency of Cuban surnames! But today, of course, Cuba has the necessary infrastructure to 'operate from home', so to speak.

An example of this is eye surgery. Over the last 3 years alone (from 2004 to 2007), according to a report by Cuba Solidarity,[10] Cuba has provided eye surgery free of charge to 700 000 patients. Most of these have come from Latin America and the Caribbean, but some have come from much further afield. Due to the enthusiastic reports from patients returning to Brazil, this programme was dubbed by newspapers there as 'Operation Miracle', and that name has stuck.

As the Cuban article describes it, Dr Mercelino Rio Torres, Director of the Havana Ramon Pando Ophthalmological Institute, where the first Venezuelan patients were treated, stated that Fidel Castro himself visited the centre in July 2004. He formally launched the project at that time, although of course it was already up and running. During its first year after that formal inauguration, it provided surgery for 14 000 people.

The aim of Operation Miracle is to reduce blindness, primarily in Latin America and the Caribbean, by treating 6 million people by 2014. Some of these operations will be carried out by centre staff in the home countries of the patients, using local facilities. To support such a vast undertaking, Cuba has constructed nearly 40 specialist units in Bolivia, Ecuador, Guatemala, Haiti, Honduras, Mali (in Africa), Nicaragua, Panama and Venezuela. As of 2007, about 600 Cuban health professionals are working in these units.

Yet another extraordinary contribution has been the elaboration of vaccines. Several significant contributions could be mentioned, but perhaps the single greatest impact has been that on meningococcal meningitis. Even parents in the First World are filled with terror at the prospect of their children acquiring this disease, as the onset is usually sudden and the outcome is often fatal. In fact, it is now the biggest killer of children under 4 years old in the First World.

However, according to BBC News,[11] Cuba has (after 7 years of research) been developing a vaccine against meningitis B since late in 2003, and routinely vaccinating babies under 1 year of age with it. Since that time Cuba has had no deaths from the disease. The Cubans developed their vaccine after the country suffered its worst death rate from meningitis B in 1986. Some would say that fortune has smiled on Cuba in this regard because – in contrast to most of the First World countries – there happened to be fewer variants of the B virus in Cuba, and this made it easier to isolate samples for vaccine production.

Since the focus of the WHO, from its inception, was to be creating global equity in primary healthcare, it is of interest to study Cuba's success in this regard – both in its own country and, more recently, on a global scale. The issue has attracted worldwide interest among medical researchers. Dr Francisco Onchoa, a Professor at the National School of Public Health in Havana, produced a summary of the details in 2003, which was published in 2004.[12]

He comments that a coherent approach to primary healthcare had not really been feasible before the revolution, but proceeded very quickly after that. The Cuban government passed the necessary legislation (Law 723) in 1960, which created Cuba's Rural Medical Services (RMS). It offered new medical graduates a contract to work in the rural context. The contract required a minimum commitment of 6 months, on the promise that a broader range of medical posts would then be made available to them. A total of 318 graduates (out of 330) signed up. In subsequent years, about 400 graduates participated, while 347 medical graduates plus 46 dentists were involved in the third period, once Law 919 for Rural Dental Services had been passed. In 1973, a total of 1265 professionals were registered in this service for a 2-year period. By then, 100% of the graduates had joined this service, as it had become a tradition since 1965 to renounce private practice in the graduates' oath.

From the very start, the primary healthcare functions of the RMS assigned to a hospital or doctor's office (called a Rural Medical Post) were directed to medical care, epidemiological surveillance, vaccination, health inspection, health education and forensic procedures. Note the early intention to integrate services.

The RMS was the first programme to have an impact in relation to primary healthcare and public health in general. The reasons why this was made a priority include the long abandonment (in terms of healthcare and other services) endured by the rural population through the years of Cuba's colonial and republican history, the clear awareness of this situation by the Revolution's leaders, due to their close interaction with farmers during their fight in the mountains (against Bastista), political commitment to the farmers who had themselves been fighters in the Rebel Army, and the fact that these health (and educational) services would be a perfect complement to the Agrarian Reform, which was the central policy in the Revolution's early years, and the engine for economic development.

Simultaneously with the implementation of the RMS, Health Units were set up in the small towns that were the seats of each municipality. These carried out primary healthcare tasks, including ambulatory care for patients in the programmes for tuberculosis, leprosy, venereal diseases, pregnancy, children's acute diarrhoeas, and malnutrition in children. They conducted vaccination drives, administered waste disposal services, and carried out health inspections. These units integrated some vertical programmes which had existed since the previous administration, such as those for leprosy, cutaneous diseases and syphilis prophylaxis (LCDSP) and tuberculosis control. All of these Health Units later took up all primary healthcare functions in the urban areas of their municipalities, managing the First-Aid Houses that still existed and also the Children's Dispensaries of the National Children's Dispensaries Organization (NCDO), which had been dissolved and integrated into the Ministry of Public Health. This confirms the fact that the idea of service integration was applied from very early times.[13]

In those early years, the primary healthcare movement, closely coordinating its work with health services and prompted by health education activities, generated community initiatives for health. These initiatives were first expressed in the Rural Health Posts, then in the Volunteer Collaborators of the National Service to Eradicate Malaria (NSAP), and later in the Health Coordinators of the Committees for the Defence of the Revolution and the Health Brigades of the Cuban Women's Federation. Social workers from the Ministry of Welfare in each rural area supported primary healthcare services for as long as this ministry existed.

Primary healthcare also naturally includes midwifery services. The first unit devoted exclusively to this was created in 1962. Local Cubans regarded them with a high degree of warmth and good humour. This author was puzzled by the fact that lay people referred to them as 'Casas de las Trocas' ('Houses of Tricks'), and when he asked why, the answer was 'Because only two go in, but three come out!'

The next major breakthrough in primary healthcare, and community-based medicine generally, occurred only a few years later.

In 1964, the comprehensive polyclinic was created, an institution that was to become the core of primary healthcare in the years ahead. There were already some units described as polyclinics, but their scope was limited to doctors' visits with outpatients. These new polyclinics were put to the test by having to minister to a population of 45 000 inhabitants over a 9 km$^2$ area. Furthermore, innovations were introduced in the polyclinics, including keeping family records as an expression of the proposed comprehensive family care policy, making population groups, implementing damage or disease-oriented programmes (e.g. for tuberculosis, venereal diseases, infant mortality and acute diarrhoeic diseases), encouraging community participation, and carrying out immunization programmes and health education. Doctors' offices services were also strengthened.

The proposition was made to generalize the comprehensive polyclinic experiment on the basis of the results achieved at the Aleyda Fernández Chardiet Polyclinic under the leadership of Dr Roberto Fernández Elias. Polyclinics were defined as:[14]

❑ medical institutions which develop activities for the promotion, protection and recovery of health for the population of a geographically determined area, by means of services that cover the whole family

❑   institutions whose main goal is to offer basic health services, extending across their communities by means of their field personnel, within certain geographical limits which are called 'health areas.'

Polyclinics are found in most countries, but in Cuba they are the fulcrum of community health, not only looking after medical cases as such, but also providing outreaches into health promotion, child psychology, etc. In many ways they are one of the jewels in the crown of Cuba's elaborate and multi-faceted healthcare system. By 1964, comprehensive polyclinics were the action point in healthcare – the next step after the family doctor's surgery.

However, even they became a focus for wide and critical public scrutiny. Indeed, one of the distinguishing features of Cuban society policy is that it is very much a bottom-up phenomenon. Cubans can (and do) complain, and have many avenues for doing so. One of the commonest is at local meetings of the Committee for the Defence of the Revolution (CDR). It should be explained that all Cubans even children – belong to a CDR. In urban areas, there is a CDR for approximately every city block, and local participants take turns to host the regular monthly meetings and determine dates and times and agendas for the regular meetings as well as for any extra ones that might be desired.

The Cuban climate generally allows the meetings to take place outside, with people simply bringing chairs out into the street. At CDR meetings any issue of concern to anyone attending can be discussed. Attendance is not compulsory, and children drift in and out without let or hindrance. And it was at CDRs that complaints about those first comprehensive polyclinics were articulated. By 1974, five main shortcomings had been identified, and it was decided to address them by means of appropriate reforms. These categories of complaint were as follows:

1   The polyclinics were supposed to be integrated with primary healthcare and with other medical facilities, but this had not happened. They had become little clinical enclaves, often reflecting specialist interests of the staff.
2   They were too medicalized, treating social problems that caused distress too dismissively.
3   Teamwork among the staff was often conspicuous by its absence. Don't forget that the people who were making these complaints were well used to shouting the odds at CDR meetings – and could they yell!
4   The professional staff often left on the spur of the moment to work in the big hospitals.
5   Far too often the polyclinics simply got rid of awkward patients by sending them on to the local hospital.
6   Doctors received hardly any training at polyclinics, but mainly in hospital settings.

This diagnosis brought about a new model for primary healthcare, which was called community medicine, and its core institution, the community polyclinic. An experimental test was carried out at the Alamar Polyclinic, which is now named after the director who led the experiment, Dr Mario Escalona Reguera. Innovations in the new model have been described by Dr Ana M Más Hernández in her specialization thesis ('Primary Health Care in Cuba: Its Organization and Historical Evolution', School of Public Health, Havana, 1998).

These units are expected to carry out actions to implement the area's basic programmes, grouped together in a coherent manner to care for people and the environment. They are classified as follows:

**I Programmes for the Care of Persons**
Children's Comprehensive Care Programme
Women's Comprehensive Care Programme
Adults' Comprehensive Care Programme
Comprehensive Dental Care Programme
Epidemiological Control

**II Programmes for the Care of the Environment**
Urban and Rural Hygiene
Food Hygiene
Medicine for the Workplace

**III Service Optimization Programme**

**IV Management Programme**

While many people in the First World were just starting to get used to health promotion in the late 1970s, the Cubans were already sufficiently empowered by community values and the country's social policies to change the character of their polyclinics! Indeed, Cuban life reflects a multitude of such examples of 'bottom-up' initiation of policy formulation.

Another innovation in this period was the introduction of the concept of the health team, and encouraging teamwork, according to the Community Polyclinic Programme published by the Ministry of Public Health ('Foundations to a New Approach to Community Medicine.' Havana, undated, but around 1972–74). The phenomenon is described in that manual as follows:

> All polyclinic staff are part of the area's health team. The primary team is formed by a small group of specialists who act together to tackle specific tasks, with very close contact among its members. Examples of these teams are the sanitation brigades or the paediatrician and the nurse's aide. The former example would make a vertical primary team, as it is composed of individuals with the same profession or activity. The second example is a horizontal primary team, integrated by personnel with different categories or professions, thus being interdisciplinary . . . In the model proposed, these horizontal teams are composed of a doctor (internist, obstetrician-gynaecologist or paediatrician), and the nursing staff, each of which is responsible for one sector or a certain number of inhabitants.

In addition, this model defines measures that are aimed at ensuring comprehensive teamwork, coordinated by vertical teams, or carrying out actions that involve social workers. Guidelines are also given in the document for encouraging and coordinating the community's active participation in protecting the public's health, attaching particular importance to their role in health education.

In Cuba, the Alma Ata spirit had really taken root and the government's social policies prevented it from being swamped by neoliberalism.

## CUBA'S MEDICAL USE OF NEOLIBERALISM

As Tom Fawthrop[15] points out, Cuba has not been reluctant to use neoliberal methodology to generate money – both for its medical activities in Third World countries and for its domestic health needs. For one thing, it exports its pharmaceutical products, vaccines and biotechnology quite openly in countries that can afford to pay for them, including Brazil and Argentina. For instance, its vaccine against meningitis B (discussed above) has been licensed to GlaxoSmithKline. They will market it in Europe and, they hope, eventually in the USA itself.

Cuba has also been a target of health tourism since the early 1960s. This author has described elsewhere[16] his rather amusing discovery that, as early as 1961, Cuba was selling cosmetic surgery to Americans who were anxious to have it but unable to pay the high US prices. Typically the 'patient' would arrive and stay in a motel in Havana for one night and then undergo the requisite surgery the next day. They would spend a few days in hospital and then return to the comforts of the motel, from where they would report daily for a medical check-up for about another week, before returning to the USA. The price all in, including the motel stay and meals, was often only a fraction of what the medical treatment alone would have cost back home.

Fawthrop's paper[15] reports that health tourism remains a lucrative source of US dollars. He observes that in 2006 in excess of 5000 people travelled to Cuba for a whole range of medical treatments, including eye surgery, neurological disorders such as Parkinson's disease and multiple sclerosis, and orthopaedic surgery. In particular, Cuba's controversial treatment for the eye condition retinitis pigmentosa has attracted large numbers of patients from the EU countries. In total, health tourism generates about US$40 million a year.

However, US authorities have been extremely energetic in trying to cut off this source of hard currency. Neoliberalism will not remain inactive in the face of Cuba's inventiveness. For instance, the US Helms-Burton Act not only prohibits US firms from trading with Cuba, but also interferes directly with other countries that are trying to sell goods or services to Cuba. For instance, the Helms-Burton legislation rules that any country trying to do business on a commercial basis with Cuba can be barred from trading at all with the USA, or the USA with it. In the face of such draconian intervention, most important sources of much needed hard currency cave in. Even the UK, companies that organize tours to Cuba for British people have been blocked in this way and the survival of their businesses threatened. Barclay's Bank, to cite another example, is prevented from mediating financial transactions between UK professionals who want to offer services – including medical services – in Cuba. In this regard, Hilton Hotels, a US-owned firm, has famously refused to accede to this intimidation. At a recent international conference held at a Hilton Hotel, the hotel management was threatened with legal action if they allowed Cuban delegates to stay there. However, the hotel argued that for them to follow this order would put them in breach of UK anti-discrimination legislation! At the time of writing (2007), the stand-off has not yet been resolved.

Despite all of this, though, there still remain many examples of how Cuba profits by selling its medical technology abroad. Indeed, its now multi-million-dollar biotechnology industry is attracting renewed opposition and legal resistance from US corporate sources. If such opposition succeeds, Cuba's economy really will be seriously threatened, for it benefited immensely from this industry from 1990 onward. For instance, Heber Biotech SA (Semi Autonomous) is a public-private company created in 1991 by the Cuban government for the sole purpose of marketing high-tech pharmaceuticals. By 1998 it was marketing an indigenous interferon (for cancer treatment), the above-mentioned hepatitis B vaccine and an advanced streptokinase drug that dissolves coronary clots.

Extraordinarily, another Cuban biotechnological invention which – although not itself of any direct medical significance – has generated huge sums for Cuba's public health system is a method for cloning food fish that 'will grow twice as fast as the usual variety.' In November 1998, this 'transgenic fish' was Cuba's centrepiece exhibit at a 5-day biotechnology conference held in Havana.

Much of this activity was reported in an article in the *Miami Herald* in Florida,[17] from which much of the following detail is derived.

> High-Tech Pharmaceuticals is now selling products in 34 countries. Among them are the afore-mentioned indigenously developed interferon, a hepatitis B vaccine and an advance streptokinase drug that destroys coronary clots.
>
> With annual sales as high as $290 million a year, Heber, Sotolongo's Finlay Institute and other centres in Cuba's biotech industry, by 1998, ranked behind only tourism, nickel production and tobacco as the country's largest export earner. And it is poised for even bigger growth in the years ahead.
>
> The Finlay Institute's high-tech Plant No. 3 is the cornerstone of that expansion effort. Packed with more than $100 million in state-of-the-art imported equipment, the factory has the capacity to produce 100 million doses of vaccines every year – more than double what it has marketed in the past. And the institute has prepared slick brochures and marketing campaigns to advertise its potential worldwide.
>
> The Biotechnology Habana '98 Transgenesis conference scheduled to open on November 16 was subtitled 'From the Laboratory to the Market', and it included commercial endeavours once unthinkable in this communist state. Exhibit space, for instance, rented at US$50 per square foot. And Heber Biotech,

marketing itself under the slogan 'Approaching Horizons', in 2000 had offices or direct business relations in more than 50 countries, and it boasted that its sales increased more than sixfold between 1992 and 1996.

Through much of its 50-year revolutionary history, Cuba's biotechnology research industry focused almost entirely on preventing and curing diseases at home – an island nation where medicines were scarce, largely because of the USA's punishing trade embargo.

However, after the collapse of the former Soviet Union, Cuba lost billions of dollars that kept its socialist economy afloat. The government was forced to inventory its state industries for potential exports to raise money that it needed to continue subsidising food and providing free education and healthcare. Its biotechnology industry emerged near the top of the list.

In recent years, the government has invested hundreds of millions of dollars in biotechnology facilities and research. This has created something of a technology gap – scientists using advanced genetic techniques to clone fish in a land where the US embargo has made antibiotics scarce on hospital shelves, and smoke-belching, 1950s-vintage Chevy's and Buick's commonplace on the streets!

Dr Mario Pablo Estrada, who heads the above-mentioned fish transgenetic project, explains the phenomenon with simple mathematics: 'With $7 million, we couldn't even begin to produce our own basic medicines.' He said that the latter are far more costly to mass-produce than highly specialized 'niche' products such as vaccines.

'But with a $7 million investment here at the genetic research centre', he said, 'we made by 1998 $30 million in sales, and we can use that to buy a lot of basic medicines.'

Estrada conceded that the European and US biotechnology markets are highly competitive, and that Cuba will need 'very strong joint-venture partners' such as SmithKline to penetrate them. US market analysts, who confirmed that Cuba does have state-of-the-art research and production capability, agreed that Cuba's entry into the global biotechnology market will be an uphill battle.

Still, US–Cuba trade experts, backed by the US scientists familiar with Cuba's work, say that the key to Cuba's success so far in biotechnology has not been the financial incentive. They credit the talent of Cuba's mostly young scientists – along with the ability of a one-party state to minimize internal competition and bureaucracy – as the chief reasons for the medical breakthroughs.

The US scientists said that the Cubans' safety and research standards equal or even exceed those of the US Federal Drug Administration and the European Union. And if a poor Third World country could do so much, just imagine what the WHO could do! However, it is Cuba's extensive network of medicine services that really illustrates the eminent feasibility of a global application of the Alma Ata principles.

Cuba's contribution to the developing world's health workforce has been essentially a practical one, focusing on healthcare delivery and medical education.

Since 1960, over 100 000 Cuban health professionals have served in 101 countries, staffing public health infrastructures, and over 21 000 students from Africa, Latin America, Asia and the Caribbean are currently enrolled in Cuban medical schools, not counting those in nursing and allied health professions. More will be said later about a truly remarkable Cuban system for training foreign doctors.

This collaboration has evolved over time. The first Cuban medical team was sent to earthquake-devastated Chile in 1960, when the two governments had no formal relations. Such disaster-relief missions were dispatched to another 16 countries over the next decades, but were soon overtaken by a more long-term modality. By virtue of government-to-government agreements, Cuban health professionals (the vast majority of physicians) began to provide healthcare to underserved populations and regions in Africa, Latin America, the Caribbean and Asia.[18] Since the 1963 request from the Algerian government of Prime Minister Ahmed Ben Bella (bereft of physicians at the end of French occupation), a further 100 governments have initiated pacts with Cuba for a sustained presence of Cuban health professionals in their countries' healthcare delivery programmes – six in the 1960s, 22 in the 1970s, 11 in the 1980s, 47 in the 1990s, and 15 since 2000.

The fact that half of this cooperation began in the 1990s attests to developments in Cuba's own health system during that time, which made larger numbers of physicians available for international service, and also reinforced Cuban health authorities' commitment to primary care as key to improving health status. In particular, by mid-decade, the neighbourhood-based family doctor and nurse programme was in place across the country, and by 1999 it covered 98.3% of Cuba's 11 million people. The programme was the culmination of a process of embedding health services more deeply into communities, aimed at more effective health promotion and disease prevention efforts. As a result, curricula in Cuba's 21 medical schools were revised, and a residency in family medicine was created, increasing the number of graduates annually to cover needs at home and growing interest from other countries. By the end of the decade, Cuba had nearly 30 000 family physicians, and a total of some 60 000 doctors – more than all of sub-Saharan Africa. By 2005, the island's physician population had reached over 70 000.[19]

The other factor that explained the jump in cooperation during the 1990s was external. In 1998, Hurricanes George and Mitch swept Central America and the Caribbean, leaving 2.4 million people homeless. Cuban medical teams, which were initially deployed on an emergency basis, stayed on at the request of several governments under Cuba's Comprehensive Health Programme (CHP), created in response to the region's crisis and later expanded to include a total of 27 countries in Latin America, the Caribbean, Africa and Asia. By way of example, in May 2006 there were 448 Cuban health professionals in Guatemala, 426 in Haiti, 113 in Belize, 347 in Honduras, 93 in Botswana, 188 in Ghana, 109 in Mali, 134 in the Gambia, 143 in Namibia and 278 in East Timor.

Under these agreements, the host country provides accommodation and food, domestic transportation, a locale for work, and a monthly stipend (usually

US$150–200), while Cuban personnel receive their regular salaries, airfare and other logistical support from the Cuban health ministry. In arrangements outside the CHP with wealthier countries such as South Africa, the host government pays additional hard-currency salary, part of which is kept by the professionals and part of which is remitted to the Cuban health ministry.

In July 2006, a total of 28 664 Cuban health professionals were serving abroad in 68 countries. In each country, the thrust of Cuban assistance has been to bolster public health infrastructures, providing the often desperately needed staff in remote areas – some in hospitals, but mainly in primary care clinics and medical posts – where local governments have been unsuccessful in attracting local physicians to the public sector. In several countries, including Honduras, Haiti, Guatemala, Mali, South Africa and the Gambia, there are whole regions where the Cubans have been the first bearers of local physician services to rural, indigenous and other marginalized communities. They also carry with them the Cuban philosophy of combining population-based public health principles and prevention with clinical medicine.

On other levels, Cuban medical scientists and advisers have participated in the design of public health departments and systems, and in epidemiological research and campaigns aimed at tackling specific health problems (e.g. malaria in several African countries, dengue in El Salvador and Honduras, cholera in South Africa). They have also worked with health ministries to devise more reliable statistical record-keeping and information systems in many countries, especially those which have so far had the weakest infrastructures.[20]

Health professionals on the ground participate and often lead local courses for midwives and other community-based health personnel, and participate in more formal training for paramedical and allied health professionals. Most recently, Cuban biomedical engineers and technical support have been increasingly in demand, repairing nearly 55 000 pieces of medical equipment since 1999.[3]

Cuban coverage has resulted in an increase in patient care levels in poor communities, according to statistics kept by the medical teams. For the 22 countries in the CHP by 2004, from November 1999 to February 2004 this translated into 36.7 million doctors' visits, 917 381 surgeries, 397 636 deliveries, 11.9 million health promotion activities, and medical education courses for 910 120 local health personnel, including midwives. Health status has also improved in areas where Cuban doctors serve. In Guatemala, the infant mortality rate dropped from 45 to 16.8 deaths per 1000 live births, in the Gambia it dropped from 121 to 61, and in Haiti it dropped from 59.4 to 33, between 1999 and 2003.[21]

Recently, Cuba has taken a more proactive role in initiating trilateral collaboration, in which a third country or agency donates resources for health programmes developed between Cuba and another nation. This was the case for the 2001–2002 vaccination drive in Haiti, when Cuban epidemiologists and family doctors teamed up with Haitian health authorities to immunize 800 000 children against five childhood diseases. Funds from the French government and 2 million doses of vaccines from the Japanese government completed the triangle. The

German government contributed to Cuban projects in Niger and Honduras, the South African government donated US$1 million for Cuban medical cooperation with Mali, and the WHO has supported Cuban collaboration in the Gambia and elsewhere. According to the Cuban government, 95 non-government organizations worldwide contributed to CHP projects between 1999 and 2004.[22]

Since 2000, Cuba has launched four special cooperation initiatives. One focuses on HIV/AIDS in 19 countries, through joint projects in prevention and treatment (Botswana, Honduras, Mali and Haiti among them), and in 2001, Cuban officials offered African countries 4000 doctors and other health professionals, medical school professors, a stock of antiretroviral drugs and diagnostic equipment to help to combat the epidemic.

The second initiative, begun in 2003, makes a major commitment to Venezuela, a country with one of the greatest discrepancies between rich and poor in South America. The Venezuelan government's 'Barrio Adentro' programme relies on around 20 000 Cuban family doctors to provide health services and health education in medically underserved communities ranging from the shanty towns of Caracas to the jungle riverbanks of Amazonas State. The agreement falls under the ALBA accords (Bolivarian Alternative for the Americas), offered as a South-South alternative to the Free Trade Area of the Americas (FTAA), in which several Latin American and Caribbean countries now participate – the principle being that each brings to the table the resources at its disposal to be used for social programmes bilaterally and throughout the region. Thus in the case of Cuba and Venezuela, the arrangement is often referred to in the international press as 'oil for doctors.'

The third initiative is a vision restoration programme, begun in mid-2004, which addresses the condition of the estimated 6 million people in Latin America and the Caribbean who have reversible blindness or vision loss due to cataracts and other conditions, but who are too poor to pay for the surgery in their own countries. From the inception of the programme in 2004 through to July 2006, a total of 317 489 patients from 27 countries had been treated (including 69 000 Cubans). Ophthalmology centres have also been opened in Ecuador, Bolivia and Mali under this programme, which receives support from local governments as well as the ALBA accords.[23]

The fourth new initiative is the Henry Reeve Disaster Response Contingent, originally consisting of around 1500 physicians offered to the USA in the wake of Hurricane Katrina. When the Bush administration turned down the offer, the contingent was established as a permanent volunteer corps and given special training, ready to be dispatched to disaster areas within 24 hours. Their first mission was in October 2005, when 2500 health professionals travelled with 32 field hospitals to earthquake-stricken Pakistan, where they remained for 5 months. Since then, the contingent has also been dispatched to Guatemala, Indonesia and Bolivia. The contingent builds upon earlier Cuban cooperation in disaster relief since the 1960 earthquake in Chile, which took Cuban health professionals to Nicaragua, Honduras, and several other countries thereafter. The treatment in Cuba of over 17 000 children of the Chernobyl nuclear disaster is also part of this history.

Over time, Cuba's South-South cooperation has faced endless challenges – the political and social instability besetting many developing countries, the sheer size of the effort and resources needed to make a dent in the poorest countries' health status (sometimes straining domestic health facilities), barriers to access and treatment found in the various health systems staffed by Cubans, initial concerns from in-country medical associations fearful of job displacement, the need to expand the skill set of Cuban physicians serving abroad (who confront circumstances and infectious diseases long absent from the Cuban health picture), and the unabating effects of the US embargo (which continue to generate barriers for Cuban healthcare at home and abroad).

## CUBAN DISASTER TEAMS IN ACTION WORLDWIDE

Natural disasters are horrors that do not respect borders or political ideologies. They seem to happen at random and usually without adequate warning. One only has to recall such recent ones as the tsunami in December 2004, the earthquake in Pakistan in October 2005, and the horrific catalogue of hurricanes, mud-slides, etc., mainly in Latin and Central America and the Caribbean. These disasters are the natural arena for WHO health teams, and indeed they were involved. For the moment, let us briefly consider the Pakistan earthquake. It attracted a vast and impressive display of worldwide compassion and desire to help. The major countries, both at government level and at the level of private citizens, virtually competed with one another to send aid. Not mentioned much (except sneeringly on Fox News) was Cuba's response, but in fact Cuba's initial aid input *and* its maintenance over time beat those of much richer nations hands down. It just wouldn't be decent to admit that a country that describes itself as 'communist' could do such a thing, so we don't speak of it as we doze off in front of our mind-cleansing TVs. The earthquake itself claimed 75 000 lives and caused at least 120 000 serious injuries that required surgical intervention, all within the first fortnight. The *real* disaster of lingering deaths from pneumonia and other illnesses then set in. Cuba sent 2465 medical workers, including 1430 qualified doctors. While most of the aid teams from the big countries had left within 5 weeks, and dropped off the TV news (a case of compassion fatigue), the Cubans stayed for 8 months. Some teams were still there in November 2006. They had treated just over 1 million people for injury and/or disease, and carried out 12 400 surgical interventions. More importantly, they left behind 32 fully equipped hospitals. No other country had done so much!

How can tiny Cuba organize such massive responses so quickly? It takes an incredible level of managerial skill, and can only operate in the kind of context which Kofi Annan called for in launching the MDGs. As discussed above, he observed that the MDGs could only work if individual governments could learn to put global needs ahead of national advantage. However, in a world dominated by the neoliberal canons of competition, it is asking rather a lot for any nation to put anything at all ahead of its own desperate clawing for a 'place in the sun.' Self-advantage will dominate its thinking. It is conspicuous, especially in the light of the following, that Cuba is not unduly hampered by such an impediment.

## CUBAN RESPONSES TO GLOBAL DISASTERS

Conner Cory has produced a through analysis of the incredible phenomenon of Cuban international medical involvement with two Third World countries, namely Pakistan and Guatemala.[24] This author has come across such teams in Angola, Mozambique, South Africa, Malawi, Ghana, Nigeria, Nepal, India, Grenada and many others. Moreover, while teaching postgraduate healthcare students, he has heard large numbers of students from all over the world comment on their positive memories of Cuban health teams building clinics, giving advice about public health and – more often than not – linked up with literacy teams teaching reading and writing to huge classes of hitherto disempowered adults.

Consider the following quote from Cory's paper:

> Mothers swing pick axes and claw at the mud, searching for loved ones buried in the rubble. Rotting corpses and shortages of food, water and medicine threaten survivors, while relief efforts are hampered by impassable roads or inclement weather. This same, desperate scene is repeating itself from Guatemala to Pakistan, where catastrophic natural disasters have shaken these nations to the core.
>
> The aftermath is horrific, with entire communities entombed in Guatemala and Pakistan, while nearly 1,000,000 are displaced in Mexico, and a dengue outbreak grips El Salvador in separate post-disaster scenarios. To help save survivors of such events is the goal of Cuba's Henry Reeve International Team of Medical Specialists in Disasters and Epidemics.
>
> Units of this specialized, rapid-response volunteer team of health professionals are now serving in Guatemala and Pakistan, their expenses assumed by the Cuban government.

Cory goes on to describe how Cuban teams proceeded. These teams are called Henry Reeve teams. The history behind this is that Henry Reeve was an American, born in Brooklyn in 1850, who fought in the US Civil War and then went to Cuba to fight on their side against the Spanish colonialists in 1869. He was killed in battle in 1976, and is revered in Cuba today as one of their heroes. By attaching his name to its overseas medical brigades, the Cuban government – never slow to miss a good piece of propaganda – illustrated the social significance of the courageous work of these brigades.

The specialized rapid health brigade alluded to in the last sentence of Cory's quote above was a Henry Reeve Brigade. It was drawn up initially in response to Hurricane Katrina, which so dominated the media in 2005 because of the devastation it inflicted on New Orleans. However, that hurricane also wreaked havoc in a number of other areas. The Cuban mobile team was staffed by 1586 medical professionals, each carrying about 20 kg of medicines, in addition to their other equipment.

In a ceremony on 19 September 2005, Cuba formally constituted the International Team, the founding members of which collectively possess an average of 10 years' clinical experience and service in 43 countries. Predictably, the USA rejected Cuba's offer to send these medical professionals to the Gulf States during the ongoing post-Katrina relief effort.

Now 3000 strong, the team's members are required to speak at least two languages, take postgraduate courses in epidemiology, and be physically fit. They also receive specialized training in medical assistance during epidemics and pandemics, and HIV prevention methods and treatment for people suffering from HIV/AIDS.

'We're ready and willing to go anywhere we're needed', said Dr Dayane González, 'whether it's Cuba, the United States, wherever.' Dr Gonzalez' colleague and fellow team member Dr Alexander Martínez echoed this sentiment when asked to which country he preferred to travel. 'We're trained to serve and help save lives; wherever that's necessary, I'm willing to go.'

And what a need there always is. Several hundred specialists are currently serving alongside local and other international health workers in post-earthquake Pakistan, and in Central America in the wake of Hurricanes Stan and Wilma. Although each disaster scenario presents specific challenges, the circumstances in which the Henry Reeve Teams are working to save lives are both tragic and extremely difficult.

Guatemala, with over 840 people missing and 650 dead following Hurricane Stan, was the first country to accept the Henry Reeve doctors, 300 of whom began arriving on 8 October, each carrying medicine-filled backpacks to treat acute diarrhoea, respiratory illnesses, skin afflictions, malaria, dengue and other illnesses. By the end of October 2005, the Cuban Henry Reeve volunteers in Guatemala numbered 600.

Among their ranks are surgeons, paediatricians, internists, vector specialists and epidemiologists. These professionals supplement the 235 Cuban doctors on long-term stints in Guatemala, providing rural primary healthcare services as part of the ongoing Comprehensive Health Programme (CHP). The CHP was established between Cuba and several Central American countries following Hurricane Mitch in 1998, as a more sustainable way of addressing the underlying health problems of these countries.

Speaking from Guatemala, Dr Yoandra Muro, head of the Cuban CHP team there, said that 'the situation is very difficult and our main goal now is to prevent epidemics, which we have done, despite outbreaks.' The Cuban doctors have also been going from house to house as part of a prevention campaign in which they inquire about general health – particularly fevers and diarrhoea – and talk to families about measures such as the need to boil drinking water. The strategy has paid off according to Muro, who believes that basics like this have saved many lives, especially among children.

As new Cuban volunteers arrived in Guatemala on 8 October 2005, an earthquake measuring 7.6 on the Richter Scale ripped across northern Pakistan, killing upwards of 73 000 people and seriously injuring another 69 000, according to Pakistan's Chief of Disaster Response. The death toll was predicted to rise as relief teams made their way into previously inaccessible areas.

As many as 3 million people were instantly made homeless – three times the number in Asia's tsunami of December 2004 – as the bitter winter approached. Relief officials announced recently that there were not even enough winter-weather tents in the world to house these people! Into this situation arrived 200 Cuban doctors – including surgeons, anaesthetists, internists and trauma specialists – one of the largest groups of foreign doctors to come to Pakistan's aid.

Later, planeloads of physicians dramatically increased the original number, so that eventually there were over 900 Cuban doctors serving in Pakistan. Further supplies pledged by Cuba to the Pakistan relief effort included three field hospitals and hundreds of winterized tents.

By January 2006, the Cuban team had divided among three hospitals, one in central Islamabad, which received patients airlifted to the capital for care. 'We're working very intensely in 12-hour shifts', said one Cuban volunteer at the time. 'It's astonishing the number of children we're treating, especially for trauma.'

Cuban medical teams have been providing international disaster aid for 45 years, beginning in 1960 when the twentieth century's most violent earthquake struck Chile, killing 5000 people. Since then, Cuba has provided post-disaster medical and technical assistance to nearly a dozen countries.

Recognition of Cuban expertise in preparation for and response to disaster prompted the UN Development Programme (UNDP) and the Association of Caribbean States to select Havana as the headquarters for the new Cross-Cultural Network for Disaster Risk Reduction, to facilitate regional cooperation in disaster management.

Keeping a universal public health system with such international solidarity underpinnings as Cuba's well staffed in terms of both quantity and quality is an ongoing challenge. On 19 September 2006, in the same ceremony officially constituting the new international disaster and epidemics team, 1905 new doctors graduated from Cuban medical schools across the country.

Increased opportunities to study health science careers have also boosted enrolment. In the academic year 2005–06, 95 595 Cuban students were enrolled in medicine, nursing, dentistry, clinical psychology and university-level allied health sciences.

Impressive as all of the foregoing may be, it fails to consider what must be one of the world's most impressive public health enterprises, namely ELMA (Escuela Latinoamericano de Medicina). This 'Escuela' is like no other medical school, for all of its students are drawn from other countries, and not only pay no fees, but are fully provided for during the 6 years that they spend in Cuba on the course. The students, in turn, agree to return to their own countries and donate their services to improving public health.

However, just before we consider this remarkable innovation, readers can gain some insight into the selfless internationalism expected of Cuba's medical graduates. The following is an extract from the Cuban Medical Graduates' Oath, taken on 19 September 2005 by the graduating class in Havana.

> **Cuban Medical Graduates' Oath, 2005**
>
> **We pledge:**
> To strive always to be worthy representatives of Cuban health professionals, devoting ourselves with true love to our profession, with a profound respect for human life, feeling the pain of others as our own, seeing in each patient and their family our own loved ones, and working tirelessly towards excellence in health services.
>
> **We pledge:**
> To make every effort, every day to improve ourselves professionally, politically and culturally, so as to offer the highest quality care to our people, based on the principles of medical ethics and revolutionary values that reject commercialization, corruption, and the mistreatment of people wherever we may find ourselves.
>
> **We pledge:**
> To serve the revolution unconditionally wherever we are needed, with the premise that true medicine is not that which cures, but that which prevents, whether in an isolated community on our island or in any sister country of the world, where we will always be the standard bearers of solidarity and internationalism.

By the 1990s, the vast experience that Cuba amassed in sending individual brigades long distances, either to establish primary healthcare facilities in poor countries or in response to catastrophes, had made feasible the idea of actually setting up a medical school to teach students from far-flung countries. In fact, tradition has it that Che Guevara (himself a medical doctor) suggested the idea to Fidel Castro, who then implemented it in 1999.

## CUBA'S MEDICAL SCHOOL FOR THE WORLD

Cuba's extraordinary undertaking in setting up a medical school with the specific aim of training foreign students to become doctors represents a major step forward from its already famous policy of sending doctors abroad. However, even now there is some confusion about these two policies, and specifically about the names used to describe them. The medical brigades which went to areas of the Third World – either to set up primary healthcare programmes as part of general aid, or in response to medical emergencies arising from natural disasters – became known collectively as La Escuela de las Americas. Thus this initiative was never centred at a specific location, campus or 'school' in the usual sense. The brigades were drawn from a wide variety of Cuban medical schools on a voluntary basis for each project. And the new name 'Escuela de las Americas' is still used to describe the initiative, even though the brigades are now sent all over the world. As noted previously, they played a huge rôle in both the aftermath of the tsunami of December 2004 in Indonesia, Sri Lanka, India and other Asian countries, and the earthquake of October 2005 in Pakistan.

However, Che Guevara and others had long thought that a more effective procedure might be to actually set up a special medical school in Cuba itself and specifically train medical students from abroad. Most of these, it was suggested, should come from Third World countries, and would be required to return to their own countries at the end of their training to set up clinics and establish primary healthcare programmes for their own people. In 1999, as stated above, such a school was set up at an old naval hospital in Girón, not far from Havana. It is at this point that the above-mentioned confusion with names began!

At first the new medical school was called Escuela Latinoamericana de Ciencias Medica (ELCM). However, shortly afterwards its name was changed to Escuela Latinoamericana de Medicina (ELAM). Its medical course is identical to the one for Cuban doctors, and has been thoroughly inspected and validated by the WHO. To understand the discourse, it is important that the reader appreciates the functional difference between Esculela de las Americas (ELA) and ELAM (formerly ELCM). Both ELA and ELAM/ELCM still exist. It was originally assumed that ELAM/ELCM would render ELA redundant, but this has not happened. Indeed, some of the volunteers who served in the medical brigade that was sent to Pakistan in 2005 were ELAM students.

ELA is still active in carrying out the kind of interventional medical work that the WHO so vigorously prosecuted from 1948 to 1988, before it gradually became progressively undermined by neoliberal pressures. However, the WHO has never set up a free-of-charge medical school with the objective of training doctors from Third World countries for them to return to serve their own countries at the end of the course. In fact, the ELAM idea is virtually unique to Cuba. The reader will probably be aware that, in the 1960s, the former Soviet Union set up its Friendship University in Moscow, for Third World students, but it was not primarily, and certainly not exclusively, for training doctors.

It is interesting, and the author feels significant, to note the way in which the world's media reported and interpreted this Cuban initiative. Although the overwhelming majority of its students were drawn from less developed countries (LDCs), a few were attracted from the USA. Most of that small cohort were attracted for financial reasons (as reported below), while some came out of a mixture of curiosity and idealism. However, to read (and listen to) reports from the USA, the UK and the EU, one could be forgiven for assuming that the whole enterprise had been set up to embarrass the USA! To gain a broader perspective, one usually has to check other sources.

## ELAM GRADUATING CLASSES

On 24 July 2007, at the Higher Institute of Medical Sciences in Havana, 1806 new doctors graduated, including eight from the USA. To put that figure into perspective, at the same ceremony 664 Cuban doctors from various other medical schools in Cuba received their diplomas. Nationwide, 7078 other types of medical workers also graduated. At that graduation, the Cuban Health Minister José Ramón Balaguer commented that 53 000 students, from Cuba and 88 other countries, were at that time studying medicine in the country.[25] Balaguer proudly added that Cuban doctors – as of 2007 – are treating 60 million people worldwide.

Also present was the Reverend Lucius Walker, leader and founder of the Pastors for Peace organization. He was quoted as referring to the graduation as a 'significant and unprecedented event.' The Pastors for Peace are famous for circumventing the blockade by getting vital medical and technical equipment into Cuba – partly by relentless pressuring of public figures and partly by various clandestine methods.

The US graduates, like many young Latin Americans who have become doctors at the Cuban school, plan to return to their country and provide healthcare in poor neighbourhoods and communities. 'Cuba offered us full scholarships to study medicine here. In exchange, we commit ourselves to go back to our communities to provide healthcare to underserved people', said 30-year-old Carmen Landau, of Oakland, California, as quoted by Reuters news agency.

'We have studied medicine with a humanitarian approach', said 29-year-old Kenya Bingham, of Alameda, California. She added that 'healthcare is not seen as a business in Cuba. When you are sick, they are not going to try to charge you or turn you away if you don't have insurance.'

'The future is ours – the Americas and Africa are waiting for us', said Chilean graduate Katia Millarai Riviera as she spoke on behalf of all foreign graduates.

The graduation ceremony, held at Havana's Karl Marx Theatre, was also attended by Cuban Vice President Carlos Lage and other Cuban Communist Party Politburo members, including Jose Ramon Machado Venturea and Concepción Campa.

In total, 91 new US students enrolled for the academic year beginning in September 2007. The views of US students, both before and after training, suggest a number of things. Almost all of them were impressed by the focused nature of the course, with little time spent on overtly political issues or anything that could be regarded as 'propaganda.' Cuba's free and universally accessible healthcare system amazed many. Some of them found life in Cuba 'austere' (e.g. the lack of hot water for showers, etc.), but for the majority – from economically deprived backgrounds in the USA – such matters were of minor concern. Many of the US students were worried about the two sets of exams they will have to face on their return to the USA to be allowed to practise there – the State Board Exams and an exam in basic medicine. These must both be passed at 70% or better, and are required of all foreign medical graduates, not just the Cuban ones!

However, it is this author's view that they have little to worry about, because the course is well up to standard and includes all of the rigorous coursework found in the best medical schools worldwide. Not all of these students have an undergraduate degree (a requirement of all US medical schools), but they work hard, are highly motivated and have first-rate teachers. The US students were generally only given a week's notice that they had been accepted before having to be present for the first day of classes! However, they all accepted, dropping everything to do so, and those with children leaving them behind with parents.

One can say that they had all desperately wanted to attend medical school, but to do so back home they would have needed up to US$250 000. This was the deciding factor for some of them. Having to learn Spanish, as all instruction is in that language, was a worry for some, but did not prove to be a barrier for any of those who graduated in 2007. This is because during the first year they do an intensive course in Spanish for 8 hours a week.

It was not anticipated at the outset that US students would be applying. The change of policy came about as follows.[26,27]

In June 2000, a US Congressional Black Caucus (CBC) delegation visited Cuba to meet with Castro. Representative Bennie Thompson (D-Miss.) mentioned to Castro that his district had a shortage of doctors, and Castro responded by offering full scholarships for US nationals from Mississippi at ELAM. Later that same month, in a meeting with the CBC in Washington, DC, the Cuban Minister of Public Health expanded the offer to all districts represented by the CBC. At a speech event at Riverside Church, New York City, in September 2000, Castro publicly announced a further expanded offer which was reported as allowing several hundred places at ELAM for medical students from low-income communities from any part of the USA. Reports by the US press of the size of this offer varied – 250 or 500 places were suggested, with perhaps half reserved for African-Americans and half for Hispanics and Native Americans. The ELAM offer to US students was classified as a 'cultural exchange' programme by the US State Department in order to avoid the restrictions of the US embargo against Cuba. The first intake of US students into ELAM occurred in spring 2001, with 10 students enrolling in the pre-medical programme.

In 2004, the legality of the presence of US students at ELAM was threatened by tightened restrictions against travel to Cuba by US nationals under the administration of President George W Bush. A CBC campaign led by Representatives Barbara Lee (D-Calif.) and Charles Rangel (D-NY) with 27 other members of Congress persuaded Secretary of State Colin Powell to exempt ELAM from the tightened restrictions.

Applications from US citizens are administered through the New York City-based Interreligious Foundation for Community Organization (IFCO), headed by the noted human rights activist and critic of the US embargo of Cuba, the Reverend Lucius Walker, mentioned above as leader of the organization Pastors for Peace.

Naturally there is also a high degree of cooperation between Cuba and the new Venezuelan government of Hugo Chavez in training medical staff for that country. Some of those students are enrolled at ELAM, but most of them are attending ordinary Cuban medical schools. Considering foreign students from countries other than the USA, we learn that – initially in response to devastating hurricanes – Cuba set up a Comprehensive Health Programme (CHP) to help neighbouring countries which couldn't protect themselves in the way that Cuba itself could from the negative impacts of such hurricanes.

That is, CHP aimed to build in sustainability to Cuba's international health cooperation, and training foreign medical students in Cuba seemed to promise to replace the need for Cuban doctors to take over such post-disaster medical services.

By 2004, enrolment in the programme topped 9000, and by 2005 it hit the 10 000 mark. Government-to-government agreements have expanded the programme to 29 countries, and in the case of the USA, attracted students even in the absence of a bilateral accord. In all cases, the basic curriculum consists of a 3-month to 1-year pre-medical bridging course, which includes Spanish language for those who need it, 2 years of basic science at either the Havana or Santiago campus, followed by 4 years of clinical rotations, when students are dispersed to Cuban medical schools in all 14 provinces and train alongside Cuba's future physicians.[28]

However, as we have seen, the ELAM idea could be very much expanded by similar actions, with their more extensive resources, by the WHO. How will Cuba's initiative pan out in meeting the needs anticipated in selling it up? Will the majority of these graduates be the harbingers of a fundamental shift in the profession of medicine for the Third World, in desperate need of their services and commitment? Will they live up to their communities' expectations? Will they find jobs and make a difference? Or will they simply add to the internal and external migration of the developing world's professionals?

The answers – and the onus – lie more with the forces and structures outside Cuba than with those within it. Some of the region's public health systems are providing for the insertion of the new graduates, offering them posts in poor and especially indigenous communities. However, in others the IMF legacy freezing public health jobs makes it tougher for them to practise, and in yet others, local medical societies simply fear this new breed of public health doctor.

Yet one thing is absolutely clear – the need for these new physicians could not be greater, as indicated by the sobering statistics from the first graduating class of 2005. Factoring in both the Latin American Medical School and other foreign graduates in Cuba that year, the number of new doctors for the 47 countries of the developing world plus the USA totalled 1800. Those 47 countries, many of them in Africa, have an average ratio of 9.8 physicians per 10 000 inhabitants, compared with an average ratio of 30 in Europe and the USA, and nearly 60 in Cuba.[29]

Cuba provides us with so many more socially constructive responses to health problems than seem to be available under neoliberalism that this author often feels that – quite unintentionally – Cuba's social policies have become an embodiment of the Alma Ata spirit. One could cite hundreds of examples, but let us consider just one – although it is of very great relevance globally.

## CUBA CONFRONTS HIV/AIDS – AND CHANGES!

When Cuba was first faced with HIV/AIDS among its own people, its reaction was one familiar to many of us who have lived or worked in the Caribbean, and one that is still strongly evident in Jamaica today. It was a response based firmly on a fear and detestation of homosexuality. In 1985, when this author took a group of Australian teachers to Cuba, one of the group – during a visit to a large Cuba hospital – asked about the management of homosexuality and the newly emerging issue of AIDS in California. The response was that 'Homosexuality does not exist in Cuba because it is the product of capitalist social relations!'

How quickly and dramatically they changed their views and their social policies with them! This is yet another example of Cuban social policy often being a result of a 'bottom-up' (no pun intended!) approach, rather than the professionally led 'top-down' approach characteristic of the neoliberal context. In 2005, UNAIDS declared that Cuba had the lowest HIV incidence in all of Latin America, Central America and the Caribbean.[30]

When Cuba discovered its first AIDS case in 1986 among soldiers returning from Angola and Mozambique, alarm bells went off among the island's communist leadership. The virus was largely unknown, and 300 000 Cuban soldiers who had fought in Africa over a decade could have been exposed. The authorities scrambled to test all military personnel who had been in Africa, and quickly found dozens of cases.

HIV-positive Cubans, at first mainly heterosexuals but later increasingly homosexuals, were shut away in a sanatorium – a controversial policy that attracted international criticism. Cuba stopped quarantining in 1993, and now allows people with HIV to stay at home after attending a course to teach them how to look after themselves and not spread the virus.

Universal free access to locally made generic antiretroviral drugs has kept the number of AIDS cases and deaths very low, according to the UNAIDS program.[31] Almost 20 years later, Cuba has one of the lowest rates of HIV infection in the world, with a prevalence of less than 0.1% of its sexually active population. This is six times lower than the prevalence in the USA, and a big exception in the Caribbean, which is the second most affected region in the world after sub-Saharan Africa.[31]

Cuba, which has a population of 11 million people, now focuses heavily on prevention, and marks World AIDS Day annually by sending out volunteers to distribute free condoms on the streets of central Havana to encourage safe sex. Since 1986, only 6782 Cubans have tested positive for HIV, and 2784 have developed AIDS, with 1314 deaths, according to the Health Ministry.

'The quarantine was very effective in stopping the first wave of the epidemic that came from Africa, given the amount of people we had over there', said Cuba's top AIDS expert Dr Jorge Perez, a director at Havana's Pedro Kouri Tropical Medicine Institute.

'Of course, it was painful for the people interned', he said.

Cuba still requires mandatory HIV testing for pregnant women, blood donors, army recruits, prison inmates and all adults with sexually transmitted diseases. However, at the Los Cocos sanatorium in a mango and coconut grove on the outskirts of Havana, the 300 resident HIV patients are there because they want to be. They live in bungalows with room-mates or their partners. Pets are allowed, there is a basketball court, and the food is better than in the average Cuban household. In addition to 24-hour medical care, Los Cocos gives gay patients a refuge from the rapidly diminishing levels of homophobia in Cuba's society.

'I've been here eight years and decided to stay. I have everything I need – food, medicine, housing and the doctor right there', said 36-year-old Josue, who lives with his gay lover.

Another resident is Maria Julia Fernandez, an anti-AIDS health worker and widow of the first AIDS case detected in Cuba, Reynaldo Morales. He was a soldier who returned from Angola in 1986 and died at the age of 45, after 11 years at Los Cocos. Fernandez has lived with HIV for almost two decades without developing AIDS, and does not take antiretroviral drugs.

When Cuba adopted its outpatient programme for people with HIV in 1993, only 15% of the patients left the sanatoriums.

'We were surprised. We thought the sanatoriums would empty', said the Director of Los Cocos, Rigoberto Lopez.

Mass testing allows Cuba to detect 80% of HIV cases in their first year of infection, according to public health officials. The virtual absence of intravenous drug use in Cuba has also helped. Cuba's big advantage in the fight against AIDS is that its biotechnology industry produces six antiretroviral drugs – ZDV, DDI, D4T, 3TC, DDC and IDV.

'The manufacture of generic drugs brought an extraordinary turnaround in the lives of people who live with HIV, giving them a better quality of life, clinically and psychologically', said Lopez.

Deaths at Los Cocos have dropped from 25–30 per year to 4 or 5 a year. Cuba currently treats 1900 AIDS cases with generic drugs that cost the state US$350 per person per year, and will soon start producing protein inhibitors to replace imports. Dr Jorge Perez expressed concern about a steady increase in HIV-positive cases among gay men, commenting that 'We have done a lot in controlling the impact of AIDS, but we cannot sit back contented.'

The total change in Cuban attitudes towards homosexuality is almost unbelievable, especially in the context of the Caribbean, Central and South America, to say nothing of many African countries. How did this happen? And can the WHO learn anything from it? Possibly, but it didn't happen as a result of such now famous Cuban films as *Chocolate and Strawberries* – or other cultural inputs. Instead, such cultural sensitivities have arisen from Cuba's flexible and responsive socialist social policies. The WHO, the UN and indeed all of us have much to learn from the alternatives that these offer to neoliberalism.

## REFERENCES

1 MacDonald R. An inspirational defence of the right to health . . . (book review). *Lancet*. 2007; **370**: 379–80.

2 MacDonald T. *Developments in Cuban Health Care Since 1959*. Queenston, NY: Edwin Mellen Press; 2005.

3 MacDonald T. *Making a New People: education in revolutionary Cuba*. Vancouver: New Star Books; 1986.

4 Ibid., p. 28.

5 Ibid., p. 37.

6 Sloan D. First of all – health. *Public Affairs Magazine*. 2000; **27 April**: 103–4.

7 Aleksandrov A. *The Secrets of Cuban Medicine*; www.worldpress.org/Europe/1659.cfm (accessed 7 August 2007).

8 MacDonald T. *Developments in Cuban Health Care Since 1959*. Queenston, NY: Edwin Mellen Press; 2005. pp. 17–50.

9 Fawthrop T. Cuba's struggling economy has been boosted by the successful export of its medical technology abroad. Broadcast on *BBC News 24*, 6 January 2007; http://news.bbc.co.uk/2/hi/business/3284995.stm (accessed 16 July 2007).

10 Cuba Solidarity Campaign. Third anniversary of Operation Miracle. *Cuba Si Magazine*. 2007; **summer issue: 7**.

11 BBC Radio 4. *Meningitis: prevention*. Broadcast 8 February 2003; http://news.bbc.co.uk/1/hi/health/medical_notes/278346.stm (accessed 16 July 2007).

12 Oxchoa F. *Origins of Primary Health Care in Cuba*; www.medic.org/publications/medicc_review/1104/pages/cuba (accessed 16 July 2007).

13 Ibid., p. 4.

14 Ibid., p. 5.

15 Fawthrop T, op. cit., p. 1.

16 MacDonald T. *A Developmental Analysis of Cuba's Health Care System Since 1954*. Queenston, NY: Edwin Mellen Press; 1999. pp. 2–5.

17 Fineman M. Little-known biotech industry vital to Cuba's economic future. *Miami Herald*, 14 August 1998, p. 4.

18 Jiménes Y. Mirando al Future desde la Cooperacion Internacinal (Looking at the future for international cooperation). Unpublished Power Point presentation, Medical School, Habana, 26 June 2006.

19 Pan American Health Organization (PAHO). *Health Human Resources Trends in the Americas: evidence for action*. Washington, DC: PAHO Human Resources for Health Unit; 2006. p. 6.

20 Bagley R. From Pakistan to Rotherham – spreading the word on Cuba's humanitarian work. *Morning Star*, 9 July 2007, p. 8.

21 Medical Education Cooperation with Cuba (MEDICC). *Cuba and Global Health*; www.saludthefilm.net/ns/cuba-and-global-health.htm (accessed 21 August 2007).

22 Ibid., p. 3.

23 Ibid., p. 4.

24 Cory C. *Cuban Disaster Doctors in Guatemala and Pakistan*; www.medicc.org/meic_review/0905/international-cooperation (accessed 21 August 2007).

25 UK Indymedia. Internationalist doctors graduated in Cuba. www.indymedia.org.uk/en/2007/07/377039.html (posted by F Espinoza on 27 July 2007).

26 Mullan F. Affirmative action, Cuban style. *NEJM*. 2004; **351**: 27–35; www.ifconews.org/MedicalSchool/articles/NEJM.Article122304.pdf (accessed 21 August 2007).

27 Reed GA. Where there were no doctors: first MDs graduate from Latin American Medical School. MEDICC Rev. 2005; **7**; www.medicc.org/Medical/School/documents/LAMSbrochure.pdf (accessed 21 August 2007).

28 Pan American Health Organization (PAHO), op. cit., p. 7.

29 Ibid., p. 8.

30 Cuba Solidarity Campaign. *Cuba Fights Aids With Free Drugs, Not Quarantine*; www.globalexchange.org/countries/americas/cuba/3613.html (accessed 18 July 2007).

31 Ibid., p. 1.

# Chapter 9

# Summary and recommendations

## USES AND MISUSES OF THE UN

If there is one 'credal' statement, one 'dogma' if you like, on which the UN was founded, and explicitly stated by them, it is the Universal Declaration of Human Rights (UDHR). Likewise, if there is one such 'credal statement' or 'dogma' implicit in the mandate of the WHO, it is the Alma Ata Declaration. What both the UN and the WHO within it testify to, then, is that human values transcend business efficiency and finance, and that the paramount value is human rights. We have the means to implement these ideals, and few can claim not to have at least a rough grasp of the knowledge that they are urgently called for.

What, then, is stopping us? We have had international conferences, pledges to help the poor nations, Jubilee 2000, Live 8, and so on, so there has been no shortage of declared will. However, out of all that effort and enthusiasm nothing like enough actual improvement has taken place – and what improvement *has* taken place is in no way proportional to the number of words spoken, the volume of paper expended or the huge bureaucratic structure of the UN or its agencies. In previous chapters we have seen some examples of how the UN has been sold out to neoliberalism. As Share the World's Resources makes clear,[1] few literate people (other than the contemptuously over-wealthy) can deny that the plight of most of our fellow humans becomes more dire by the day. According to the World Bank, the 'good news' is that the number of people living in absolute poverty (earning equivalent to less than 1 US dollar a day) has dropped to less than 1 billion. However, that kind of reassurance from the UN is not really good news, because almost half of the world's population are now trying to survive on less than 2 US dollars a day![2]

Moreover, as data from previous chapters have shown, the poverty of the mass of people, including the miserable deaths of around 30 000 children a day,[3] is enabling the already obscenely rich to become even richer. That is, global inequity is increasing, and yet the whole idea of the UDHR, the primary purpose of the UN, was to decrease the equity gap. The UN is not fulfilling its purpose. It has now become complicit in extending financial aid to countries so that they can arm militia to keep a desperate citizenry from rioting.[4]

The extent to which the UN, despite its stated ideals and World Bank rhetoric, had become compromised is unambiguously illustrated by the statistics. While billionaires begin to dominate the new capitalist economies of China, Russia, India and Brazil, major uprisings are now becoming commonplace. For example, the 'new rulers' in China have had to increase the number of armed special anti-riot militia 100-fold. The numbers are just as stark for the developed world. There the richest 50 million people, safely ensconced in Europe and North America, have the same income as 2.7 billion poor people worldwide. However, in the First World itself the top 1% income share has risen dramatically in recent decades, to levels not seen since before World War Two. The pay of an average CEO has risen 821 times since 1978, and even a few hundred millionaires own as much wealth as the world's poorest 2.5 billion people. However, the wealthiest country in the world, namely the USA, is also the most unequal. Between 1990 and 2000, worker pay and inflation remained approximately equal, while corporate profits rose by 93% and CEO pay rose by 571%.[5]

The conclusions, however cursorily the figures are reviewed, are incontestably clear. All around the world, the inordinate gap between rich and poor is getting wider both between and within countries, more poor people are sick and needlessly dying than we can even imagine, and despite the affluence enjoyed by the highest echelons of the richest countries, the vast majority are working longer hours with less pay, less creativity, less happiness and more debt.

All of the above are the fruits of neoliberalism – and the situation is, of course, exacerbated by the environmental crisis, which is itself to a large extent a result of unrestrained neoliberalism. And the UN has not only been complicit in this in a general way, but also specifically in such antisocial activities as the sale of arms.[6,7] Not only that, but the corporate brains behind neoliberalism, working through the UN, have not been innocently ignorant of the implications. They anticipate both nuclear war and serious environmental degradation.

Other cheerful predictions from eminent commentators on the possibility of a future war, and even a global nuclear catastrophe, require no further introduction. US military spending is at its highest inflation-adjusted level since 1946, surging by 25% over the past 5 years, with China proudly contending itself as a 'major power' in the global arms race, not to mention Israel, North Korea, Pakistan and Iran. In January 2007, the infamous Doomsday Clock moved its minute hand forward to indicate that the world has edged closer to Armageddon than at any time since the most precarious moments of the Cold War in the early 1980s.[8]

The Doomsday warnings naturally take into account the second greatest threat to humankind's continued existence. If the forecasts from the Intergovernmental Panel on Climate Change come anywhere close to fruition, then a 'near apocalyptic vision of Earth's future'[9] will be the inheritance of the coming generation – sea level rises, increased droughts and crop failures, more diseases and species extinctions, and a 'great climate change divide' that ravages even further the poorest countries. To add the consequences of an intensely speculated stock-market crash would paint such a terrible picture that we might be forgiven for placing all newspapers aside and never opening them again. As Lao Tze once said in his oft-quoted apothegm, 'If we do not change direction, we are likely to end up exactly where we are headed.'

However, we must contend with the simple psychological truth that most people – deep down – fear change, and apologists abound to confirm the legitimacy of this attitude. For every statistic that begets the imperative need for economic reform, dozens of others can be used to justify continuing on the present course. 'The protesters and do-gooders are just plain wrong', writes Robyn Meredith in his new book on the boons of free-market capitalism:[10] 'It turns out globalization is good – and not just for the rich, but especially for the poor.' It seems that public opinion in the Occident is divided into three opposing categories – the 'for', the 'against', and the 'I do not care to know.' As summed up by the Peruvian economist Hernando De Soto, one of the most celebrated proponents of the first group: 'I am not a die-hard capitalist . . . But for the moment, to achieve those goals [of freedom, equal opportunity and compassion for the poor], capitalism is the only game in town.'[11]

The presumption that free trade through liberalization and privatization has 'overwhelming benign effects' is taken as a marker in establishment thinking for distinguishing between 'those who understand economics and those who don't.' To question the opposite is not just to challenge the dogmas of orthodox economics, but also to challenge the fundamental belief system that underpins the consciousness of democratic society – that to usurp is to be happy, to compete is to succeed, to succeed is to win, and that to consume is to be free. A rejection of unfettered, globalized market forces does not mean a rejection simply of certain systems and institutions such as the IMF, the World Bank and the WTO, but of a whole centuries-old history of aborted ideologies and diametrically opposed 'isms' and creeds. No wonder that 'Another World is Possible!' is the current slogan of most campaigners, when defining the 'other world' requires a quantum leap of faith into the complete unknown.

And it is a leap which we have no realistic choice but to make. It is no longer a question of 'Will it happen?', or even 'Who's fault is it?', but 'Given that it has happened, what do we do now?'

For example, one comfortable counsel of advice goes along the following lines. The more money that accumulates at the top and the less at the bottom (in other words – the greater the inequity becomes) the more likely it is that the richest – in hiring the necessary labour to support their lifestyle – will ensure that money 'trickles down' the hill, eventually enriching those at the bottom. In other words, 'Don't worry – greed is good.' However, all the evidence shows that the 'trickle-down effect' does not equalize things – it simply fractures communities more effectively, as we have shown in previous chapters.

In fact, faith in the trickle-down theory differs very little from a number of other irrational beliefs. The foremost dogma of free-market theory is the blind belief in economic growth. 'Trickle-down' economics, or the textbook premise that increasing the size of the economic 'cake' will eventually lead to some falling 'crumbs' for the poorest of the poor, is not only unsupported by either theory or evidence, but is also dependent on the same model of human behaviour that favours selfishness over the public good. People respond only to incentives, argue the theorists, leading to inordinate tax breaks for the highest earners, and a decline in after-tax wages for the remaining majority. In the USA, chief executives of large companies earn more than 10 times what they did in 1980, with the justification from the White House that higher taxes on top earners would cause them to work fewer hours and take fewer risks, thereby stifling economic growth. Besides, even if the average person feels poorer, they say, it will provide them with an incentive to recoup their income loss by working harder than before.[12]

Only with such a cut-throat and egotistical vision of life could the World Bank release its latest poverty statistics this year and not even defend a continuing rise in inequality among citizens in almost every country. So long as the gross domestic product is still expanding, a rise in inequality is quietly seen to be positive. Income disparities, say the trickle-down theorists, strengthen the aggressive motivation to 'get ahead.'

The one question that they don't answer is when the 'growing' will be forced to stop. Economic growth, which translates as a continual increase in the production and consumption of goods and services, is obviously predicated on increasing population and per capita consumption. As the public begins to recognize that economic growth is the root cause of climate change and environmental damage, the foundation stone of Western economic policy for the past 200 years is gradually washing up on the shore. It requires no theory or philosophy to realize that the lives of most people are governed by more than 'income' or 'expenditure' measures, even though such concerns as health, education, social cohesion and food security are currently not even considered important when assessing the 'development' of any country.

## WHAT CAN GOVERNMENTS DO?

Of course, it is freely acknowledged that for the UDHR to work, governments of member states of the UN must individually think in terms of coordinating their policies (e.g. on trade) with those other countries for the maximum global good to be achieved, rather than only representing their own advantage over other nations. ActionAid,[13] a well-known non-government organization (NGO), argues that governments of richer nations are indifferent to the causes of global hunger, widespread infant mortality in other countries, etc., and that some way has to be found to change this attitude. Although we have mentioned a number of UN agencies, one that we have not mentioned much is the Food and Agriculture Organization (FAO). Through it, the UN could do much more to promote the kind of international attitude alluded to above. However, it too has become very much a creature of neoliberal interests – as reflected in both EU and US protectionist agricultural policies.

Reading the Action Aid comments, as reported on the website of Share the World's Resources, it is surprising to find how neoliberalisation policies actually prevent governments from working together to address the food crisis.

The causes of hunger are being ignored by governments, manifested in the final declaration of the World Food Security Committee meeting at the FAO in Rome, 30 October 2006.

More than 100 organizations, including farmers, indigenous people and fishermen, government delegations and NGOs met to review progress towards halving hunger by 2015, pledged 10 years ago at the World Food Summit.

'The US, Canada and some members of the European Union are ignoring the major causes of hunger – lack of access to natural resources and services to farmers', said Francisco Sarmento, head of food rights at the international development agency, ActionAid. Consider the following three comments as well.

'But no progress was made on these key demands or on women's access to land, despite the final declaration reaffirming the key rôle played by women in food security', said Alejandra Scampini, ActionAid's women's rights coordinator in the Americas.

'We need to strengthen our coalitions in order to make governments accountable to the promises they've made', averred Marta Antunes, ActionAid global coordinator of the international food security network.

'Southern governments and civil society need to work together to challenge the current balance of power in the FAO so that we don't come together in another 10 years and find that hunger is still increasing', stated Nancy Kachingwe, adviser to ActionAid's women's rights team, based in Zimbabwe.

The factors that actually prevent the FAO, the WHO and the UN as a whole from effectively mediating solutions to these problems stem – as we have seen in previous chapters – from the degree to which policy formulation of accepted procedures in the latter has been allowed (since the late 1980s in particular) to become subject to the 'needs' of First World cooperation engaged in creating infrastructure in the Third World for 'development.' However, in 2006 this process became official UN policy under the then Director General of the UN, Kofi Annan.

Joe Lauria[14] reports that Kofi Annan, as well as stressing the desirability of public and private cooperation in mediating development projects in the less developed countries (LDCs) – including provision of healthcare by private insurance schemes, as described in previous chapters – expressed his intention of outsourcing the UN's Department for General Assembly (DGA) and Conference Management. That is, it was his intention to privatize the very heart of General Assembly business. The DGA issues about 200 documents a day in six languages. As we shall see later, when studying a report by Alison Katz, even these six languages have not been recognized equally since privatization. Readers will recall that Annan's decision came as the 'oil for food' scandal erupted, in which UN officials were accused of taking bribes from Saddam Hussein's regime in Iraq.

At the end of February 2006, Annan reported on management reforms to the General Assembly. According to an internal UN document previewing Annan's report and obtained by *The Business*,[15] he will include 'proposals to outsource or off-shore select administrative processes' – suggesting that its New York headquarters may shed staff. Annan is reviewing the study conducted for the UN by the two US consulting firms Epstein & Fass Associates and Faulkner & Associates. Their preliminary study, which *The Business* has seen, makes no firm recommendations. However, it examines three privatization possibilities, from the most conservative to the most radical:

1 maintain the status quo of in-house operations, but save money and create efficiency through greater use of technology and eliminating more than 200 jobs through attrition by 2009
2 retain a core of in-house functions while outsourcing some operations, along the lines of a similar exercise by the World Bank and the IMF
3 spin off the General Assembly Department entirely as a for-profit, private company or an independent unit with some control by the secretariat.

The study gives frank assessments of the risks with privatization, especially guarding privileged information and interrupting projects if new contractors are hired. It concedes that privatization may not save money: 'Outsourcing does not guarantee reduced cost . . . [which] depends on market factors, and also . . . on how outsourcing is managed.'

This greatly increases the probability of improper financial pressure determining policy. The Bush administration has made an overhaul of management a centrepiece of its UN reform programme. John Bolton, US ambassador to the UN, once said that if the New York headquarters lost 10 of its 38 floors, 'it wouldn't make a bit of difference.' He is leading an effort to move the UN towards the efficiency of a private company, including transforming the Deputy Secretary General into a Chief Operating Officer, and demanding that tasks are done by merit, not geography.

Christopher Burnham, a former Bush State Department chief financial officer, was named UN Under-Secretary General in charge of management in June 2007, and declared that the UN needed to 'refocus on those areas where we have a competitive advantage.'

Rick Grenell, spokesman for the US mission, told *The Business* that the Bush administration had no position on outsourcing:

> Our position is that the UN needs to function better. We need to look at all ways to make that better. No one is talking about cutting jobs or turning out lights. Talking about outsourcing is way ahead of the game.

However, the UN has been under growing pressure from Washington to cut costs.

The USA pays 22% of the UN's general budget, France pays 6.4%, the UK pays 5.5%, China pays 1.53% and Russia pays 1.2%. All five countries can wield a veto on war-making decisions. Congressman Henry Hyde's proposed UN Reform Act of 2005 would withhold 50% of US dues unless at least 32 of 39 proposed reforms are adopted – a clear indication of pressure intended to break the deadlock.

Some staff fear that privatization would cause a cultural shift within the organization where international civil servants have been chosen through competitive examinations for more than 60 years.

This is exactly the point raised by the above-mentioned Alison Katz,[16] who served with the UN, devoting her attention particularly to the HIV/AIDS crisis in Africa. In her paper she deals especially with the speed with which the WHO fell prey – often only too willingly – and the highly damaging effect that it has on staffing, policy formulation, morale, effectiveness and research. The paper is entitled 'Implications of the work stoppage involving 700 staff of the WHO in November 2005.'

## THE WHO: BEING UNDERMINED BY NEOLIBERALISM

Alison Katz argues that over the past quarter of a century the traditional workplace rights of international civil servants have progressively been eroded in many UN agencies (including the WHO) by managerial acquiescence with the neoliberal agenda. The paper explores some of the strategies in which management has created divisions and an atmosphere of mutual mistrust among staff engaged in crucial technical health work. For instance, managerial staff are increasingly appointed without the participation of other staff – not even the progressively psychologically disabled Staff Association. Other neoliberal techniques, widely used in cut-throat competitive business practice, involved discouraging employee solidarity by a variety of forms of alienation – inducing high levels of insecurity.

In addition, the funding for WHO research and other programmes, which was originally plainly reported on a regular basis, is now increasingly opaque. This, for instance, has pleased wealthy member states – with large-scale access to corporate funding from corporate sponsors and powerful banking interests with no obligation to the Alma Ata principles supposedly guiding WHO policies. Ideally, of course, principled policies demand that those who implement them are free from external constraints in applying their skills and insights to promoting global equity access to primary healthcare.

Although the bulk of Katz's paper is devoted to her own involvement in a 1-hour work stoppage by staff in her department in protest at the way that they were being browbeaten, for instance, by insecure short-term contracts, she was able – during 17 years with the organization – to gain considerable insight into how neoliberal techniques, profitable to bodies outside the WHO, damaged crucial WHO work in the field. Her entire paper is highly recommended to the reader as clearly indicating what is really happening within the international organization in which the world's people have invested such hope and expectation.

Her seminal paper is forcefully summarized, though, in the epilogue which constitutes the final few paragraphs. In it she shows explicitly how the WHO readily sacrifices human life – especially among the most economically disadvantaged people in the LDCs – to the financial benefit of bloated First World corporate interests. Katz, in this regard, is particularly exercised by the rôle of the IAEA and the WHO (as discussed in Chapter 6) in restricting access to the truth about the Chernobyl disaster in 1986. The UN, and the WHO along with it, and the powerful nuclear lobby, have all cooperated in this endeavour – to the great advantage of the latter. More will be said about the rôle of the nuclear power industry, and why it is so important to its interests for civil society to think of nuclear power in benign terms, later in this chapter. However, the WHO is supposedly both our advocate and our mediator with regard to protecting the health of all of us.

As Katz comments, 'Today, WHO stands accused of twenty-one years of silence, complicity and lies. Since 1986, under pressure from private interests, it has actively participated in u cover-up of the health consequences of the world's most serious industrial accident.'[17]

How did the WHO become involved in this atrocious deflection of legitimate popular concern? In answer to this, Katz refers to an agreement that the WHO made with the IAEA, preventing the former from investigating and reporting on the health consequences of nuclear accidents.[18] That, of course, is one of the WHO's cardinal duties.

As stated in Chapter 6, the IAEA is a bona fide UN agency which is supposed to report to the UN Security Council (the Permanent Five Member States) in promoting use of the atom. This author (unlike Katz and many others) would argue that the UN's mandate to 'forestall international conflict' is not only legitimate, but necessary. In 1948, when the IAEA was established, it would not have been necessary to modify the phrase 'use of the atom' to 'peaceful use of the atom', because the UN was already committed to 'promote peace', and this could not condone military use of atomic energy. As will be explained later, though, we now have good reason to suspect that 'peaceful use of the atom' is much riskier than the nuclear industry wants the public to believe. This suggests to the author that one of the required reforms of the UN is that it should outlaw *any* use of the atom, at least until we have developed a secure system for disposing of the used rods.

However, even so, if the WHO had not lied to the public about what was known about Chernobyl – only 9 years after the accident – even peaceful use of nuclear energy would have been highlighted as too potentially dangerous to health. In June 2007, the WHO lied by claiming that the proceedings of the International Conference on the Health Consequences, in Geneva, *had* been published. This just is not so, and those proceedings and those at a similar conference in Kiev in 2001 have never seen the light of day. A former Director General of the WHO, Dr Hiroshi Nakajama, even admitted this in a Swiss TV documentary broadcast in 2004.[19] Furthermore, the film-maker himself even published a book about it[20] 2 years later! It seems extraordinary that he would publicly lie about something so well documented. Does common sense decline with loss of principles?

Dr Hiroshi Nakajama explained that if the WHO had conducted studies on the possible implications of nuclear accidents for health, starting after the two A-bomb attacks on Japan, and for the subsequent years of heavy experimentation with nuclear weapons, there could well have been an international demand for the use of atomic energy to be banned outright.

What is even more problematical, under the present arrangement, is that the WHO/IAEA relationship can be terminated without notice by either party. This means that neoliberal influences can soon reach the point at which any WHO control over the potential health risks associated with the use of nuclear power can be taken from it. As we have seen in Chapter 6, there is ample independent evidence that the effects of the Chernobyl accident have been vastly and deliberately underestimated at the behest of the nuclear industry.

Katz ends her admirable paper as follows:

> WHO's abdication of its responsibilities in radioprotection of populations will be qualified as a crime against humanity. If staff and directors of the technical departments dealing with ionizing radiation in WHO were supported in their independence as international civil servants and were held accountable to the world's people for their interpretation of WHO's mandate, the cover-up of the crime of Chernobyl (and the real health consequences and crimes of Hiroshima, Nagasaki, weapons testing and the use of depleted uranium in weapons today) would have been revealed years ago, many lives would have been saved, and responsible decisions on energy options for the future would be possible.

In other words, neoliberalism is not only bad for your health, but it also represents an outright menace to all human values and civic life. We need to find an alternative to it.


## HOW PEACEFUL IS THE USE OF NUCLEAR ENERGY?

For several years now, some in the Green Lobby, in their determination to find a source of energy that is free of carbon emissions, have been recommending nuclear energy. In the context of the IAEA's consistent cover-up of the aftermath of the Chernobyl disaster, many thinking people have become so open-minded about the issue that their brains have fallen out! The Non-Nuclear Proliferation Treaty (NPT) has, since the collapse of the former Soviet Union, become increasingly flagrantly violated. Not only is the UK sufficiently confident that its people are sleeping that it is moving forward to replace and update Trident nuclear submarines, but other signatories to the NPT have been active in selling nuclear technology (for peaceful purposes) to countries not renowned for their political stability or democratic credentials – most recently France's deal with Libya. The nuclear industry is exultant.

However, the IAEA and other UN agencies have tended to cooperate in muting news reports of nuclear accidents elsewhere in the world than in Chernobyl, and involving 'peaceful' nuclear installations. Obviously if a country is reliant on nuclear power for domestic and industrial use, it would be a prime target for any agency attacking that country. This not only renders the nation concerned more likely to be attacked, but such an attack (even with conventional arms) would have the potential, in destroying the nuclear plant, to release lethal amounts of radioactivity. However, leaving aside military uses of nuclear energy, the panoply of accidents that can render nuclear power plants instruments of widespread death is huge and varied.

Consider such an accident, very much played down by the corporate-owned media, which occurred in Japan on 14 July 2007. It received one brief mention on the BBC Radio World Service, and was almost completely ignored by the mainstream broadsheets. It was reported more fully in the *Morning Star*[21] in the UK, but there has been no further comment on how much leakage occurred or what the health risks, both for the Japanese and for others, might be. The accident happened as a result of an earthquake which struck Japan early on that Monday morning. It shook the world's largest 'peaceful purposes' nuclear reactor, precipitating a radioactive leak.

We are told that the Japanese nuclear industry initially glossed over the true impact, assuring people that there was no danger of a leakage at all. However, it subsequently emerged that 1230 litres of radioactive wastewater had entered the Sea of Japan. The international health implications of this, in relation to Japan's flourishing fisheries industry, could be enormous, although they probably will not be noted for some months. However, in addition the Japanese Communist Party Chairman Kazuo Shii visited the reactor, and noted visible widespread damage outside the plant, including large cracks in the roads, toppled concrete fences and buckled pavements.

Even after Kazuo Shii had taken the Tokyo Electric Power Company's Deputy Superintendent to task for misinforming the public, the company was very reticent about the details of 100 drums containing low-level nuclear solid waste that were toppled at the plant's warehouse. The company has finally had to admit that it has been confirmed that the barrels had split, releasing nuclear waste. The article goes on to discuss Green Party reactions to the accident.

The Executive Director of the US Friends of the Earth, Norman Dean, said that the accident highlights the fact, of which people need to be reminded, that nuclear power is 'hardly the safe panacea that its supporters claim it to be. Energy conservation and wind and solar power are cleaner and safer than nuclear power, and they are a better way to fight global warming.

Greenpeace nuclear campaigner, Jan Beranek, also warned that there is 'a real risk in Japan, and globally, of larger earthquakes and other natural disasters, as well as of terrorist attacks that could lead to far more serious nuclear accidents.' Mr Beranek pointed out that the Japanese and global nuclear industry has been marred by a series of accidents and cover-ups.

He claimed that nuclear power undermines the real solutions to climate change 'by diverting resources away from the massive development of clean renewable energy sources the world urgently needs. What's more, climate change will increase natural disasters, in turn, posing a greater risk to nuclear power plants and to our safety.'

The Kashiwazaki-Kariwa plant has been plagued by mishaps. In 2001, a radioactive leak was found in a turbine room. Residents filed lawsuits claiming that the government had failed to conduct sufficient safety reviews when it approved construction of the plant in the 1970s. However, in 2005 a Tokyo court threw out a lawsuit filed by 33 residents, saying that there was no error in the government safety reviews.

The cover-up continues, with the complicity of the WHO, the IAEA and other agencies of the UN in its drive to neoliberalize smoothly and without upsetting important corporate interests. However, the leaking of information about such incidents into the media is not part of the plan, and one can only wonder about all those accidents we may never hear about. But not all of the effects of neoliberalization of the UN are so spectacular, although they are still real enough.

Physicians for Social Responsibility – Nepal (PSRN), a highly proactive Nepalese-based NGO, has listed 10 reasons for being extremely wary about the use of nuclear power, even for peaceful domestic purposes. At present there is nothing 'peaceful' about taking risks like this with the environment – and with the lives of people.[22]

1   Almost all mined uranium (more than 99%) is uranium-238, which is highly toxic and too dirty.

2   The mining of uranium is itself 'dirty', causing long-lasting and in some cases permanent damage to the environment. Mining is often done in indigenous land belonging to or inhabited by disempowered or voiceless communities and peoples. Too much waste or slag from such mines seriously pollutes land, air and water resources. The soil soon becomes unfit for agriculture and forestry, the air becomes too toxic and ionized with radioactive radiation, and water resources become unfit to drink or to use for irrigation. Such contamination may persist for thousands of years. Many miners will eventually get lung and other organ cancer, and many of their children may have birth defects with a more than 1500% increase in the risk of ovarian and testicular cancer.

3   The heavy vehicles and equipment used in mining operations are heavily polluting – discharging numerous and frequent actual flame shoots, toxic fumes, 'greenhouse' gases and dusts, as these are excessively fossil fuel intensive. These scar the land permanently, leaving ugly and barren sites of eroded or splintered rock, mud and slime.

4   Supervision and monitoring systems to ensure the safe operation of nuclear power plants are never cheap, and are still not completely accident proof. Clean-up and decontamination operations and processes of after-accident plants are far too expensive and too traumatic in terms of human cost. Chip Ward reports that 'To make a difference (if at all) in global climate change, we have to immediately build . . . at least as many as 2000 nuclear power plants

worldwide. This is simply impossible, as the global uranium reserve wouldn't suffice to feed these . . . The partial meltdown at Three Mile Island in the USA taught investment bankers how a two-billion-dollar investment can turn into a billion-dollar clean-up in under two hours.'

5   The uranium enrichment process is also polluting, as it involves too many energy-intensive processes, including the use of dirty coal-fired plants, and highly dangerous, as the end-product is extremely fissionable, immensely radioactive and can produce nuclear weapon grade uranium-235. The same thing can be said about the production of heavy water for so-called 'cleaner' nuclear reactors.

6   Huge quantities of depleted nuclear waste are produced by the nuclear reactors. This places a great burden on the country's resources and environment. Often such waste is dumped in under-developed countries. This practice itself is immoral and puts the people in such sites at great risk with regard to their health and security. Furthermore, misunderstandings among communities can lead to armed conflict and the subsequent effects of corruption.

7   Reprocessing the spent nuclear fuel is another dirty and deadly trap which is prone to too many radiation leaks, the danger of waste mismanagement and, of course, diversion to nuclear bomb development operations. Substantial amounts of weapons-grade plutonium may be produced during the reprocessing. A glaring example of this is the shutdown of Sellafield experimental nuclear reprocessing plant because there were too many episodes of leaks into the surrounding ocean, land and air.

8   When some nuclear plants are, from time to time, employed to produce materials for military contracts, too many safety variables enter the equation and accidents can all too easily occur. This is so even when conventional weapons are sent to such domestic nuclear power stations to be 'radioactively tipped.'

9   Nuclear power plants are targets for terrorists. The capacity of international terrorists to penetrate and attack is increasing rapidly. Untold catastrophes are obvious if they ever succeed. Another danger is that the terrorists may gain access to nuclear-bomb-grade material by 'stealing', or through the black market, or by developing these materials themselves to make 'dirty' nuclear bombs. They can even produce 'back-pack' nuclear bombs that can be easily concealed while transported, and then used. Increasing the numbers of nuclear power plants and reprocessing 'spent fuels' would increase these risks.

10  Lastly, a nuclear power plant is always a mega-project. It ultimately becomes time and resource intensive, energy intensive, and too risky in terms of natural and human-related accidents, and complicated operational and nuclear waste management systems. Nuclear power plants require a complex management system, which is too easily suborned at various levels.

As has already been pointed out by the author in Chapter 6, we can only count on a future in which nuclear power becomes a safer and realistic option for the supply of energy for domestic and other civil use when – at the very least – we can dispose of the used rods and dismantle redundant nuclear facilities without risk.

We could cite many more examples, but the link between neoliberal/corporate interests and UN agencies supposedly acting only in compliance with their stated mandates, without outside interference, is now clear for all to see. The catalogue of specific incidents is immense. But let us now, in passing, consider a very dramatic human right (defined as such in the UDHR), namely, the right to adequate and secure shelter.

## THE UN AND OUR RIGHT TO ADEQUATE SHELTER

The growing inequities of income generated by the worldwide influence of neoliberalism on UN policies and activities have greatly increased the number of people without adequate and secure housing. This, combined with the neoliberalization of basic commodities such as water, exacerbates a whole gamut of other human rights, including maternal and child health, access to primary healthcare, etc. Miloon Kothari[23] reported on the matter as of 2003:

> The human rights of people and communities to housing, water and sanitation – guaranteed under international law and commitments of development targets made at global summits including the Millennium Summit and the World Summit on Sustainable Development – continue to erode as the process of privatization deepens and accelerates. It is time to rethink the current global economic and social policies and to recommit ourselves to the human rights principles and standards that offer the only real paradigm for improving the lives of millions of the poor.
>
> It is estimated that 600 million urban dwellers and over 1 billion rural persons now live in overcrowded and poor-quality housing without adequate water, sanitation, drainage or garbage collection. More than 1.2 billion people still have no access to safe drinking water, and 2.4 billion do not have adequate sanitation services. This grave situation puts lives and health continually at risk. It also threatens a range of human rights, including the right to adequate housing. Globalization policies have accelerated the trends towards privatizing human rights, such as water, often leading to the violation of the rights of the poor.

Tremendous effort has been expended in attempting to strike some kind of workable balance between the meeting of human rights under the UDHR, and economic constraints on support services imposed under the IMF and World Bank development agendas. The latter faces poor people with four alternatives to degradation and ill health. Under a privatized UN, human rights count for little in the equation. There are three reasons for this.

1   Private businesses emphasize profit and cost recovery. This is even true of programmes of private health insurance, and uneven access to primary health-

care because of IMF-imposed verticalization and WTO policies on GATS.

2 This means that there is a grotesque difference in the number and quality of services available to vulnerable sub-groups and those with more economic power.

3 Above all, private operators are not accountable, either to the public they are ostensibly serving or to the WHO that is commissioning them.

## WHAT NEEDS TO BE DONE?

In the light of all that has gone before, it is clear that the UN's rôle as an international mediator of international peace (consider World Bank financing of the arms trade) and as an advocate of global human rights is now widely recognized as inadequate. As this book has shown, much of this is due to the fact that it has – in so many respects – sold out to the highest bidder to run its services, and that highest bidder is global neoliberalism. However, as the author has made clear in previous publications,[24] before neoliberalism made itself felt in a big way, the UN was internally compromised for four basic reasons. These can be summarized briefly as follows.

1 Composition of the original committee. As World War Two drew to a close in 1944, a committee made up of the UK and its allies met in Bretton Woods, New Hampshire, USA, to plan for a replacement for the League of Nations. The latter, of course, had conspicuously failed to prevent World War Two. The main states represented at Bretton Woods were the UK, the USA, France, the former Soviet Union and China (the Big Five). These, of course, represented the victorious nations. Thus the UN's values tended to reflect allied, generally eurocratic democratic traditions. At the start this did not seem to be a problem, because the defeat of fascism was the very basis for world peace. However, it increasingly became a problem. In fact, the USA – as by far the richest of the five and the least physically damaged by the war as it drew to an end – wielded immense moral and financial power. For various associated reasons, between then and now, UN resolutions have often been little more than US foreign policy writ large, but with the moral authority of the UN behind it.

2 Power of the veto. Every state is a member of the UN, with 52 of those other than the 'Big Five' constituting the General Assembly, and the Big Five being called the Security Council. However, only members of the Security Council have the power of the veto. What this means is that, even if all of the nations in the General Assembly vote for a proposed resolution, along with four of the Security Council, a single Security Council member voting against the motion (vetoing it) can prevent the proposed resolution from becoming UN policy. In addition, the membership of the General Assembly is decided by elections every 2 years (run in such a way that every region of the world is represented), while the Big Five of the Security Council are permanent members. They have not changed since 1944. Obviously the former Soviet Union no longer exists, so Russia holds that seat, and the People's Democratic Republic of China

now represents China. The little island of Taiwan originally represented all of China!

3   The UN, by virtue of some of its agencies working at cross-purposes with others (e.g. the IMF and the World Bank being able to block WHO decisions on health) is compromised. This came about because some of the agencies – such as the WHO and UNICEF – were formed to support the UDHR, whereas agencies such as the World Bank, the IAEA and the IMF were simply added on to the UN. In theory, all member states are duty-bound to 'promote and defend' the values of the UDHR but, as we have seen, this does not work out in practice. Thus, in a sense, the UN is often rendered indecisive and ineffective because of these structural contradictions.

4   When the UN was formed, most geographically defined 'countries' could also be considered as ethnic entities. However, in the 60 years since the UN's formation, speed and ease of travel, etc., have rendered us all more multicultural. The word 'nation' no longer has the same connotations that it had in 1944. The UDHR's mandate requires the UN to 'uphold, protect and promote' the integrity of each member state in order to prevent international war. Changing attitudes towards 'nationhood' mean that it is often impossible for the UN to fulfil the first and second mandates simultaneously. For example, what about the human rights of the people of Darfur in the Sudan, or of the Karen people in Burma?

Therefore the UN can only become less effective as we move into the future unless we take immediate steps to reform it, as summarized below.

1   We need to prevent the veto from only being exercised by the same five powers. If we do need a Security Council, its five members should be elected by the General Assembly or, better still, by all of the member states.

2   We need to slim down the tasks of the UN. The UDHR needs to be its major concern. Agencies like the IMF and the World Bank need to carry out their analyses for financing developments as a separate entity, and then bring their suggestions to the UN. The UN can then consider the proposals in the light of their health and human rights implications, adding guidance when necessary. The UN has to have the final say.

3   Before infrastructural intrusion can be made in an LDC, for example, an International Health Impact Assessment (IHIA) should have to be carried out by health experts nominated by the WHO to establish what safeguards need to be in place to protect the human rights of the citizens of the target country.

4   Trade needs to be rationalized by a WTO much along the lines suggested originally by Maynard Keynes. Financial transactions between nations using bancors (or some equivalent) would prevent any one nation's banking system, or fluctuations in its currency or its balance-of-payments problems, from having a prevailing influence on a just decision-making process.

5   The present WTO – as formed in 1995 – has very little to recommend it. It enshrines neoliberalism exclusively, forcing it to promote 'free trade'

rather than 'fair trade.' Its apparatus of TRIPS, GATT and GATS, etc. ties it unequivocally to the neoliberal competitive context, seriously undermining the UDHR. There simply is no moral way in which the WHO should have to base its recommendations on the patenting of various foods and medicines. It has to be free to deploy the world's resources (either physical or intellectual) so as to optimize global health. As far as trade is concerned, a much more rational approach – as suggested in a previous book by this author[25] – should involve some system of 'Regional Fair Trade', especially between small nations in similar geographical/climatological 'zones' (rather than between states). These 'zones' would not be geographically fixed, but could be varied regularly by the UN, in consultation with the affected people and in accordance with changing environmental circumstances.

None of the above suggestions require a violently revolutionary upsurge. In fact, masses of people, because of the environmental crisis, are beginning to realize that if we try to bury our heads in the sand (produced aplenty by desertification and global warming!) we shall all be lost. Only an enlightened sense of 'thinking globally in order to act locally' holds out the promise of centuries more of civilization.

One of the strangest repositories of neoliberalism and its malign impact on the UN is the 1995 WTO. The WTO is not an agency of the UN, but it works so closely with the IMF and the World Bank that it is effectively part of the UN. The IMF and the World Bank would be unable to act without it, and it would have no means of controlling global trade without them. Let us then consider the possibility of getting rid of it altogether, unless we can restructure it along the lines originally suggested by Keynes.

## DISBANDING THE WTO

Obviously some people, especially in economically powerful nations, already want to get rid of the WTO, but for reasons of nationalistic self-interest. For instance, the author has often encountered this view in certain communities in the USA and the EU. There should be a world oversight of trade, but one that allows capitalist nations to make the decisions governing such trade! Those who oppose the WTO, on the other hand, do so out of the belief that civic values informed by respect for human rights and environmental sustainability should take precedence over the 'right' of a few to amass great power and wealth. The WTO speaks constantly about 'protecting trade rights', but the real issue is to protect more vulnerable people and communities from the ravages of competition between opposing business interests. This has been well pointed out in an essay by the Z-Net team:[26]

> The critic's theoretical understanding of the WTO as a vehicle only moved
> by corporate profit-seeking logic is borne out from that organization's history

to date. In every case that has been brought to the organization challenging environmental or public safety legislation on behalf of corporations, the corporations have won. When foreign commercial shrimp fishing interests challenged the protection of giant sea turtles in our Endangered Species Act, the turtles didn't stand a chance. When it was Venezuelan oil interests versus the US Environmental Protection Agency's air quality standards for imported gasoline, the oil interests won. When it was US cattle producers against the European Union's ban on hormone-treated beef, European consumers lost. The list goes on.

As mentioned before, we do have to live under some kind of global regulation of trade if war and pandemic disease are to be prevented, but the WTO is not the appropriate instrument to mediate this, being based on cut-throat competition involving commercial rights to valuable medicines and much needed agricultural varieties. As the Z-Net essay[25] notes, there are 10 major reasons for disposing of the WTO – or at least for drastically altering its present form.

1   The WTO prioritizes trade and commercial considerations over all other values. WTO rules generally require domestic laws, rules and regulations designed to further worker, consumer, environmental, health, safety, human rights, animal protection or other non-profit-centred interests to be undertaken in the 'least trade restrictive' fashion possible – trade is almost never subordinated to these non-commercial concerns.

2   The WTO undermines democracy by shrinking the choices available to democratically controlled governments, with violations potentially punished with harsh penalties.

3   The WTO actively promotes global trade even at the expense of efforts to promote local economic development and policies that move communities, countries and regions in the direction of greater self-reliance.

4   The WTO forces Third World countries to open their markets to rich multi-nationals and to abandon efforts to protect infant domestic industries. In agriculture, the opening to foreign imports will catalyse a massive social dislocation of many millions of rural people on a scale that only war approximates.

5   The WTO blocks countries from acting in response to potential risk – impeding governments from moving to resolve harms to human health or the environment, much less imposing preventive precautions.

6   The WTO establishes international health, environmental and other standards at a low level through a process called 'harmonization.' Countries or even states and cities can only exceed these low norms by winning special permission, which is rarely granted. The WTO thereby promotes a race to the bottom and imposes powerful constraints to keep people there.

7   WTO tribunals rule on the 'legality' of nations' laws, but carry out their work behind closed doors. The very few therefore impact on the life situations of the many, without even a pretence at participation, cooperation and democracy.

8 The WTO limits governments' ability to use their purchasing dollars for human rights, environmental causes, worker rights and other non-commercial purposes. The WTO requires that governments make purchases based only on quality and cost considerations. Not only must corporations operate with an open eye with regard to profits and a blind eye to everything else, but so also must governments and thus whole populations.

9 WTO rules do not allow countries to treat products differently based on how they were produced – whether they were made with brutalized child labour, with workers exposed to toxins, or with no regard for species protection.

10 WTO rules permit and in some cases require patents or similar exclusive protections for life forms. In other words, the WTO does whatever it can to promote the interests of huge multinationals. There are no principles at work, only power and greed.

## LET'S BUY BACK THE FARM!

During the dust-bowl years of depression in the 1870s and again in the 1930s in many parts of the prairie land in the USA, one often heard the phrase 'Let's buy back the farm.' It was usually uttered by share-croppers and tenant farmers who had once held mortgages on farms which were recalled by the banks when drought and economic depression combined to turn once proud farmers into share-croppers on land that they had farmed for years as their own. However, during the late 1950s and early 1960s this author, while working in North and South Carolina, Georgia and Mississippi (in the USA), heard the expression again and again uttered this time by black agricultural workers. It was rarely uttered as a real proposition, but as a lingering expression of a pride long trampled down by penury, racism and insecurity – or more often as a plaintive cry over a drink, called out into the uncomprehending dark night.

As we have seen, much the same situation still prevails globally, and it is with good reason that the Third World (which is associated with poverty, corruption and exploitation) is often called 'The South', while the wealthy, powerful industrial nations are referred to as 'The North.' Much of the Third World *is* in the tropics, and was the playing field of contending European nations carving out empires. The USA, as we know, did the same in Central and South America.

Therefore, when we set about addressing the issue of the UN being brought out by neoliberal corporations and banks in the First World, we must – if we wish to prevent the loss of the UN's initial noble purpose – join with those share-croppers and resolve to 'buy back the farm' so that all of us can live in peace, brotherhood and plenty.

## REFERENCES

1 Share the World's Resources. *The Globalization of Justice: human values beyond economic theory*; www.stwr.net/content/view/1954/37 (accessed 25 July 2007).

2 World Bank. *Global Monetary Report 2007: confronting the challenges of gender equality and fragile states*. New York: World Bank; 2007. p. 11.

3 UNICEF. *The State of the World's Children*. Geneva: UNICEF; 2007. p. 1.

4 Petras J. *Global Ruling Class: billionaires and how they 'made it.'* Published on-line by Global Research on 23 March 2007. www.globalresearch.ca/index.php?context=view/Articles&code=PET2007323articled=5159 (accessed 13 December 2007).

5 Buchheit P. *The Income Gap: profits up 93%, CEO pay up 571% – worker salaries stagnant*; www.CounterPunch.org (accessed 25 July 2007).

6 World Policy Institute. *Contractors Win in the War: arms sales, cluster bombs*; www.worldpolicy.org/projects/arms/updates/032307.htm (accessed 25 July 2007).

7 WTO and Global War System. *The World Trade Organization and the Links Between Economic Globalization and Militarism*; www.ratical.org/co-globalize/WTOandWar.html (accessed 23 July 2007).

8 Cornwell R. The Doomsday Clock: nuclear threat to world 'rising.' *The Independent*, 17 January 2007, p. 6.

9 McCarthy M, Castle S. How the worst effects of climate change will be felt by the poorest. *The Independent*, 7 April 2007, p. 4.

10 Meredith R. *The Elephant and the Dragon: The Rise of India and China and What it Means to US*. New York: WW Norton and Co.; 2007.

11 De Soto H. *The Mystery of Capital*. London: Black Swan; 2001.

12 Etebari M. *Trickle-Down Economics: four reasons why it just doesn't work*. www.faireconomy.org/research/trickledown.html (accessed 17 July 2007).

13 Share the World's Resources. *Governments Indifferent to Causes of Hunger, Says ActionAid*; www.stwr.net/content/view/1270/36 (accessed 27 July 2007).

14 Lauria J. *Annan Prepares for Privatization of UN*; www.globalpolicy.org/reform/topics/general/2006/0212privatization (accessed 25 July 2007).

15 Burchart N. Annan reports on General Assembly management reforms. *The Business*, 31 August 2006, p. 7.

16 Katz A. *The Independence of International Civil Servants During the Neoliberal Decades*. www.i-sis-org.uk/LUALTD.php-29k (accessed 13 December 2007).

17 As amply testified to by documents on the website of the group 'Independent WHO'; www.independentwho.info

18 World Health Organization. *Agreement Between the International Atomic Energy Agency and the World Health Organization*; www.who.int/gb/bd/PDF/bd46/en (accessed 25 July 2007).

19 Tchertkoff W. *Nuclear Controversies*, a film made for Swiss-Italian TV and edited by E Andreoli, Fedal Films, 2004. It was widely distributed, with subtitles in English, French, German, and Italian! It can be downloaded from the website of Independent WHO; www.independentwho.info

20 Tchertkoff W. *Le Crime de Tchernobyl: le goulag nucléaire*. Paris: Actes Sud; 2006.

21 Mellen T. Japan quake 'caused nuclear leak.' *Morning Star*, 19 July 2007, p. 3.

22 Physicians for Social Responsibility, Nepal (PSRN). *Global Solidarity Against Nuclear War*. Published for PSRN by Mathura P Shrestha, President of PSRN, Kathmandu, 20 July 2007.

23 Kothari M. *Privatising Human Rights: impact of globalization on access to housing, water and sanitation.* Habitat International Coalition; 2005. www.hic-net.org/-21k (accessed 13 December 2007).

24 MacDonald T. *The Global Human Right to Health: dream or possibility?* Oxford: Radcliffe Publishing; 2007.

25 Ibid.

26 Z-Net. *Q&A on the WTO, IMF, World Bank and Activism.* Prepared by Michael Albert from Elaine Bernard, Peter Bohmer, Jeremy Brecher, Dorothy Guellec, Robin Hahnel, Russell Mokhiber, Mark Weisbrot, Robert Weissman and Michael Albert's own work. www.zmag.org/zmag/articles/jan2000albert.htm (accessed 23 July 2007).

# Index